The Middle English Version of *De Viribus Herbarum*

(GUL MS Hunter 497, ff. 1r-92r)

Late Middle English Texts

2

LMET

Javier Calle-Martín
Antonio Miranda-García

The Middle English Version of *De Viribus Herbarum* (GUL MS Hunter 497, ff. 1r-92r)

Edition and Philological Study

PETER LANG
Bern · Berlin · Bruxelles · Frankfurt am Main · New York · Oxford · Wien

Bibliographic information published by die Deutsche Nationalbibliothek
Die Deutsche Nationalbibliothek lists this publication in the Deutsche Nationalbibliografie; detailed bibliographic data is available on the Internet at ‹http://dnb.d-nb.de›.

British Library Cataloguing-in-Publication Data: A catalogue record for this book is available from The British Library, Great Britain

Library of Congress Cataloging-in-Publication Data

Macer, Floridus. [De viribus herbarum. English] The Middle English version of De viribus herbarum : (GUL MS Hunter 497, ff. 1r-92r) : edition and philological study / Javier Calle-Martín, Antonio Miranda-García.
p. cm. -- (Late Middle English texts ; 2)
Study and transcription of the manuscript version held at the Glasgow University Library.
Includes bibliographical references.
ISBN 978-3-0343-0697-3
1. Materia medica, Vegetable--Early works to 1800. 2. Medicine, Medieval. 3. Didactic poetry, Latin (Medieval and modern) 4. English philology--Middle English, 1100-1500. 5. University of Glasgow. Library. 6. Macer, Floridus. De viribus herbarium. I. Calle Martín, Javier. II. Miranda García, Antonio. III. University of Glasgow. Library. IV. Title.
RS81.M1613 2011
615.1--dc23

2011045421

This book stems from the research project P07HUM02609 entitled "Reference Corpus of Late Middle English Scientific Prose", funded by the Autonomous Government of Andalusia and from the project FFI2008-02336 entitled "Compilation of an Electronic Corpus of Middle English Scientific Manuscripts" funded by the Spanish Ministry of Science and Innovation.

ISBN 978-3-0343-0697-3
ISSN 2235-0136

Hochfeldstrasse 32, CH-3012 Bern, Switzerland
info@peterlang.com, www.peterlang.com

Printed in Switzerland

To my wife Ana…

Contents

Chapter 2. The language

Chapter 3. The text

Chapter 4. The glossary

Acknowledgements

The present research has been funded by the AUTONOMOUS GOVERNMENT OF ANDALUSIA (grant number P07HUM02609) and by the SPANISH MINISTRY OF SCIENCE AND INNOVATION (grant number FFI2008-02336). We are also grateful to the generous funding of the CALEDONIAN RESEARCH FOUNDATION – the Royal Society of Edinburgh (2006 European Visiting Research Fellowship). These grants are hereby gratefully acknowledged.

We are particularly indebted to the Keeper of Special Collections and Assistant Director at Glasgow University Library, Mr David Weston, for his assistance in the digitisation process, and for granting us permission to use this unique collection of manuscripts.

We are also grateful to Dr David Moreno Olalla (Department of English, University of Málaga) for his help and scholarly advice in the making of the glossary and to Joaquín Garrido Garrido (Computer Manager), for the design of an *ad hoc* tool for the retrieval and handling of linguistic data.

Abbreviations and symbols

a.	Adjective
AF	Anglo-French
Angl.	Anglian
Arab.	Arabic
adv.	Adverbs
c.	Conjunctions
e-MED	Electronic *Middle English Dictionary*
f.	Folio
fem.	Feminine
ff.	Folios
Gr.	Greek
GUL	Glasgow University Library
H497	GUL MS Hunter 497 (V.7.24)
L	Classical Latin
LALME	*Linguistic Atlas of Late Middle English*
masc.	Masculine
ME	Middle English
ML	Middle Latin
MS	Manuscript
MSS	Manuscripts
n.	Noun
neut.	Neuter
OE	Old English
OED	*Oxford English Dictionary*
OF	Old French
p.	Prepositions
p.	person
PDE	Present-day English
plur.	Plural
pres.	Present (tense)

prob.	Probably
S	Subject
sb.	Somebody
sing.	Singular
sth.	Something
Sp.	Spanish
V	Verb
v.	Verb
WS	West Saxon
ON	Old Norse
#	Footnote number
*	Reconstructed or hypothetical form

Preface

This welcome new edition of materials from Glasgow University Library MS Hunter 497 (V. 7. 24) makes available for the first time the only Middle English version of the Latin verse *De viribus herbarum* by Macer Floridus not previously edited by modern scholars. It is a pleasure to be able to read the text in an accessible scholarly format, supported by full notes and glossary and a detailed and informative introduction. Such works of practical guidance have recently been receiving much welcome scholarly attention, and the secondary resources for their study have developed very significantly in the last thirty years, thanks to the work of scholars such as Linda Ehrsam Voigts, Patricia Deery Kurtz, Peter Murray Jones and George R. Keiser.[1] But, no matter how magisterial the overview, and no matter how comprehensive the calendaring and finding aids, there is no substitute for the experience of sitting down and reading through these materials.

As is typical of the English vernacular translations of practical works in this period, the hexameter verse is translated into serviceable,

1 For an overview of recent scholarship and helpful bibliography, see George R. Keiser, 'Scientific, Medical and Utilitarian Prose', in *A Companion to Middle English Prose*, ed. A.S.G. Edwards (Cambridge: D.S. Brewer, 2004), pp. 231-47, and his indispensable 'Scientific and Practical Writings', in *A Manual of the Writings in Middle English*, 1050-1550. Vol. 10: Science and Information, gen. ed. Albert E. Hartung (New Haven, CN: Connecticut Academy of Arts and Sciences, 1998), and the bibliographical references in this volume. See also Peter Murray Jones, 'Medical Libraries', in *The Cambridge History of Libraries in Britain and Ireland*, vol 1 to 1640, ed. Elisabeth Leedham Green and Teresa Webber (Cambridge; Cambridge University Press, 2006), pp. 461-71, and other mentions by index; and the relevant chapters by Keiser, Murray Jones and Nicholas Orme in *The Cambridge History of The Book in Britain*, vol 3 1400-1557, ed. Lotte Hellinga and J. B. Trapp (Cambridge; Cambridge University Press, 1999); Lisa H. Cooper, 'The Poetics of Practicality in Middle English', ed. Paul Strohm, Oxford Twenty-First Century Approaches to Literature, 1 (Oxford: Oxford University Press, 2007), pp. 491-505.

if often necessarily formulaic prose. The efflorescence of such translations in the last quarter of the fourteenth century and throughout the fifteenth, culminating in the appearance of many similar texts from the early printing houses, is tribute to the growing pragmatic literacy of lay readers and book owners, as well as the ongoing need for religious and educational institutions to be able to make practical and local provision for the needs of their members. The rapidly expanding readership for vernacular works of this kind was often locally and idiolectally inflected, and works of particular utility and popular appeal were often translated on several occasions, independently, in geographically diverse locations, and in ways that reflect the particular needs or interests of the target audiences. In religious writing, for example, no fewer than seven different independent vernacular translations were made of Richard Rolle's useful compendium of spiritual guidance, the *Emendatio vitae*, originally targeted at a male monastic readership but later made extensively available for mixed lay and religious audiences. Similarly, it is useful to have a complete array of the now more than a dozen known Macer Floridus translations available for scholarly perusal, comparison, and analysis. Frequent translation not only suggests the utility that such texts were felt to have in a variety of social, institutional and domestic contexts, but also reminds us that, even in the face of a rapidly expanding lay market for vernacular books, much book production was local, occasional, amateur, and pragmatic. Gentry and clergy, householders and scholars, medics and manciples, monks and merchants, all needed and wanted to be able to consult herbals and to apply their conventional and proverbial wisdom to the needs of their clients, customers, and colleagues. Although the medieval provenance of Hunter 497 cannot be ascertained, dialectally the editors locate it in the south of the county of Essex, close to the metropolitan centres of London and Westminster, with their burgeoning mercantile and professional readerships and their lively institutional life, and also home to many significant religious foundations. The Macer Herbal is only one of a series of popular herbal taxonomies, but its separate translation on many occasions suggests both its penetration into the marketplace, and its appeal and efficacy as a compendium of lore. It is striking that the *Corpus of British Medieval*

Library Catalogues to date records sixteen copies of the Latin Macer Floridus in the catalogues and *registra* of institutional collections so far published, and only three of a vernacular version, all three at Syon Abbey, the Birgittine double house founded by Henry V in 1415, one of the last major monastic foundations of the English Middle Ages, and itself a notable centre for vernacular translation and the transmission of vernacular materials.

* * *

The peculiar mixture of calm menace and hair-raising peril recorded in the various recipes is a fascinating insight into the routinely hazardous business of self diagnosis and self-treatment, where the application of the wrong herb at the wrong time in the wrong strength and to the wrong part of the body is likely to produce spectacular outcomes of an unforeseen and potentially uncontrollable nature. These herbals are often soberingly gruesome, cataloguing a gleeful glossary of riotously unpleasant symptoms and side effects. An alarming number of these herbs produce in one or more of their applications emetic or enematic effects, and reveal the ease with which Pertelote in Chaucer's *Nun's Priest's Tale* would have been able to find in her farmyard 'tho herbes...The whiche han of hire propretee by kynde/To purge yow bynethe and eek above' (VII. 2951-3).[2] Indeed the very versatility of commonly found herbs in their different applications bespeaks not just the flexibility of their users but also the bravery and versatility of those who experimented to extend the range. One example, from early on in this herbal, reveals quite how versatile a single herb might be:

> Southernewode as yt ys y radde ys hoot yn te thyrde degre . & drye yn te same . hys seed ys moor feruent . yt ys bytwene Þe thrydde degre . & Þe fourthe degre . Make þer of a plaster and yt shal hele synowes þ*a*t ben bolle*n* yf yt be leyde þer to . A noþer . Drynke þe cocc*io*n

2 *The Riverside Chaucer*, ed. Larry D. Benson, 3rd ed. (Oxford: Oxford University Press, 1988), p. 255. All other Chaucer quotations from this edition.

> of þ*ys* herbe yt doth good to all þe synowes & to streynesse & to all other causes of þe brest . A nother drynke yt ofte raw wit*h* wyne & yt doth good to þe cowhe & to þe chynke & to ache of þe ludes & to þe greuance of þe p*re*ue me*m*ber . And makyth þe to pysse & destroyth þe stone & wormes yn þe bely . It clensy thentrall . & dryueth oute womans floures . It purgyth passyons & dysseses . þ*a*t fallen yn te whyrlebone of þe hype . It dyssoluyth þe festre & destreth yt . Thys herbe {chasyth} away serpentes thorugh hys odour . Drynke southerwode & yt wol destroue þe uenym of serpentes . If þow haue þe cold feuer . or þan þe dyssese come upon þe drynke þe Ius of southernewod wit*h* wat*er* medle yt wit*h* comou*n* oyle & wit*h* þ*a*t oyle anoynte þy leymes . Take þe Ius of þ*ys* herbe . & put yt yn þe eere luke warme of hym þ*a*t ys deffe & he shal soon heere . Take southerwode cromes of bred & apples þ*a*t me*n* calle quynsys & sethe hym to gyder yn water & leye yt þan to thyne eyes yt destroyth and helyth þe bocche & teache & þe hete of þe eyen . Make of southernewode a playster by yt self . or medle yt wit*h* grece . & yt wol draw oute a shafte or torne styked yn te body . Leye þ*ys* herbe only under þy pylowe atte thyne heed & yt wol scure þe hugely to lecherye . Also drynke þe same herbe & yt wol quenche þe lust of lechery . And yt helpyth ayenst þe goute (see below, pp. 71-72).

This astonishing catalogue of cures and palliatives is all effected by different preparations of a single herb. But the ability to prevent lechery in one of its forms, and to extract impaled objects, or ward off snakes in others reveals the flexibility of imagination as well as of medical applications that medieval readers found in (and needed to bring to) such texts. The modern reader notes the range and frequency of the ailments that such herbs address: menstrual problems, urinary problems, stones, worms, earache, damaged limbs, muscle strains and other everyday trials are addressed in many of the recipes. Variants on the phrase 'It brekyth þe ston . & makyth þe to pysse & yt purgyth wommens floures' (p. 107, here in relation to 'Synuey') recur throughout the collection, suggesting that the likely failure of one herb would simply encourage the sufferer to move on to another.

The Macer Floridus text is very catholic in its range of sources, even, for example, recording the differences of opinion between physicians about the uses and utility of onions and the disadvantages of their application. It is hospitably far-reaching in the range of effects and formulations that particular herbs are found to provide. Poppy, for example, is said to have twelve different powers ('uertues'), depending on its preparation and application. The twelfth is that if an ointment is laid 'under þyn erse' it will encourage sleep 'And as yt ys trowed yt wol do þe same by hys sauor oonly' (p. 113). Some familiar plants and vegetables turn out to have medicinal properties: lettuce (which is 'colde and ryght moyst') works both when eaten and when applied as a plaster, an encouragement to salad-dodgers everywhere. As Beatrix Potter's Peter Rabbit discovered to his cost in Mr McGregor's garden, lettuce has a soporific effect when eaten, and, according to our text, makes those who consume it to excess go blind (p. 90). More moderate consumption can cure problems of nocturnal pollution in men, and encourage the production of milk in nursing women. Clearly credulous consumers were walking a tightrope of unforeseeable consequences when judging how much to consume. Descriptions of how to prepare infusions of herbs do not encourage belief in the exactness of the method or the precision of its application: one recipe involves soaking thirty fresh leaves in wine overnight, grinding them up and resolving them into the wine to make a drink, reporting that thirty leaves is enough for 'fatte and stronge men' but should be reduced for others 'after her myghte and age' (p. 134). Rose petals, in a variety of forms, could cure excess menstruation, stop diarrhoea, heal festering wounds, and a plethora of other positive outcomes: no wonder the text affirms it as 'floure of all floures' (p. 90). Hemlock is acknowledged for its dangers as 'a colde venym', and its role in the death of Socrates and in Athenian executions is recounted, along with the symptoms and telltales of its effects so that they can be recognised. But the text understandably resiles from giving instructions about how the poison should be made 'for þy þat no thynge shold be tolde here oute neþer y taught þe wyche myght noye but only thylke þat shal helpe & profyte to man' (p. 118). There is, however, a suspiciously straightforward (and pleasurable) antidote ('Drynke he stronge wyne chaufed & he shal a scape þe perell'), which no doubt encouraged many readers in the regular application of apotropaic doses of mulled wine, just to be on the safe side.

* * *

'Have ye no mannes herte, and han a berd?' What the correct strength for herbal administration to chickens might be is hard to deduce from Macer Floridus, but the most famous Middle English account of herbal remedies is of course that found in Chaucer's *Nun's Priest's Tale*:

> Ye been ful coleryk of compleccioun;
> Ware the sonne in his ascencioun
> Ne fynde yow nat repleet of humours hoote.
> And if it do, I dar wel leye a grote,
> That ye shul have a fevere terciane,
> Or an agu that may be youre bane.
> A day or two ye shul have digestyves
> Of wormes, er ye take youre laxatyves
> Of lawriol, centaure, and fumetere,
> Or elles of ellebor, that groweth there,
> Of katapuce, or of gaitrys beryis,
> Of herbe yve, growyng in oure yeerd, ther mery is;
> Pekke hem up right as they growe and ete hem yn.
> (VII. 2955-67)

Like so many other aspects of this mercurial tale, Chaucer's use of herbals blends domestic realism with magical realism to create a heady and intoxicating brew of farmyard wisdom and medical absurdism. Critics have pointed out that not only would the herbs she recommends not all be available at the same time or at the season of the tale, but also that they would have had conflicting and potentially fatal consequences if taken together.[3] But an attentive medieval reader of Macer Floridus would soon have worked out that Pertelote's prescriptions for her husband's wellbeing would have created a toxic blend of reactions that would be more likely to carry him off than to cure what ailed him, and they would have probably revelled in the poisonous comedy of her wifely solicitude, which would have resulted in a purgation that was potentially purgatorial. More sedately and reflecting a more ordered and Platonically choreographic view of the universe, John Gower's linkage of the fifteen major stars with stones and herbs in book VII of his *Confessio Amantis* is based on the account said to have been given by Nectanabus to Alexander the Great:

> Of certein sterres what thei mene;
> Of whiche, he seith, ther ben fiftene,
> And sondrily to everich on
> A gras belongeth and a ston,
> Wherof men worchen many a wonder
> To sette thing bothe up and under.
> (*Confessio Amantis*, VII, 1303-8)[4]
> [...]
> The seconde is noght vertules;
> Clota or elles Pliades
> It hatte, and of the mones kinde
> He is, and also this I finde,
> He takth of Mars complexion:
> And lich to such condicion
> His ston appropred is cristall,

3 Paula Aiken, 'Vincent of Beauvais and Dame Pertelote's Knowledge of Medicine', *Speculum* 10 (1935): 281-287; Corinne E. Kauffman, 'Dame Pertelote's Parlous Parle', *The Chaucer Review*,4 (1969): 41-48.

4 John Gower, *Confessio Amantis*, Volume 3, ed. by Russell Peck, with Latin translations by Andrew Galloway, TEAMS (Kalamazoo, MI: Medieval Institute Publications, 2004), available online at <http://www.lib.rochester.edu/camelot/teams/cav3b7fr-fifteenstars.htm>.

And ek his herbe in special
The vertuous fenele it is.
(*Confessio Amantis*, VII, 1319-27)

Gower's account reflects the sort of knowledge of natural magic found in encyclopaedic works like the *De proprietatibus rerum* of the thirteenth-century Franciscan Bartholomaeus Anglicus, which was translated into the English vernacular by John Trevisa in the second half of the fourteenth century. But whereas encyclopaedias were always likely to be a recherché taste, largely restricted to religious and educational institutions, the upper classes of the laity, and the professions, texts like Macer Floridus also provided a more portable and accessible compendium of herbal lore 'þat techyth and oponly shewyth the uertues of many dyuerse herbes' (p. 61). Vernacular versions of texts such as this would have given generations of provincial Pertelotes the confidence to diagnose and prescribe for their households:

Though in this toun is noon apothecarie,
I shal myself to herbes techen yow
That shul been for youre hele and for youre prow.
(VII. 2948-2950)

What alarming consequences may have followed from such leech craft is hard to know but easy to imagine. The welcome availability of editions like this can only deepen our understanding of an important and still under researched aspect of popular socio-medical lore.

Vincent Gillespie
University of Oxford
October 3rd, 2011

Chapter 1. The Manuscript

1.1. Source

GUL MS Hunter 497 (V.7.24.) (henceforth H497) contains a mid-to-late 15th century English translation of Macer Floridus' *De Viribus Herbarum*, a Latin poem written in hexameters with a total of 2269 lines (and 77 plants). According to Frisk's own estimation (1949: 13), the Latin source is thought to have been written some time between 849 and 1112, on account of a series of cross-references found.

The author of the Latin version is Odo de Meung, a medical practitioner from Meung (on the Loire), who compiled this medical lore from those sources to which he had a regular and handy access, particularly the works of Pliny and Galen. However, we have no information about the adding of *Macer Floridus* as the subtitle of the poem, and any attempt to justify its adding is but a conjecture. Frisk (1949: 13-14) argues that Odo de Meung himself added it, plausibly with the following objectives. On the one hand, *Macer* may be a pseudonym after the Latin author Aemilius Macer, a contemporary of Virgil and Ovid, so as to imitate the classical writer's didactic poem, which dealt with similar material. On the other hand, Odo de Meung might have coveted the name and popularity of the Latin writer, a fact leading him to cite the authority in the subtitle of his work.

1.2. Parallel manuscripts

Odo de Meung's *De Viribus Herbarum* was widely known in the latter Middle Ages, both among general practitioners and laymen. The mediaeval appraisal of the poem may be corroborated on account of the number of translations available into the different European vernacular languages, such as French, German and Danish (see Frisk 1949: 15)[1].

In the case of mediaeval England, the level of estimation of the Latin original was such that we observe a proliferation of vernacular Macers, particularly throughout the 14th and 15th centuries. The crucial problem here lies in the fact that many of them are what Frisk calls "false English translations of Macer" (1949: 16), the bulk of ME herbals wherein the name of Macer is spuriously added to gain a wider acceptance among their readership. BL MS Sloane 5, and BL MS Sloane 963, for instance, are good examples of this attributed authorship.

According to Voigts and Kurtz (2000), there is a long list of English MSS arising from Macer Floridus' *De Viribus Herbarum*, some of them complete and some others fragmentary, or simply excerpts. The main drawback of Voigts and Kurtz's account is that they do not distinguish between real and false Macers, thus being of little help to investigate the textual tradition of the Latin source. In addition, their list is incomplete because they do not mention the existence of the ME version of *De Viribus Herbarum*, housed in two Sloane manuscripts (*i.e.* 2269 and 2527).

In light of this, we have largely benefited from Frisk's own readings of the actual manuscripts, a fact leading him to postulate a total of eight parallel manuscripts, all of them from the second half of the 15th century, forming the basis of his 1949 critical edition. The manuscripts are listed below (Frisk 1949: 17-26):

- Stockholm Royal Library X.91, ff. 1r-45r (X).
- Bodleian Rawlinson C. 81, ff. 18r-57r (R).

1 For a complete description of these translations in the vernacular, see Frisk (1949: 15).

- Bodleian Digby 95, ff. 10r-80v (D).
- Bodleian Hatton 29, ff. 1r-55v (H).
- CUL Ee.1.15, ff. 24v-65r (E).
- BL Add. 37786, ff. 2r-42v (A).
- BL Sloane 2269, ff. 81r-112v (S1).
- BL Sloane 2527, ff. 251r-293v (S2).

Frisk's compendium has been supplemented with Keiser's (1998: §235), which adds one complete and other five fragmentary versions of this same text:

- BL Sloane 393, ff. 88r-145v.
- Bodleian Selden Supra 73, ff. 75v-82r.
- Bodleian Rawlinson A.393, ff. 88v-89r.
- BL Sloane 1571, ff. 17, 20v-22v, 31v-33r.
- BL Sloane 2187, ff. 45r-48v.
- BL Sloane 3866, ff. 12r-13r, 73v-77v (conflated with other material).

Notwithstanding the meritorious labour of Frisk to get hold of every mediaeval English version of Macer's text, there is one manuscript which escaped his attention, GUL MS Hunter 497 (V.7.24), possibly because he carried out his research during the war when most manuscripts were evacuated from libraries to ensure their preservation. In light of this deficiency, H497 is the only English version of a Macer's text which remains so far unedited.

Therefore, the present edition of the Hunterian text, basically diplomatic, has been especially thought of to complement Frisk's critical edition of the extant manuscripts of *De Viribus Herbarum*. The immediate objective is therefore to offer an accurate transcription of the original text, which can be used as a primary source for subsequent linguistic insight.

Besides, the edition also contributes to offering an alternative link to survey the relationship among the various manuscripts. Frisk initially postulates the existence of two independent groups, the first containing

X, R, H, and S1 and the second D, E, S2 and A. As far as we have been able to investigate, and given the close parallelism between the Hunterian and the Stockholm texts, the former would be, in principle, ascribed to the first group of manuscripts, even though the matter still awaits the labour of further inspection.

1.3. Contents

H497 exclusively houses the above-mentioned version of Macer's *De Viribus Herbarum*, running from f. 1r through f. 92r. The treatise is divided into three books which, according to the writer, correspond to the organization of the Latin original. The first book (ff. 1r-61r) deals with the properties of a total of 66 herbs; the second (ff. 61r-79v) accounts for the remedies of other twenty plants; and finally, the third (ff. 79v-92r) is devoted to the healing properties of twenty common spices.

In addition, the volume also houses a total of five prescriptions. Two of them are displayed on the verso of a vellum flyleaf at the beginning with a legible 18th-century hand. The other three are found on f. 92v. All these are recipes especially recommended for the treatment of digestive and urinal problems.

1.4. Codicology

1.4.1. Material, dimensions and ink

H497 is written in a relatively coarse and defective vellum. It is worn out by the passing of time and its top and edges are somewhat charred (Young and Aitken 1908: 409; Cross 2004: 33-34). F. 11r perfectly illustrates the level of coarseness of the parchment, plausibly as a result of innate malformation, which has eventually produced the blurring of a great part of the text.

Written in an *octavo* size, the volume's dimensions are 167mm x 120mm, thus complying with the standard proportions of that particular type of folding in the period (Johnston 1945: 69).

Black ink is systematically employed for the running text, whilst red is used as a macro-textual device to signal a new section or subsection. In this fashion, the copyist exploits vermilion in the following situations: a) in the opening lines of the book to refer back to Aemilius Macer as the author of the text; b) in rubricated initials to signal the actual beginning of a new herb or spice; and c) in initials (just touched with vermilion) to spot the different virtues within a given herb.

1.4.2. Quiring and collation

According to Young and Aitken's collation of the volume under scrutiny (1908: 409), the 104 ff. of the manuscript are distributed in thirteen quires with the following characteristics:

> Two modern buff paper fly-leaves (i^{2}), I, I. attached. One original vellum fly-leaf (ii^{1}). || 1^{8}-11^{8}, $15^{5(8)}$, $13^{1(8)}$. || One modern buff paper fly-leaf (iii^{1}), attached to the remains of 13, 7. 13, 8. attached in lieu of fly-leaf. The following leaves are lost: 12, 6. 7. 8; 13, 1-7. ii, I. originally attached.

There are no signs of pagination to grant the correct sequence of quires after writing. The scribe, in turn, recurs to the use of quiring catchwords "whereby the first word of a quire was written at the bottom of the last leaf of the preceding quire" (Petti 1977: 6). H497 presents the characteristic *octavo folding* wherein quires consist of eight leaves each (Johnston 1945: 68). Therefore, catchwords are found in f. 8v (*mor strongly*), f. 16v (*uyolet*), f. 24v (*trowe be*), f. 32v (*to be moyst*), f. 40v (*þat þey wol*), f. 48v (*kerneles*), f. 56v (*blod*), f. 64v (*uij uertu*), f. 72v (*euer*), f. 80v (*cancres*) and f. 87v (*takyth*).

1.4.3. Ruling

Drawn with brown crayon, some of the manuscript folios present some traces of frame-ruling, according to which the writing surface consistently measures 114mm x 88mm.

As a result of such a careful planning of the writing surface, there is also a consistent dimension of the margins. In a folio recto, the upper and lower margins measure 20mm and 40mm, respectively, while the left and right margins, in turn, amount to 15mm and 25mm. According to Johnston (1945: 72), the margin dimensions are in most cases a matter of convention in early English manuscript composition insofar as the foot margin is usually twice as wide as that at the top and the side margins are greater than the top and less than the foot. By doing this, mediaeval scribes pursued that "the height of the written space equalled the width of the page" (de Hamel 1992: 21).

H497, however, partially complies with these conventions. Even though it is a fact that the inferior margin measures twice as much as the superior margin, the left margin never equals the size of the top margin. In addition, de Hamel's prerequisite is also ignored since the height of the written space (88mm) does not tally with the actual width of the page (120mm).

Contradictory as it may be, the author of H497 cold-shoulders the use of line-ruling, which becomes so frequent in other mediaeval prose compositions, to secure a visually appealing layout of the text. Instead, the scribe is at all times meticulous so as to provide a consistent number of lines per folio, ranging from 21 to 22, though the latter overwhelmingly prevails.

1.4.4. Foliation

Foliation in H497 is systematically positioned at the top right corner of every folio recto. The text gives evidence of two foliation systems and, unlike other mediaeval manuscripts where a double foliation is often the result of different bindings, in H497 they coincide.

The first foliation is just partial, running from f. 1r through 35r. F. 36r, in turn, only shows the use of number <3>, giving the impression that the person in charge of foliating the text was interrupted therein and never concluded the task. This foliation, according to Young and Aitken (1908: 409), dates back to the 16th century on account of the particular form of some figures. Of these, number 3 stands out, fairly rounded and resembling a cursive <z>; number 4, already with its modern appearance; number 5 showing a square top; and number 9 with its tail curved back (Tannenbaum 1930: 155-157).

The second foliation, on the other hand, is complete, running from ff. 1r-92r. It is written with a 17th-century hand insofar as the shape completely coincides with that of their modern counterparts (Young and Aitken 1908: 409).

1.4.5. Binding

According to Young and Aitken, H497 shows an early 15th-century binding consisting of bevelled oak boards covered with sheep skin, now stained and discoloured (1908: 409; see also Cross 2004: 33). It measures 195mm x 140mm so as to exceed the actual dimension of the folios for the sake of a better preservation. To some extent, the volume demands a re-binding process because the quires are now torn from the spine, a fact which may lead to the eventual splitting of quires and/or folios.

The volume shows traces of the existence of a former leather strap and a buckle to secure a tight fastening of the folios (see Pollard 1976: 61). Even though repaired before the publication of Young and Aitken's catalogue in 1908, the pin is now fallen (Cross 2004: 33).

1.4.6. Flyleaves

According to the collation provided by Young and Aitken (1908: 409), the volume shows the existence of two buff paper fly-leaves at the beginning (i^2), which are accordingly followed by another vellum fly-leaf (ii^1), originally attached. In its present state, however, there is no trace of these paper fly-leaves, which have been plausibly lost as a result of the deficient condition of the binding.

The vellum fly-leaf contains the reference to the scientific authority of the treatise, the prestigious practitioner Aemilius Macer, with relatively legible 18th-century hand in the following terms (quoted from Young and Aitken 1908: 409).

> Opusculum Æmilij Maceri | Medici Italiensis . vixit Centuria | prima ante | Galenum Ames (¿) | vide pleen Hystoria Medicin.

The remains of this same fly-leaf also show two 16th-century prescriptions. The volume also includes another blank paper fly-leaf at the end (iii^1), which is attached in-between ff. 92 and 93, the latter used as the inside back cover.

1.5. Palaeography

1.5.1. Letterforms

With the exception of section titles and marginalia, H497 is written with a fairly legible 15th-century secretary script (Petti 1977: 14-15), also termed as *Gothic littera cursiva secretary media* (Roberts 2005: 230-231). Of Italian provenance, this script was imported from France throughout the 14th century and, in view of its swiftness and cursiveness, it soon gained the acceptance of 15th-century scribes.

Roberts (2005: 211) argues that this script underwent a three-stage chronological process: heavy; splayed; and eventually tall and narrow. H497 is observed to belong to the incipient variety of this script wherein letters are mostly characterised by their rounded and angular appearance. In this vein, thin and thick strokes combine together with horns on the heads and sides of bowls, thus contributing to the accessible reading of the text (Petti 1977: 14).

Figure 1 below contains a reproduction of the minuscules used by the scribe of H497. For reference purposes, the letters are numbered. Formally speaking, the scribe is meticulous as to the use of the secretary hand insofar as all the letters, with the only exception of letters <s> (18) and <w> (23), conform to this orthographic standard of the 15th century.

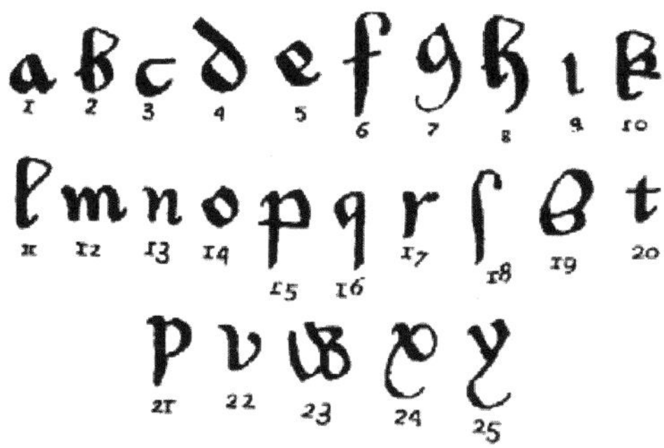

Fig. 1 Catalogue of minuscules in H497

As shown, the secretary hand is witnessed in the use of particular letter-forms, such as the following: single-lobed <a> with a pointed head (1); two-lobed <b> (2); the letter <d> consisting of a shank with a somewhat oblique ascender (4); <g> with a pointed head and a small tail (7); the letter <f> showing a shaft with an arced head-stroke (6); the letter <l> with a lobed arm (13); right-shouldered <r>, footed and sitting on the script line (17); and cursive <x> written with a single stroke (24), among others. The letter <þ>, in turn, consists of an infra-linear letter rendered by a vertical and clubbed stroke with a curved serif at the top of the backbone (21), thus preventing the likely association with the letter <y>.

There are some letters which show alternative forms depending on their relative position within the bounds of a word, either initially, medially or finally. As in other late mediaeval manuscripts (Calle-Martín 2004a: 83), double-length long <s> is consistently used word-initially (18), which may be deemed a direct influence of the 14th-century *Anglicana Formata* (18 above). If in a medial or final position, on the other hand, it consists of a small *B* or a *c* and *3* run together, as in (19) (Petti 1977: 14).

As mentioned above, letter <w> is the only item which cannot be properly ascribed to the catalogue of the *Secretary* hand. Instead of a double <v>, H497 presents the combination of two looped *l*'s and a *3* (see 23), a letterform which typifies the late 14th-century *Anglicana Formata* script.

In view of all this, in spite of the overwhelming primacy of the 15th-century standard, the script of H497 may be defined as a hybrid script, wherein the *Secretary* script is softly blended with the *Anglicana Formata*. Petti argues that, in the particular case of the secretary script, these borrowings were more than common in the early part of the 15th century, "both in features of general style and in use of graphs" (1977: 15).

1.5.2. Section titles

Section titles show a different type of script, a somewhat bigger formal hybrid hand, agglutinating features of the *hybrid Anglicana* and the 15th-century *Secretary*. The former has been found in the representation of the double-lobed <a>, the single-shanked <d> with a perpendicular ascender, letter <w> consisting of two looped *l*'s and a *3* along with letters <e> and <h>. The secretary hand, in turn, is noted in the letter <k> with a rightwards looped stem, lobe-armed <l>, right-shouldered <r> and the letter <g> with a pronounced head-stroke. As above, the letter <s> shows two alternatives, word-initial long <s> and beta-like <s>, preferred in medial and final positions.

1.5.3. Numerals

Orthographically speaking, the Middle Ages is a key period in the development of numerals insofar as it is a landmark in the transition from the Roman to the Arabic system. Even though of sporadic use in English in the 12th century, Arabic numerals gained considerable ground throughout the 13th and 14th centuries, particularly when numbering the quires and folios of a manuscript. Hector (1966: 43) maintains that Arabic numerals do not become really common in English documents as mere graphic alternatives for Roman figures until 1530. Before that date, however, the use of one or the other was basically a matter of scribal choice.

Despite a 15th-century composition, H497 discards the use of Arabic numerals. Instead, Roman figures are systematically used and, according to the mediaeval practice, they are reproduced by using the same cursive form as the rest of the letterforms. In the light of this premise, the mediaeval system developed a set of intrinsic characteristics which differed from the Roman usage, all these are found in H497.

On the one hand, numerals are consistently rendered as small-case letters and, as such, they share the same orthographic convention as to the use of <u> and <v>. Number five, for instance, is represented in H497 as <u> in view of the overwhelming preference for this letter to the detriment of its counterpart <v>. On the other hand, final and isolated units are reproduced with the *j-longa*, a practice which avoids the likely confusion of the figure with the following word, as in <j, ij, iij, uj> and the like. Third, there may be more than three figures in a sequence, as in <iiij>, <uiiij>, etc.

Ordinal numbers, in turn, are quite frequent in H497 to enumerate the different virtues of a particular herb. The first three numbers (*fyrste*, *seconde* and *thrydde*) are always spelled out, whilst the orthographic representation of the other numerals is twofold: either with a superscript <e> as in <x^{e}>, <ix^{e}>, <xij^{e}> or without it, as if a cardinal number, like *the iiij uertu*, *the u uertu*, *the uj uertu*, etc. The latter, however, are by far the most recurrent practice of the scribe.

1.5.4. Marginalia

Marginal notes in H497 show the use of three different hands. Hand A, on the one hand, corresponds to the scribe's actual handwriting, who uses the margin as a visual aid for the reader to point out the beginning of a new herb by means of the corresponding Roman numeral. These are accordingly underlined in vermilion.

Hands B and C, on the other hand, are written with a 16th-century *Secretary* script, with features of the Early Tudor *Secretary*. Even though some of them are in a dim greyish ink, it is possible to see the use of some letterforms which characterise these scripts, such as the open reversed <e>, the <h> with a double-looped shaft, the 2-like <r>, the long <s>, the hybrid <g>, or the <x> looking like *v* with an enclosing tail (see also Petti 1977: 17). The information contained therein serves as an index for the reader who may find the remedy of a particular pain or malady just by a quick turning of the pages, with phrases like the following: *for the breste*, *for the spleen*, *for podagre*, *for the feuer of coler*, etc.

1.5.5. Punctuation

Punctuation practice in early English manuscripts is not as consistent as modern punctuation, a fact which explains why this area of palaeography has been traditionally disregarded in the literature owing to its high level of arbitrariness (Jenkinson 1926: 154; Denholm-Young 1964: 77; Arakelian 1975: 614-615). In the last decades, there has been a proliferation of studies arguing the existence of a conventional system of scribal punctuation, with a more or less restricted set of rules, both grammatical and rhetorical, which the scribe skilfully uses for the correct understanding of the message (Alonso-Almeida 2002: 207-232; Calle-Martín 2004: 407-422; Calle-Martín and Miranda-García 2005a: 95-113; Calle-Martín and Miranda-García 2007).

From a formal standpoint, scribal practice varies across centuries and scriptoria. According to Parkes (1992: 42-45), the general repertory of punctuation symbols in the latter Middle Ages was based on the following components: the *punctus*, the *punctus elevatus*, the *punctus interrogatiuus* and *littera notabiliores*, as well as the *virgule*, the *paragraph mark* and the *positura*. Notwithstanding the currency of these punctuation symbols in the period, every scribe is ultimately free to imprint his own repertory of symbols, each developing an intrinsic set of rules. In the case of H497, despite being a 15th-century piece of *Fachliteratur*, it shows a reduced repertory of punctuation marks, as it is just limited to the use of three main components: the *punctus*, the *paragraph mark* and the *double hyphen*, together with coloured initials which may be deemed as punctuation marks insofar as they signal macro-textual relations.

a) Coloured majuscules and initial shading are macro-textual devices used by the scribe to facilitate skimming and identify the major sections within the flow of writing, having the effect of a punctuation mark (Lucas 1971: 11; see also Calle-Martín and Miranda-García 2005b: 32). This is, as a matter of fact, the only sign of decoration in H497, and it consists in the use of a vermilion majuscule to highlight the beginning of a new herb or spice within the flow of writing. Likewise, the author also makes use of black-inked initials, touched with vermilion, to highlight the different virtues within a given herb.

b) The *paragraph mark* (represented here by means of ¶) only appears twice in the treatise with the form of a capital letter <C>, red-hued in both cases. As in other recipe books of the period (Alonso-Almeida 2002: 225), the *paraph* is a visual device used by the scribe to indicate that one or more words run over from the previous line. For instance, the use of that symbol in the following examples informs the reader that what comes next actually belongs to the information contained in the previous line.

> [...] Ant yt helpyth ayenst þe goute
> Wermode . ys hoot yn þe fyrst ¶ þ*at* preuy .
> degre & drye yn þe seconde . (116-18).

> Thys seed eten w*ith* hony wol staunche
> þe cowe & do muche good to þe streytnes
> Popye ys colde & drye ¶ of þe brest
> & as yt ys seyde þer ben iij ma
> neres of yt ffor þe floure of one ys
> wythe of a noþer yt ys reed [...] (1319-22).

c) The *punctus* (·), or period, is the only mark of punctuation used in H497, amounting to 2,439 instances. This mark presents two different positions, the raised and the low period, albeit the former notably prevails. It is consistently ornamented in the conclusion of every major section.

Functionally speaking, the lack of other punctuation symbols in the treatise (*i.e.* the *virgule* and the *punctus elevatus*) directly influences the level of specialisation of those used, in such a way that the less number of punctuation symbols in a text, the greater the versatility of those consistently used. In light of this, the *punctus*, therefore, is the device used by the scribe to signal all types of textual relations, both at sentence and at clause level.

At sentence level, on the one hand, the period is used to signal several kinds of relationships, particularly the beginning of a new statement, juxtaposition, coordination and adverbial subordination, as shown in the corresponding instances below:

> The fyrst u*er*tu þe decocc*i*on of þys her be drunke yn wyne curyth all deedly by tynges . The ij u*er*tu þe decocc*i*on drunke w*ith* mulsa . (1910-12).

Wasshe & bathe þe matryce . And so shalt thow clense wome*n* of her floures . Also take þe same herbe grene as she growyht & stampe yt & bynde yt to þe wombe . And she shal delyuery þe werplynge þ*at* ys þ*er*yn . Also drynke moderwort . or make þereof a subfumygacio*un* . (61-65).

Also stampe yt & leye yt to þe fresshe wondes . for yt helyth he*m* fayre . (154-55v).

Nominal and adjectival subordination, in turn, are usually left unpunctuated unless punctuation serves to clarify the actual meaning of the utterance, as in the following instance:

The u uertu wyse men sayn þat þe wyne þat þys herbe hath leyen yn . wol kepe þe stryngthe of a mans mynde yf he drynke yt . (1902-4).

At clause level, on the other hand, the *punctus* is consistently used to signal the following relationships between the constituents: to enumerate items in a sequence, to introduce coordinate phrases, tag phases such as *þat is to say*, appositions, as well as to highlight a particular clause constituent, as in the following cases:

Stampe to gyder wermode . narde & þe tre þ*at* ys called syler te*m*pre yt w*ith* uenyger & dry*n*ke yt . (130-31).

Ssho wol stampe wormode w*ith* uynegre & anoy*n*te hym þer w*ith* . hym dare not drede of gnattes flyes . ne flees . (137-39).

The u u*er*tu grene ysope stamped & melde w*ith* oxiniel . þ*at* ys to say w*ith* amaner of drynke þ*at* ys made w*ith* uenygre & hony . (858-60).

Mugworte or moderworte ys cleped . Arthemesia . yn latyn . (51).

d) Finally, the *double hyphen* (=) is the mark of punctuation chosen at the end of a line to mark off the splitting of a word into two lines (Hector 1966: 48). The use of the double hyphen in English documents, consisting in the use of two thin oblique strokes slightly curved upwards, spread from the latter part of the 15th century. Notwithstanding the increasing standardization of punctuation symbols in these contexts, they could often be left out where there was insufficient room at the edge of the folio.

In the particular case of H497, the double hyphen is systematically adopted to signal line-final division. There are just a few instances where the punctuation symbol is missing, plausibly as a result of a slip on the part of the writer. The scribe is particularly meticulous and fills most of the writing surface, thus discarding the use of line-fillers. This explains the number of word division instances in the text (954 instances).

The instances have been surveyed in terms of the particular type of splitting, whether morphological or phonological. In consequence, word division practice in H497 reveals an overwhelming preference for phonological divisions as they represent 92.38% of the instances (*clary-fye*, *her-be*, *lun-ges*, *uyne-gre*, among others) if compared with just 7.62% of instances showing morphological boundaries, like *destroy-eth*, *go-ynge*, *y-dronke*, etc. (Calle-Martín 2009: 35-53).

1.5.6. Emendations

Professional scribes were committed to revise their own compositions and, on account of the nature of the emendation, they recurred to the use of deletion, insertion or alteration. H497 may be safely deemed a valuable copy in view of several palaeographic considerations, from frame ruling to conventional margins, together with the use of a legible hand, which is represented with the utmost care for the sake of the preciousness of the composition. This fact actually explains the scarce number of emendations in the text but, when necessary, the scribe systematically resorts to deletion and insertion. Alterations, in turn, are not tracked down in the text.

Deletion, on the one hand, consists in the ruling out of a letter or word(s) of a text. There are several methods of deletion in Middle English manuscript composition, which are chosen by the writer in view of different variables, such as the ink, the level of formality of the text, and/or the visual excellence of the final product (Petti 1977: 29). As a piece of *Fachliteratur*, we have to disregard the likely participation of formality and the visual appeal of the text in the choice of a particular method of deletion in H497. The writer is mostly concerned with the perfect understanding of the message, a fact leading him to the systematic use of the *single-stroke cancellation* in the need of a particular deletion, as in the example below.

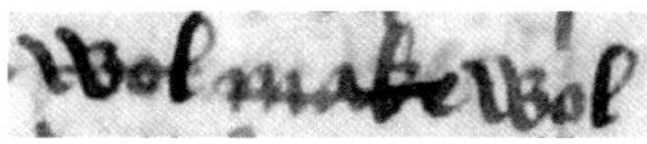

2245 '~~wol~~ ~~make~~ wol'

On some occasions, the single-stroke cancellation becomes so light that it is often overlooked during the editorial process, hence the need of a series of multiple readings to spot them. See for instance, the following example where '*we*' is ruled out with a dim criss-cross pattern.

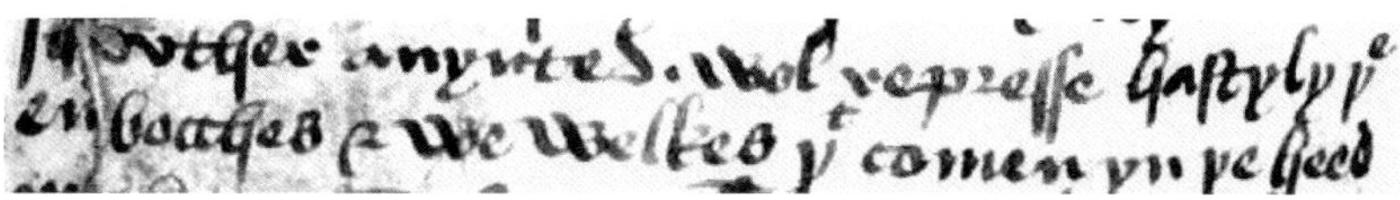

2303 'represse hastily þe bocches & ~~we~~ welkes þ*at* comen yn þe heed'

Insertions, on the other hand, consist in the actual adding of a letter or word(s) as a likely consequence of the copyist's slip. In H497, we exclusively find the use of interlineations whilst a caret is often employed to elucidate the particular point of insertion.

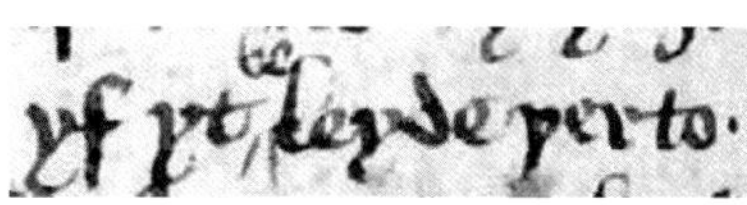

284 'yf yt ^be leyde þerto'

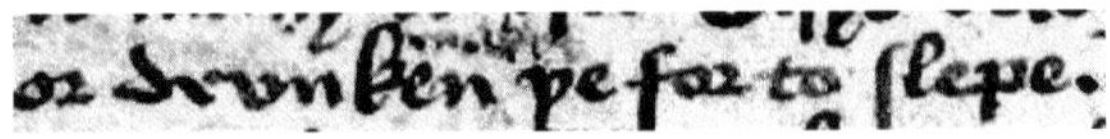

1362 'or drunken makyth þe for to slepe'

1.5.7. Abbreviations

If compared with the humble contribution of Anglo-Saxon scribes, the Middle English period witnesses the adoption of a more widespread inventory of abbreviations, particularly throughout the 13th and 14th centuries, by imitating the habits of Latin scribes (Hector 1966: 38). Mediaeval writers appropriated those symbols which were directly transferable from Latin exemplars, mostly marks of suspension and brevigraphs.

After this sudden rise, the 15th century marks off "a general diminution in the employment of abbreviations and a return to the more moderate use typical of the twelfth century" (Derolez 2003: 187), to the extent that in the 16th century its use becomes sporadic among penmen in the Renaissance (i.e. the Elizabethan proclamations housed in GUL MS Hunter 3, Calle-Martín and Miranda-García 2007).

Unlike other fields of palaeography traditionally considered erratic in the literature (word-division and punctuation, for instance), abbreviations were more homogeneous among Middle English writers in order to secure the faultless understanding of the utterances.

Complying with the standards of a 15th-century piece of prose, the scribe of H497 does not aspire to the rendering of a conspicuous shorthand, recurring instead to a fairly conventional system of abbreviations, easily interpreted by any modern reader not even acquainted with the basics of mediaeval palaeography. Therefore, the text may be considered the perfect archetype of 15th-century practice as the narrow inventory of abbreviations sheds light on the progressive obliteration of abbreviating symbols (Derolez 2003: 187). Formally speaking, manuscript abbreviations are traditionally classified in terms of four different categories:

contraction, suspension, brevigraphs and superior letters. The particulars of each in H497 are accounted for in the sections below.

a) *Contraction* is the omission of one or more letters from the middle of a word. Even though the most widespread abbreviation in mediaeval manuscripts, its use in H497 is limited to the *tittle* or the *tilde* (a straight horizontal stroke of varying length) as a substitute for letters <m>, <n>, <u> and <i>, the latter exclusively in the *-ion* suffix (Tannenbaum 1930: 120). Its use seems erratic in H497 insofar as the author prefers to spell out the corresponding word.

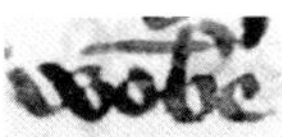

278 'wo*m*be'

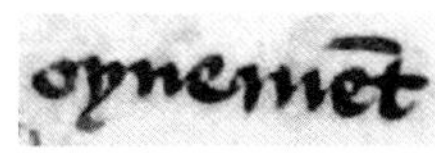

1118 'oyneme*nt*'

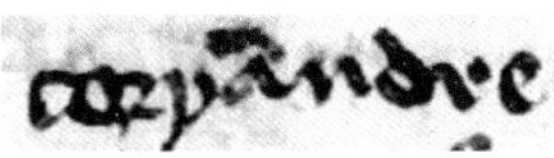

249 'corya*u*ndre'

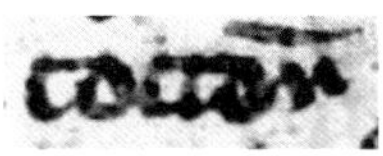

93 'cocc*i*on'

b) *Suspension*, also termed *curtailment*, is the omission of one or more letters at the end of a word (Tannenbaum 1930: 124). Unlike other 15th-century texts (GUL MS Hunter 328, for instance), the scribe of H497 is not particularly committed to the use of suspension to the extent that these abbreviations are often disregarded in favour of the actual spelling of the words. H497 gives evidence of a single form of curtailment. As mentioned above, the first is the use of the tilde as a substitute for letters <m> and <n> if in word-final positions, as in the following cases:

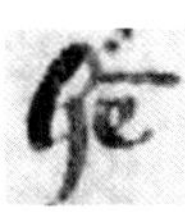

1842 'he*m*'

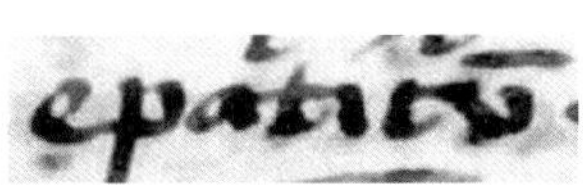

2623 'epaticu*m*'

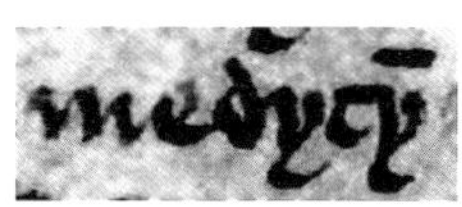

1355 'medycy*n*'

Otiose strokes, in turn, are also systematically avoided, thus preventing the editor's confusion as to whether there might be an intended abbreviation in these environments.

c) *Superior letters* consist in the raised position of one or more letters of a word, as if a superscript. This category of abbreviations was "coined for use in English-language writing" (Hector 1966: 39), being particularly conspicuous in the case of vernacular words. H497 shows a recurrent use of superior letters in three native words such as *þ*^{t} 'þat', *w*^{t} 'with' and *w*^{t} *oute(n)* 'without'.

Note, however, that the use of a superior letter does not always imply an actual abbreviation, being a matter of habit rather than omission in itself. This is typically the case of the determiner *þ*^{e} 'þe' and ordinal numbers like *x*^{e}, *xi*^{e}, *xii*^{e}, etc. In view of this, the use of italics is deprecated in our transcription.

d) *Brevigraphs* involve the use of some special signs, mostly borrowed from Latinate texts, to contract a number of frequently-occurring syllables, particularly at the beginning and at the end of a word. Medial positions, though sporadically found, become less frequent from the 15th century onwards. The brevigraphs used in H497 are the following:

- The cluster <*es*>/<*ys*> is sporadically abbreviated by means of a curved ascending stroke over the last letter of the word, irrespective of whether this is the stem or the plural morpheme, as in:

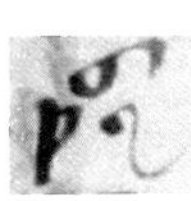

2302 'þ*ys*'

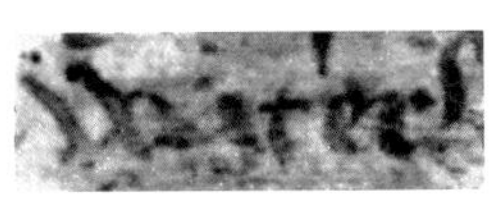

266 'water*ys*'

- The cluster <*us*> is exclusively found word-finally when the scribe recurs to using Latinate terms. This abbreviation coincides with the

<*con*> brevigraph, even though the former holds a final and supra-linear position (Petti 1977: 24). Note the use of this symbol in the following instances:

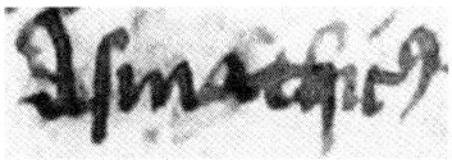

840 'Asmathic*us*'

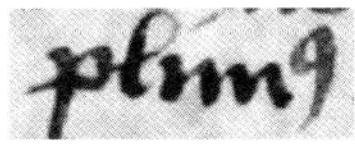

1748 'plini*us*'

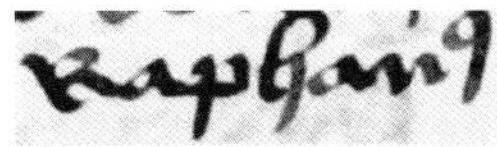

2804 'Raphan*us*'

- The cluster <*er*> is consistently represented by means of an ascending flourished stroke, curved leftwards, which is placed over the preceding letter, as in the following instances:

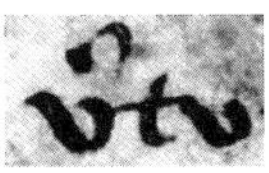

1385 'u*er*tu'

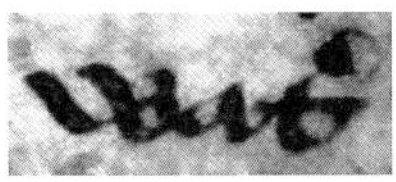

58 'wat*er*'

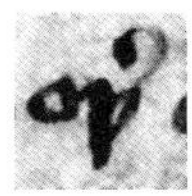

88 'oþ*er*'

- The cluster <*ur*> is occasionally conveyed through the use of a superscript letter <a>, a symbol which was widespread in vernacular compositions, as in the following instances:

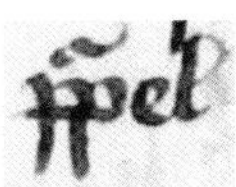

1727 'p*ur*pel'

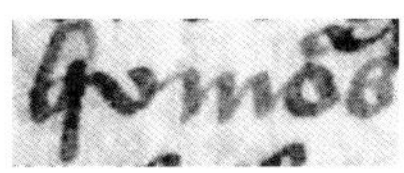

1900 ' humo*urs*'

- The other elements of the p-compendia (see Hector 1966: 39), <*par*> and <*pre*>, are abbreviated in H497 with letter <p> holding a straight bar through the stem, an abbreviation which is particularly productive in the case of Latinate derivatives, as in:

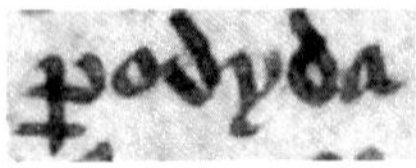

197 'p*ar*odyda'

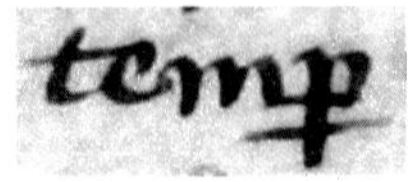

127 'temp*re*'

Note, however, that the scribe is not systematic in the use of these abbreviations insofar as the cluster *<pre>* is seldom represented by means of an ascending flourished stroke, which is the typical abbreviation of the group *<er>* throughout the text.

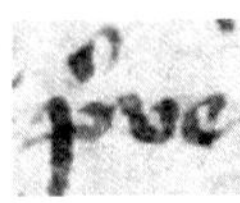

97 'p*re*ue'

- The cluster *<pro>* is represented in H497 by means of the letter <p> with a curved stroke through the descender. Unlike other manuscripts of the period, the stroke moves from left to right counter-clockwise, being made continuously with the descender, i.e. without a pen-lift (Tannenbaum 1930: 128), as in:

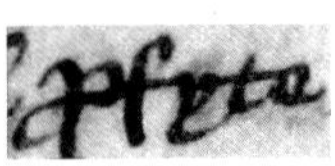

81 'p*ro*fyte'

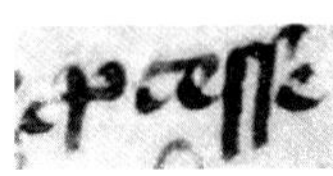

1063 'p*ro*cesse'

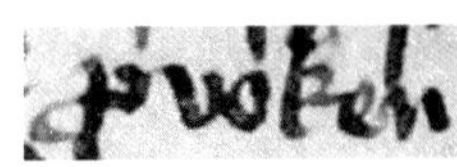

1733 'p*ro*uoken'

- The cluster *<con>* is abbreviated in initial position, taking the form of a q-like *us*-abbreviation (Tannenbaum 1930: 128), which is the typical form of this brevigraph throughout the latter part of the 15th century. Its use in H497 is just testimonial with one instance.

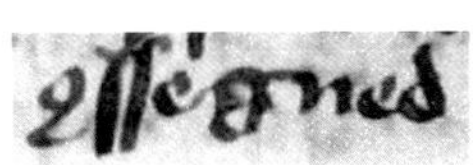

2223 '*con*ssegned'

- Even though a typical abbreviation in Latin documents, there is an example of a *q*-contraction in the Latin word *quarteyn*:

1908 'q*ua*rteyn'

1.6. A chronological note

The data obtained from the physical description of H497 serve to corroborate the dating of the text under scrutiny. From a paleographic perspective, on the one hand, the writer consistently complies with the standards of 15th-century manuscript composition, not only in terms of the script –a legible secretary hand–, but also in terms of punctuation or abbreviation. H497 may be deemed a perfect archetype of the 15th-century practice in light of the narrow inventory of abbreviation symbols and the systematic employment of the double hyphen, among others.

Codicologically speaking, on the other hand, it becomes thorny to arrive at definite conclusions as regards the particular date of composition of a given text. H497 conforms to the mediaeval convention in terms of material, ink, dimensions and ruling. Binding, however, is perhaps a more controversial aspect. Even though Young and Aitken consider it an early 15th-century binding (1908: 409; see also Cross 2004: 33), the above chronology must be tentatively ruled out on account of the palaeographic evidence. To this must be added the existence of several linguistic items pointing to a mid-to-late 15th-century composition, particularly morphological and phono-orthographic, all of them accordingly dealt with in chapter 5.

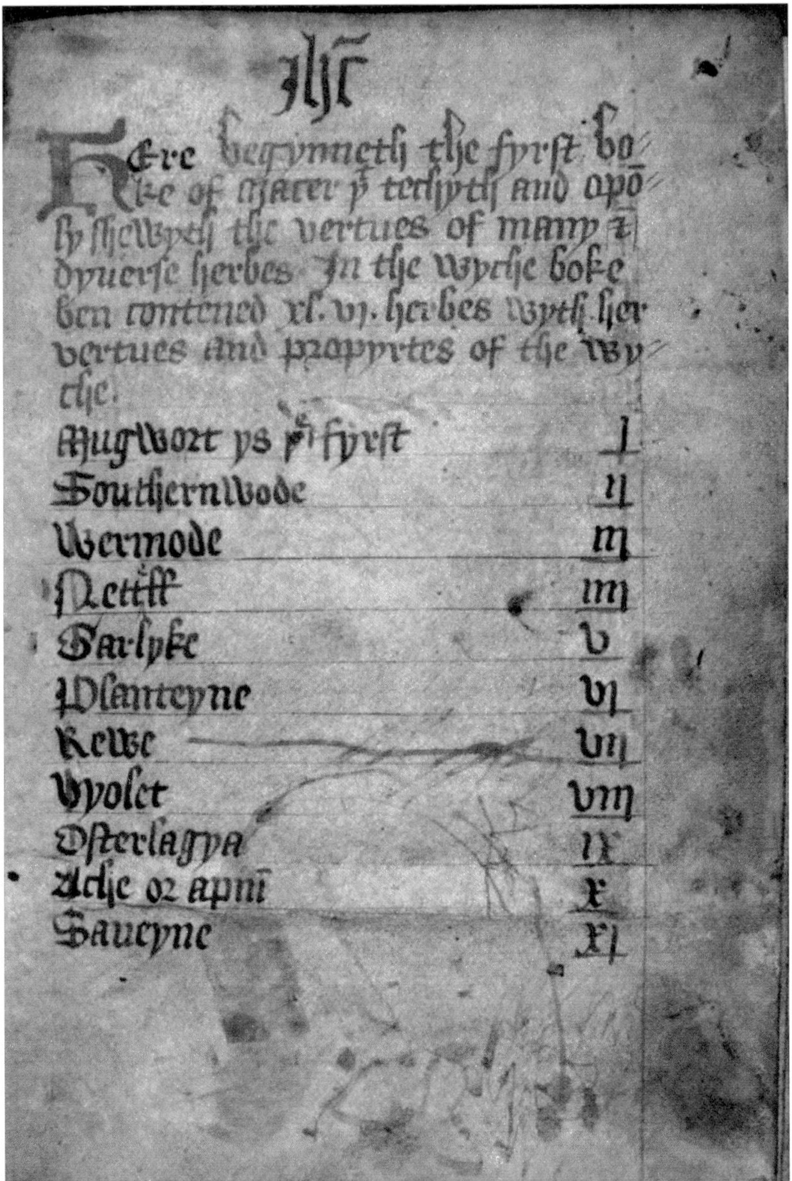

Plate 1. f. 1r

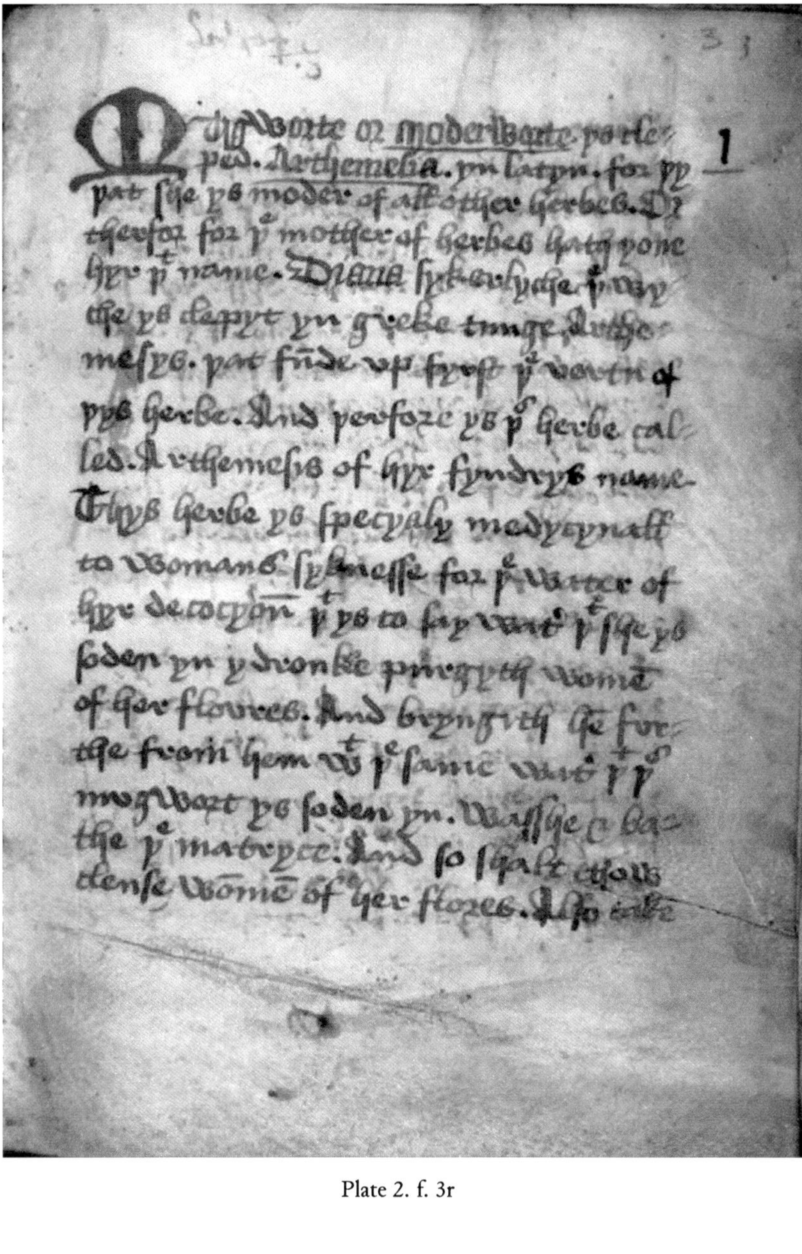

Plate 2. f. 3r

Chapter 2. The Language

2.1. Introduction

This chapter has been designed to complement the information offered in the notes to the diplomatic edition. Whilst most of the information contained therein is of phono-orthographic nature, this chapter approaches the writer's idiolect from a morpho-syntactic perspective. Our survey, however, does not aspire to a thorough examination of the text, being instead limited to considering the salient features of immediate interest for chronological, spatial or intrinsically linguistic reasons.

The chapter has been subsequently divided into three major parts. The first concentrates on inflectional morphology, thereby reviewing the accidence of the different word classes in H497. The second, in turn, succinctly approaches the syntax of the text by considering aspects such as word order, both phrasal and clausal, and the type of subordinators. The third, on the other hand, makes use of the above information to build, following the *LALME* questionnaire, the linguistic profile of H497 to conclude a likely provenance of the text.

When feasible, the occurrence of a particular token or accidence is given to determine, on a statistical basis, the factual practice of the author in every aspect, therefore allowing us to find any likely error together with the recurrent practice of the scribe, particularly at an orthographic and a morphological level.

2.2. Accidence

2.2.1. *Nouns*

As a 15th century piece of prose, H497 gives evidence of the existence of natural gender, with the only exception of several plant-names, which are usually feminine not only in classical Latin but also in OE, therefore preserving this same gender in need of a given anaphoric reference. From OE *hunigsūge* (fem.), for instance, the author consistently recurs to the feminine pronoun *she* in the anaphoric references to *honysoucle, i.e. in latyn comounly she ys cleped Baraces* (2066-67). A similar picture is observed in non-native terms, such as *uerueyne* (2280), from OF *verveine*; *letuse* (671), from OF *letües*; *wylde malowe* (924), from Latin *althaea*; and such others.

Table 1 below illustrates the nominal declension in H497, both weak and strong. Inflections are given in descending order of frequency.

	Singular	Plural
Nom/Object	-ø / -e	-(e)s / -ys / -(e)n / -(y)n
Genitive	-es / -s / -ys	-s / -(e)n

Table 1. Nominal morphemes in H497

2.2.1.1. *The nominative/objective case*

The common case in the singular is generally expressed by -ø, even though many a time the author recurs to the use of non-etymological -*e*, a commonplace among late ME scribes, as in *mouthe* (OE *mūþ*), *throte* (OE *þrotu*), *wolle* (OE *wull*), etc. The phenomenon also affects non-native words, as shown in *careweye* vs. *carewey*, *lylye* vs. *lyly*, *manere* vs. *maner*, *beteyne* vs. *beteyn*, etc.

Strong plurals, on the other hand, favour the *-(e)s* morpheme[2], amounting to 1,132 instances (84,85%). These are followed by *-ys* plurals, whose occurrence is just testimonial with 28 instances (2,09%). The plural morpheme *-(e)n/-(y)n*, on the other hand, is limited to the recurrent repetition of nouns such as *chyldryn*, *eyen/eyne*, *toon* in addition to others like *ashen*, *been*, *shone* and *hosen*, amounting to 62 instances altogether (4.6%).

Zero inflection plurals are restricted to some terms of measure, which are sporadically inflectionless after a numeral, as in *two maner of spices* (2169). This practice, however, is erratic in view of the outstanding preference for the inflected forms, *i.e. foure dragmes* (2226), *tweyne dragmes* (2542), *ij houres* (330-31), *iij maneres* (447), etc.

As a continuation of the OE system, the ME noun declension preserves a number of umlauted plurals. H497 witnesses the use of *men* (87×), *teth(e)* (9×), *women* (5×) and *feet* (3×). Foreign plurals, mostly Greek and Latin, are also found, particularly in the case of the specialized terminology, such as *asmaticos*, *orthonoici*, *euotoycy*, *exantimata*, *parodyda*, etc.

2.2.1.2. The genitive case

The singular is morphologically expressed by *-es* (46×), *-s* (45×) and *-ys* (21×), the latter as a northern reflex. There are no particular orthographic contexts governing one or the other insofar as the three endings may actually occur with a same noun. See, for instance, *a mans mynde* (1904), *a manys body* (2711) and *a manneys eyen* (993). Notably significant becomes the sporadic use of the detached genitive ending in cases like *stomake ys* (963), a scribal practice recorded in *LALME* as a charac-

2 The omission of the inflectional vowel usually takes place after a liquid consonant, paticularly <r> and <l>, as in the following cases: *autours* vs. *autores*, *brusours* vs. *bruserys*, *entrayls* vs. *entrayles*, *feuers* vs. *feuerys*, *humours* vs. *humoures*, *kernels* vs. *kerneles*, *maners* vs. *maneres*, *mesels* vs. *meseles*, *nettls* vs. *nettelles*. See also cases like *dragons* and *oynouns*.

teristic southern form, the South West in particular (McIntosh et al. 1986, IV: 322).

Strong plurals are consistent as to using *-s*, as in *wommens floures* (1981). Weak nouns, on the other hand, adopt the *-(e)n* morpheme, as in *ben mele* (1395; see also 2490). The noun *chyld* may appear either with a weak or a strong plural marker, *i.e. chyldryns kowhe* (1269) as opposed to *chyldryn helys* (1097). This fluctuation is surely the result of the on-going assimilation of the dominant pattern on the base of the strong declension.

A number of genitives are inflectionless, function being indicated by position, as in *nettell leues* (208), *þe lyfte foot sool* (440), *þys herbe root* (512), *pyone seed* (2055), etc. Words ending with *-s* and *-ch* are also uninflected in the genitive to avoid a likely euphony (Mossé 1968: 49; see also Fisiak 1968: 81), as in *gose grese* (254, 1313, etc.).

The *of*-genitive, on the other hand, which derives from an OE use of the preposition *off* to indicate the material with which something is made (Horobin and Smith 2002: 93), outnumbers the inflected genitive in H497, as in *uenym of snakes* (1687) vs. *addrys bytynges* (1690). Sporadically, the *of*-genitive may be pre-positive as in *make of nettel & of myrre a subfumygacion* (204-5).

Double genitives, in turn, are rare, being exclusively attested in the instance *of oþere autores bokes*, where the inflectional genitive *autores* occurs in-between the *of*-genitive construction.

2.2.2. Adjectives

As a 15th-century text, the only inflected adjectives in H497 are monosyllabic adjectives ending with a consonant, all the others being systematically uninflected. The strong declension, on the one hand, is unmarked in the singular whilst the plural shows ending *-e*, as in *good whyt wyne & strong* (2009-10), *þe wyche ben whyte blake & purpul* (1725-26), etc. The weak declension, on the other hand, shows *-e* irrespective of number, as in *þe whyte uyolet* (442-43), *þe blake spottes* (1277), etc.

Even when this picture holds for many monosyllabic adjectives, the line separating the weak and the strong declension is often blurred as a result of the progressive obliteration of the weak paradigm in late ME. Leaving aside the conservative London usage, the strong declension was already in use elsewhere in the 15th century (Horobin and Smith 2002: 95), a fact which explains instances like *þe blak seed* (1342), *þe red colre* (422), *þe cold feuer* (103-4), etc.

To this must be added the indiscriminate use of non-etymological *-e* among ME scribes, *Fachliteratur* in particular (Mossé 1968: 64), both in monosyllabic and, to a lesser extent, bisyllabic adjectives. This accounts for the erratic situation found in many late ME pieces, with examples such as *a newe fresshe wonde* (581), *with colde water* (2543), *whyte pepyr or whyte synuey* (1264), etc. In light of all this, the morphology of monosyllabic adjectives in H497 must be safely viewed in terms of number agreement, rather than in terms of a syntactic pattern governing the weak or the strong paradigm.

Disyllabic adjectives, on the other hand, are usually left uninflected, regardless of their origin, as in the following instances: *þe bytter akynge* (2582-83), *þys gentel & golden Rose* (739), *þe ynmoderat ache* (124-25), *uenemous bestes* (237), *þe tender bolles* (1325-26), etc.

Adjectival comparison is as follows. The degree of equality, on the one hand, is expressed by means of *as … as*, *as so … as*, and *so … as*, the latter exclusively in negative clauses. See for instance, *as thyk as hony* (2146), *þys* [*ys*] *as so good & as profytable to all þe causes before sayd as ys þe forsayd herbe* (1846-47), *she ys not so drye as she ys hote* (1265-66).

The comparison of superiority adopts *-er*, if synthetic, and *more … than*, if analytic[3]. The use of the synthetic and periphrastic models is indiscriminate in H497 inasmuch as both occur in the same contexts, regardless of the syllabic characteristics of the adjective involved, *i.e.* *moor profytable þan* (2548) vs. *profytabler* (2440). Even though it is noted elsewhere that in the late 15th century the synthetic model "occurs less

3 There are also cases of proportional comparatives to indicate parallel increase, as in *þe moor … þe sharper* (1226-27), *þe moor bred þow castyst … þe moor feble & weker* (1228-29), etc.

frequently in longer words" (Mustanoja 1960: 279), H497 purports a different picture, plausibly because it is a verbatim copy of an earlier original. This justifies the occurrence of the synthetic model by the side of comparatives like *moor feble* (1228), *moor feruent* (90), *moor sharpe* (984), etc.

The absolute superlative, in turn, makes use of *-est/-yst*, if synthetic, and *most ...*, if analytic. Note the recurrent omission of determiner *the* before the superlative, as in *hugest of alle bestes* (597-98), *gretyst of alle maladyes* (598), *most leef unto bees* (2068) in contrast with *þe most & strongyst of alle* (1727-28), *þe most conuenyent & profytable herbe* (1066-67), etc. No convention yet governs the use of the synthetic or the periphrastic models.

2.2.3. Personal pronouns

First person pronominals are singular *I* (32×) and *y* (3×) in the nominative case and *me* (4×) in the oblique case. The plural forms are *we* (3×) and *us* (5×) in the nominative and the oblique cases, respectively, forms tentatively used by the writer as plurals of majesty (Mustanoja 1960: 123-124), *i.e. yn latyn we cleped hyr Alltea* (924-25).

Second person pronominals, on the other hand, present the nominative forms *þow* (92×), *þu* (8×) and *thou* (2×) in the singular. Their distribution is still imbalanced in H497 insofar as *þu* exclusively occurs in-between ff. 5v-13v whereas variant *þow* is disseminated throughout the entire composition. The former is considered in *LALME* as a typical spelling of the north, particularly from Leicestershire, Lincolnshire, Staffordshire and Warwickshire (McIntosh et al. 1986, IV: 261) whilst *þow* is rather of southern provenance.

The objective forms, in turn, are *þe* (31×), *the* (2×) and *te* (1×), the latter witnessing the characteristic substitution of the etymological fricative consonant <th> for plosive /t/ as an East Midlands feature (McIntosh et al. 1986, IV: 320). Plural forms are missing in H497.

The third person singular witnesses masculine *he* (86×) and neuter *it* (83×) and *yt* (641×), the latter in the nominative and the oblique cases. The feminine, in turn, shows nominative *she* (165×) and *ssho* (1×) by the side of oblique *hyr* (18×) and *her* (4×). Dialectally speaking, variant *ssho* is elsewhere considered a typical northern feature (Mustanoja 1960: 130; McIntosh et al. 1982, I: 308). This spelling may be tentatively connected with the second person singular form *þu* to the extent that both, sharing a likely similar provenance, occur in neighbouring contexts in H497 (in-between ff. 5v-13v).

Plural forms are consistent as to the use of a mixed-type paradigm consisting of the Scandinavian forms *þey* (89×), *they* (2×) and *þeye* (2×) whilst Anglo-Saxon *hem* (186×) is the option in objective positions.

2.2.4. Possessive pronouns and adjectives

In the 2nd person, the possessive case agglutinates singular *þy* (15×), *þyn/thyn* (16×) and *þyne/thyne* (3×). The plural, on the other hand, is *youre* (1×) in *youre helthe* (2722). H497 is, to a certain extent, conventional as to the use of these allomorphs insofar as possessive *þy* is systematically the choice before a consonant, *i.e. þy pylowe* (114), *þy mouthe* (219), *þy tung* (1429-30) whilst *þyn*, in turn, occurs before a vowel and consonants <h> and <n>, such as *þyn ere* (255), *þyn heed* (1297) or *thyn nose* (203). Possessive *þyne*, on the other hand, may be deemed more erratic in H497 as it occurs either before consonant <h>, *i.e.* as in *thyne heed* (114) or in a plural context, *i.e. thyne eyes* (110).

The morphology of possessive adjectives in H497 is found to depend upon orthographic, rather than strictly morphemic, considerations inasmuch as variants *þy*, *þyn* and *þyne* alternate irrespective of any number agreement, as shown in *þy leymes* (106), *þy chekys* (152), *þyn eyen*

(1696), etc. Variants *þyne/thyne*, traditionally *ad hoc* plurals, occur twice in the text in between ff. 5r-7r[4].

The author's heedlessness of any number agreement in the possessive case is corroborated by the 3rd person paradigm, which makes use of masculine *hys* (70×), feminine *hyr* (62×) and plural *her* (32×). Accordingly, there is no trace of the plural marker *-e*.

2.2.5. Adverbs

The adverbial ending is generally *-ly* (76×), both with native and non-native adverbs, as in *bysely* (1816), *wysely* (1998), *coueytously* (505), etc. On the other hand, *-e* and zero inflection (14× and 5×, each) are also witnessed in H497, all of them with the same adverb, *faste* (531) and *fast* (828). Even though of minute occurrence, suffixes *-lych* (2×) and *-wise* (1×) are also found, *i.e. holsomlyche* (1164) and *plasterwyse* (401-2), leaving aside some sporadic adverbial genitives (3×) such as *attones* (1347) or *togydres* (750).

2.2.6. Verbs

Finite verbs in H497 have already lost part of their morphemic richness as a consequence of the on-going inflectional simplification which characterizes the ME period. With the exception of the present indicative, which shows a variety of verbal endings, the present subjunctive and the past indicative give evidence of an almost complete reduction, wherein inflections *-e* and *-ed*, respectively, are consistently the rule.

4 Note that possessives *þyne/thyne* appear in neighbouring ff. (in-between 5r-7r, as happens with other pronominals such as *þu* and *scho*. These are then regarded as odd forms if compared with the standard practice of the author.

2.2.6.1. *The present indicative*

The present indicative of main verbs shows the characteristic inflections of a conservative Midland dialect, *i.e.* 3rd person singular *-th* and plural *-en* (Mossé 1968: 76), co-occurring with other less frequent inflectional endings. Table 1 reproduces the different verbal morphemes for the expression of the present indicative in descending order of frequency.

Sing 1	-e; -ø
Sing 2	-e ; -est/-yst; -ø
Sing 3	-yth; -eth; -yt/-et; -th(e); -e
Plur	-en; -yn; -e; -yth; -ø; -t

Table 2. Present indicative in H497

As illustrated, the 1st person singular is outstandingly inflected as *-e* (15×) and *-ø* (1×), the latter being just testimonial, as in *moneste* (2692), *counseyle* (1229), *trow* (690), etc.

The 2nd person singular shows *-e* (21×), *-est/-yst* (5×) and *-ø* (1×), in cases like *make* (359), *makyst* (427), *underput* (129), etc.

The 3rd person singular, on the other hand, is more heterogeneous as it involves the use of the following endings: *-yth* (472×), *-eth* (64×), *-yt/-et* (98×), *-th(e)* (53×) and *-e* (6×), *i.e. makyth* (675), *claryfyeth* (2590), *dryuyt* (1306), *helpet* (1894), *sathe* (2135), *resolue* (922), etc. The inflection *-t* derives from the assimilation of <þ> when preceded by a dental consonant, being a characteristic feature of the East Midlands and the South (Jordan 1974: 186; see also McIntosh et al. 1986, IV: 324). However, the occurrence of such a morpheme in H497 is not exclusively restricted to that particular phonological environment, as it affects a wide variety of verbs, irrespective of the preceding consonant. Note, for instance, the usual assimilation in words like *puttyt* (189) together with other syncopated forms such as *destroyet* (143), *dryet* (593), *helyt* (1459), etc.

Finally, the plural endings are *-en* (156×), *-yn* (64×), *-e* (32×), *-yth* (3×), *-ø* (3×) and *-t* (1×), the latter for the reason mentioned above. See the cases of *commaunden* (2210), *akyn* (872), *calle* (109), *comaundyth* (1223), *cast* (1633) and *makyt* (1151).

2.2.6.2. The past indicative

The past indicative is restricted to a few occurrences in H497, particularly when the author refers back to the main scientific authorities of the text, such as Galen, Pliny, etc.

Morphologically speaking, weak verbs give evidence of inflectional erosion of the *-st* ending in the 2nd person singular by the side of the progressive generalization of *-ed* under these circumstances. Whilst *-de* is exclusively used in the 1st and 2nd person, the 3rd person conglomerates *-ed* (9×), *-de* (4×) and *-yd* (1×), as in *confyrmed* (2225), *radde* (1787) or *commaundyd* (2229), among others. The plural, in turn, favours the use of *-ed* (5×) to the detriment of *-den* (3×) and *-de* (2×), as in *meued* (2239) vs. *seyden* (2219) and *hade* (485).

Sing 1	-de
Sing 2	-de
Sing 3	-ed; -de; -yd
Plur	-ed; -den; -de

Table 3. Past indicative in H497

Even though amounting to no more than ten occurrences altogether, the past tense of strong verbs reveals the progressive extension of the preterite^1 to the plural, in such a way that one finds singular forms such as *yaf* (542), *wrote* (2212) and *grewe* (2130) together with *wroot* (1071) in the plural, from the OE preterite^1 form *wrāt*. There is a single reflex of a preterite^2 base in the plural form *funde* (55), derived from OE *fundon*.

2.2.6.3. *The subjunctive*

The present subjunctive is systematically formed by using inflections *-e* and *-en* for the singular and the plural numbers respectively, as in *where so euer he by come* (2267), *or þat he fele eny cold* (2282), [...] *though þey ben grete* (2161); [...] *wol make hem all mery & glad þat eten of þat mete & drynken of þat drynke* (2288-89). There is only one exception to this rule in the use of the plural ending *-e* in *yf she be rolled faste aboute yn þe mouthe so þat þe chekes sowne after* (2276-77).

The preterite subjunctive, on the other hand, is mostly attested in the case of the anomalous verb *bēn*, conjugated as *were/where*, irrespective of number, as in *þere shal noo feys byte þat person* [...] *þat he þat were anoynted with þe Iuys of ueruyne* (2309-11); *yf þe feuerys where uppon eny body anon as he were anoynted with þe Iuys of ueruenу þe feuerys shuld leue hym for euer* (2315-17). If a strong verb, on the other hand, the preterite[1] is the choice, as in [...] *but better yt were þer to yf þow sethe yt yn reyne water* (120-21)[5].

2.2.6.4. *Non-finite forms*

The infinitive of verbs makes a consistent use of *-e* (834×), irrespective of the origin of the verb, both native and non-native, as in *abate* (411), *destroye* (69), *gnawe* (183), *helpe* (523), *shewe* (964), *speke* (437), etc. Despite the outstanding preference for the *e-* ending, the infinitive is also inflectionless in a number of cases (35×), *i.e. bryng* (2222), *cast* (1370), *put* (590). Considerably less frequent is the use of *-en* (17×) and *-y* (1×), such as *purgen* (2552) or *delyuery* (64).

The present participle ending is *-yng(e)* (11×), *i.e. wassyng* (1714), *growynge* (2830), etc. There is no trace of the Anglo-Saxon ending *-end* in H497, which was progressively replaced in ME by the *-ing* ending, first in the South and Midlands and later in the North, owing to the influence of *-ing* verbal nouns (Roura 1999: 207). Final *-e* is yet arbitrarily used, being a matter of choice rather than a question of number

5 From OE *sēoþan/seaþ/sudon/soden* 'to boil, heat'.

agreement. If the verb stem ends in *-y*, *-eng(e)* is then preferred to avoid the likely occurrence of two vowels <i> in a series, as in *dryeng* (1290).

Past participles, on the other hand, are more heterogeneous insofar as a number of different morphological endings occur. If weak, *-ed* is the most recurrent morpheme (450×), followed by *-yd(e)* (117×) and *-de* (66×), as shown in cases like *resolued* (1042), *purgyd* (2654) or *cheude* (1753). Though less frequent, H497 witnesses other participial endings such as *-d* (6×), *-te* (5×) and *-yt* (3×) as, for instance, *delyuerd* (1525), *stampyt* (199), *kutte* (764).

If strong, on the other hand, the endings *-e* and *-en* are added to the corresponding stem, amounting to 318 and 197 occurrences respectively, *i.e. dronke* (87) and *knowe* (396) vs. *dronken* (193) and *knowen* (2420), among others. In addition to these, zero inflection participles constitute an important minority (30×), like *drunk* (1053), *put* (1006), etc. Finally, there are also examples with inflections *-on* and *-yn*, such as *wreton* (183) or *dronkyn* (373).

H497 gives evidence of the general obliteration of the participial prefix in the sense that it amounts to one hundred instances out of a total of 1,223 past participles in the text. Of these, the prefix is more consistently retained in the case of strong verbs (77 instances out of 550), compared to their weak counterparts, amounting to 23 instances (out of 661 weak verbs).

To finish, it must be noted the existence of some absolute constructions as a reflex of the Latin absolute ablative, showing an oblique (pro)noun functioning as the subject of the participle. This structure is rare in early ME, but spread from the second half of the 14th century, as a result of the powerful influence of French and Latin, gaining considerable ground by the second quarter of the 15th century, when the oblique case is superseded by the Nominative case (Mustanoja 1960: 114-115). Still, H497 gives evidence of the oblique case, *i.e. hym un wytyng* (166-67).

2.2.6.5. Periphrastic forms

The other verb tenses are, therefore, periphrastic. The perfect and the pluperfect, on the one hand, involve the periphrasis of the auxiliary *haven* plus the corresponding participial verb stem. The perfect is observed in cases like *I haue seyde* (481), *yt haue drawe oute* (1235-36), *men haue eten or dronken* (453), etc. The pluperfect, in turn, is exclusively found in the construction *whan þey hadde ouercome her enemyes* (500).

The future, on the other hand, is expressed by the periphrasis with *shullen* and *willen*[6]. Mustanoja argues that the future reference of the auxiliary verb *willen* spreads in the southern varieties in the late ME period, thereby co-occurring in the same contexts of *shullen* (Mustanoja 1960: 490; see also Fischer 1992: 264). Their use is basically dependent upon considerations of style insofar as *willen* is considered to be prominently popular whilst *shullen*, notoriously more common in ME, occurs in formal narrative. Statistically speaking, however, H497 differs from this statement insofar as there is a major preference for *willen* (683×), which is four times more frequent than *shullen* (136×). Among others, note the future reference of these verbs in *yt wol do away þe heed ache* (302) and *þat shal do muche profyte* (180).

Finally, the passive voice shows a narrow range in H497 in the sense that only the direct object is passivised. There is no trace, however, of other incipient ME constructions, such as the indirect object and the prepositional passives (Fischer 1992: 383). Bearing in mind that Odo de Meung's Latin original was composed some time between 849 and 1112, H497 is then a 15th-century verbatim copy of a former text, plausibly dated in the 13th century, a fact which explains why the syntax of H497 is, in many respects, conservative as to the general trends of the period. On a statistical basis, there is a total of 489 passive construc-

6 As mentioned elsewhere in the literature, it is at times thorny to discern whether an auxiliary form of these verbs expresses futurity or obligation/volition (Mustanoja 1960: 489-490). The cases implying some sort of obligation or volition constitute a minority in *H497*, and therefore have been ruled out for the present analysis.

tions in the text, all consisting of verb *bēn* followed by the corresponding past participle.

In addition, there are also cases of impersonal passives such as *yt ys seyden* (809), *yt ys sayd* (1697-98) by the side of others like *þys rose* [...] *ys seyde to hele* (933-935).

2.3. Word-order

2.3.1. Noun phrase order

The position of elements within the noun phrase does not differ much from the PDE pattern, to the extent that a given head may be pre- or post-modified according to the same set of rules. In case of premodification, the noun phrase constituents conform to the pattern already noted by Fischer (1992: 211), as shown in the examples below.

Predeterminer	Determiner	Postdeterminer	Modifier	Head
Al	þe			ache
	þe	thrydde		degree
	many		diuerse	medycynys

Table 4. Noun phrase structure

Notwithstanding the consistency of this base order, the author sporadically exploits the use of fronting and postposition, mostly for emphatic purposes. The former, on the one hand, is overtly exemplified by *of þe self grene herbe þe Ius* (193) wherein the prepositional phrase is fronted to highlight the virtue of that same herb, only if still green.

Postposition, on the other hand, consists in the stranding of a constituent within the noun phrase structure, thus displaced from its natural positioning. See, for instance, a phrase like *þat wol destroye þe frakeles alle* (526), predeterminer *alle* post-positive. This kind of ordering, however, becomes highly infrequent in late ME prose.

2.3.2. Clausal order

As a 15th-century piece of prose, H497 consistently follows the standard constituent order of S – V – O, both in main and subordinate clauses, as in the following instances, to cite but a few: *a plastre of wermode resoluyth þe hardenesse* (175), *it comfortyth þe stomak* (85-86), *Plinius sayth þe souredocke* (1868-69), etc.

Besides this commonplace order, the inverse order, *i.e.* V – S – O, is a recurrent practice of the author under the following circumstances (see Mossé 1968: 126-127): a) in questions such as *how dost þow or how faryst thow* (2291-92); b) after an adverb (of time, place, and manner, in particular[7]), as in *here begynneth the fyrst boke of Macer* (1), *þan uanysshyth þys herbe* (2139), *þus wol þys herbe do* (609-10), etc; and c) after an adverbial adjunct for reasons of emphasis[8], *i.e. of þys Rose ys made oleum rosaceum* (716), *yn þys wyse ys hyr name sette yn olde bokes* (2785-86), etc.

Object topicalisation, on the other hand, is also a frequent device in H497, in such a way that the direct object becomes the theme of the clause for emphasis. The fronting of this constituent gives rise to the base order O – V – S, thereby compliant with the V2 rule in English, as in the following constructions *alle maner unkynde hetes wol þe Rose destroy* (713-14), *þys medycyne shalt þow not do* (2837), *the same doth þe decoccion* (656-57), etc.

On other occasions the author conforms to the use of the O – S – V order on condition that the subject is a light weight monosyllable, as

7 The list of fronted adverbs causing S – V inversion is the following: *afterwarde, allone, also, as, better, elles, how, not, now, ofte(n), propyrly, so, þan, þere, þerwith, þus, unneþe* and *wherto*.

8 Compare, for instance, *but better doth þys* (863-64) with *but better yt wol do* (746), the latter considerably less frequent.

in *but þys I wot wel* (1785), *so yt wol do* (456), *thys yt doth by hem self* (1840), etc.

Finally, there are sporadic cases of S O V order, particularly when the object is a pronoun or a demonstrative (Mossé 1968: 129), *i.e. as many men yt sayn* (1318).

2.3.3. Compound sentences

Copulative coordination is introduced in H497 by *and* (1,744×), *ne* (22×), together with the correlative conjunctions *both ... and* (22×), *not only ... but also* (2×), and *neyther ... nor* (3×). Adversative coordination, on the other hand, is expressed by conjunction *but* (71×) whilst disjunctive coordination shows *or* (221×), *ouþer* (14×), *or elles* (3×) and the correlative *eyther ... or* (2×).

2.3.4. Complex sentences

2.3.4.1. Nominal clauses

Nominal clauses are consistently introduced by subordinators *þat* and, to a lesser extent, *what* and *how*, as shown in the following instances: *Zenocates seyde þat a wommans floures shulde sayle hyr as many dayes as she ete Coryaundre seed cornes* (1401-3), *I wol declare here & expowne what yt ys* (1566), *Now haue I seyde generaly how þow shalt yeue all maner herbes* (2002-3), etc.

2.3.4.2. Adjectival clauses

Adjectival clauses are introduced by relativisers *þat* (436×), *þe w(h)yche* (46×) and *w(h)yche* (5×), used irrespective of the antecedent (personal and non-personal) and clause-type (defining and non-defining). See, for instance, cases like *a good drynke for hem þat speten bloode* (547-48), *anoynte þe place þat ys swollen* (660-1) and *þe wythe Ellebur þe wyche ys moor uyolent þan þe blak ellebur* (2230-31), etc.

The relativiser *þe w(h)yche* mostly occurs in relative clauses split from their corresponding antecedent inasmuch as it allows the repetition of the antecedent, therefore avoiding any plausible misinterpretation of the neighbouring noun as the factual antecedent of the relativiser. See, for instance, *yt excytyth hugely þe hete of þe stomak & of þe mawe þe wyche heete makyth dygestyoun* (2481-83).

If a personal antecedent, however, the author sporadically recurs to the use of *who* (1×), *who* + pleonastic *þat* (1×) and objective *whom* (1×), in the following examples: *who sayth yt crepyth forthe ney by þe erthe* (1628-29), *who þat takyt þys herbe* [...] *he shal not ascape with outen an longe dyssese* (2202-3), *wol helpe hem whom eny sodeyn soor makyth for to be dombe* (1165-66).

The relativiser *whos* (3×), in turn, is used in the possessive case, regardless of the antecedent, personal or non-personal, as in *thys ys cleped comounly whyte popye but he ys best whos floure ys whyte* (1324-25) or *þe woman whos brestes aken* (2345-46).

2.3.4.3. Adverbial clauses

Temporal clauses are introduced by conjunctions *whan/whanne* (34×), *tyl (þat)* (7×), *after þat* (3×), *or þat* (3×), *syth (þat)* (2×) and *whyle* (2×). The subjunctive occurs after conjunctions *tyl (þat)* and *or þat*, as shown in *sethe yt tyl yt be as thyk as hony* (2146) or *dronke yn leuke water or þat þe colde come* (1040).

Causal clauses are headed by *for/ffor* (60×), *for þy (þat)* (12×), *for þat* (3×), *for by cause* (1×) and *for why* (1×), *i.e. yt wol destroye all uenymys ffor as yt ys sayd þe self odour of þys herbe* (1304-5), *mugworte or moderworte ys cleped Arthemesia yn latyn for þy þat she ys þe moder of all other herbes* (51-2), *a plaster of þys herbe or of þys seed ys þus profytabyle for by cause leches maken þys plaster dyuersely* (1220-22), etc.

Concessive clauses are consistently introduced by the conjunction *though* (13×) or any of its allographs *though* and *thought* (1× each). As in the case of *tyl* and *or þat*, the subjunctive is the rule in these clause types, *i.e. she wol putte oute a chylde of wommans wombe though yt be deed* (784-85). *Though* is at times accompanied by adversative particles in the main clause such as *natheles, yet*, etc. (Fischer 1992: 350). For instance, *though þys be a foule medycyne natheles yt ys holsom* (1127-28).

Final and consecutive clauses use subordinators *so þat* (5×) and *that*, as in the following instances *ryue hem on threde so þat noon of hem touche other* (887-88); *þys same onyment wol kepe þe heres þat þey shal not falle away* (1116-17). Fischer (1992: 343) notes that the line separating final and consecutive clauses is often blurred, mood being at times the clue to interpret them correctly. The subjunctive is likely to appear in purpose clauses while the indicative is largely preferred in result clauses. If the subjunctive mood is not discernible, both interpretations are plausible, *i.e. þys Iuys drunke with good wyt wyne wol helpe hem wel þat han a combred her stomak so þat þey may not wel defye* (1937-38).

Comparative clauses, on the other hand, involve the use of *as … as* for the expression of equality whilst *moor … þan* is restricted to the expression of inequality. The indicative is generally used in this type of clauses: *he þat drawyth yn as muche eyre as he puttyth oute* (839-40) or *he þat puttyth out moor of the eyre þan he resceyueth* (840-41).

Finally, conditional clauses are the most frequent type of adverbial clauses in H497 and they are systematically introduced by the subordinator *yf* (266×), even though both *whether* (5×) and *yf þat* (1×) are seldom used. For instance, *yt wol also reyse up þe moder to hyr place yf she be fallen doun* (1052-53).

2.4. Dialect

A preliminary survey of the linguistic variants in H497, particularly on a phono-orthographic basis, tentatively leads to the assumption that the text was likely to have been composed in a relatively wide area of the South East of England, comprising both the South East Midland and the Kentish dialects. There are, as a matter of fact, many characteristic items speaking for such a dialectal provenance, among which the following stand out:

- OE /y(:)/ is consistently unrounded and lowered to /ɛ(:)/, as illustrated in *kernel* from OE *cyrnel*, *felthe* from OE *fȳlþ*, etc. (see Jordan 1974: 69; 72).
- OE <eo> is rendered as <o>, thus retaining a front pronunciation /ø/, *i.e. yolow* from OE *geolu*, particularly in the East, spreading from Kent up to the North East (Jordan 1974: 96-97).
- Angl. /æ/ generally raises to /ɛ/, *i.e. helden*, thenceforth subjected to homorganic lengthening /ɛ:/.
- OE <þ> normally becomes <t>, especially if preceding a dental, affecting mostly the 3rd sing. pres. forms of verbs, as in *hat*, *staunchyt*, *drynkyt*, etc. The phenomenon is seldom witnessed word-initially, as in *te* 'thee', *tre* 'three', etc. (McIntosh et al. 1986, IV: 320).

To corroborate the South East Midland provenance of the text, the linguistic profile (henceforth LP) of H497 was built in terms of the *LALME* questionnaire (McIntosh et al. 1986). The mapping of these orthographic variants allows restricting the geography of the text (Benskin 1991: 9-26; Crespo and Lezcano 1999: 42; Calle-Martín 2000: 11). Conclusive data are therefrom obtained and show that H497 was written in a small area, north of the Thames, towards the south of the county of Essex. The resulting profile is found to have a close connection with LP's 9250 and 6350 in *LALME*, which are also ascribed to the same county (see Calle-Martín and Moreno-Olalla, forthcoming).

In addition to this, variant spellings from other dialect areas are also sporadically identified, mostly from the north and the West Midlands. The former is witnessed in the use of pronominal *sho* 'she', the past participle ending *-on*, the preterite-present verb *my* 'may' or preposition *thurght* 'through'. The western influence, on the other hand, is found in the use of the plural demonstrative *þuse* 'these', the detached genitive ending or verb *hongen* with the back sound /ɔ/.

Chapter 3. The Text

3.1. Editorial conventions

The present edition has been conceived as a textual resource for academic scholarship in a wide variety of disciplines, not only Historical Linguistics in itself, but also Codicology and the History of Medicine. Unfortunately, some modern editions are more often than not guided by the editorial principles of publishers, thus denying the reader an immediate access to the source text as copied by the mediaeval writer. Therefore, aspects such as marginalia, emendations or punctuation are a *desideratum*.

In light of these inconveniences, the principles of a *semi-diplomatic edition* have been adopted so as to provide an accurate reproduction of the source text. Our transcription is graphemic to keep the reader as close as possible to the scribal version, thus complying with the following guidelines, partially adapted from Petti (1977: 24-35).

a) The spelling, capitalization and word division of the original witness have been retained, including the systematic use of <u> for <v> and <y> for <i>. The different spellings of a same consonant, however, have been regularized, particularly in the case of the letter <s>, represented as <ß> and <ſ>. Any kind of editorial manipulation is noted between braces ({}) and accordingly recorded in one of the apparatuses. These range from simple scribal errors to omissions, the latter provided on the basis of the Stockholm manuscript.

b) The punctuation and paragraphing of the original have been retained. In addition to the period, the unusual marks of punctuation have been normalized with the use of the following convention, *i.e.* the *paragraphus* (¶), the *virgule* (/) and the *caret* (^).

c) Abbreviations have been expanded with the supplied letter(s) italicised. Superior letters are lowered to the line, as in w^{t} > wit*h* or þ^{e} > þe. Superfluous brevigraphs and otiose flourishes, in turn, have been ignored.

d) Deletions consist exclusively in the cancellation of one or more letters or even full word(s), as in ~~*wondes*~~ (291), ~~*to gydre*~~ (2766). In our edition, these appear in the textual apparatus.

e) Insertions, both of single letters and words, are above the line in the original, and they have been included in their proper sequence in the body of the text, but enclosed in square brackets, as shown in *yf yt* ˟⌞be⌟˟ *leyde þerto* (284), *or drunken* ˟⌞makyth⌟˟ *þe for to slepe* (1362), *þys oynement wol dryue away þe ache* ˟⌞of þe⌟˟ *reynes* (2464-65), etc.

f) Marginalia has been noted in the first of the apparatuses. As mentioned in chapter 1, H497 presents the use of three different hands. Hand A corresponds to the scribe's actual handwriting whilst hands B and C are written with a 16th-century *Secretary* script (with elements of the Early Tudor *Secretary*). For the sake of accuracy, the latter have been safely indicated with the use of *H2* and *H3*, respectively.

HEre begynneth the fyrst boke of Macer þ*at* techyth and oponly shewyth the uertues of many & dyuerse herbes . In the wyche boke ben contened xl . uj . herbes wyth her uertues and propyrtes of the wyche . *f.1r*

Mugwort ys þe fyrst	i	
Southernwode	ij	
Wermode	iij	
Nett⌞e⌟ll	iiij	
Garlyke	u	
Planteyne	uj	
Rewe	uij	
Uyolet	uiij	
Osterlagya	ix	
Ache or apiu*m*	x	
Saueyne	xi	
Leeke	xij	*f.1v*
Nepte	xiij	
ffenel	xiiij	
Letuse	xu	
Rose	xuj	
Lilye	xuij	
Sauerey	xuiij	
Sauge	xix	
Elycu*m*pana	xx	
Ysope	xxj	
Gladen	xxij	
Wylde malowe	xxiij	
Anyse	xxiiij	
Beteyne	xxu	
Caule	xxuj	
Oynons	xxuij	
Synueye	xxuiij	*f.2r*
Wythe pep*er*	xxix	

1 Here] IHC *top marg.*

	Kersoun	xxx
	Popye	xxxj
	Coryaundre	xxxij
	Arage	xxxiij
	Mynte	xxxiiij
	Skyrewyt	xxxu
	Cerfoyle	xxxuj
	Docke	xxxuij
	Kockull	xxxuiij
	Hemlok	xxxix
	Pilyoll	xl
	Persely	xlj
	Centory	xlij
	Camedrios	xliij
f.2v	Dragons	xliiij
	Camomylle	xlu
	Wodebynde	xluj

f.3r Mugworte or moderworte ys cleped . Arthemesia . yn latyn . for þy þat she ys þe moder of all other herbes . Or therfor for þe mother of herbes hath youe hyr þ*a*t name . Diana sykerlyche þe wyche ys clepyt yn greke tunge . Arthemesys . þat fu*n*de up fyrst þe uertu of þys herbe . And þerfore ys þ*ys* herbe called. Arthemesis of hyr fyndrys name . This herbe ys specyaly medycynall to womans syknesse for þe water of hyr decocyou*n* þ*a*t ys to say wat*er* þ*a*t she is soden yn ydronke purgyth wome*n* of her floures . And bryngith he*m* furthe from hem wi*th* þe same wat*er* þ*a*t þ*ys* mugwort ys soden yn . Wasshe & bathe þe matryce . And so shalt thow clense
f.3v wo*m*me*n* of her flores . Also take || þe same herbe grene as she growyht & stampe yt & bynde yt to þe wombe . And she shal delyuery þe werplynge þ*a*t ys þ*er*yn . Also drynke moderwort . or make þereof a subfumygac*io*n . An she

48 Dragons] Jesus *top marg. H3* **51** Mugworte] i *ext. marg.*

dyssoluyt þe hardnesse of þe moder & þe bolnyng of yt . Also take þe same herbe rawe & stampe yt & drynke yt w*ith* wyne & so yt wol do þe same Also drynke þys herbe ofte w*ith* wyne . & she wol make þe to pysse & she wol destroye þe stone . And þus also she helpyth hem þ*at* han þe Iaundyse . Also stampe þ*ys* herbe & medleyt w*ith* hennes gresse & make þer of a plastre & ley yt to þe bocche . drynke þys herbe w*ith* wyne & so shalt þow hele þe bocche . A nother yf eny euel drynkes . as ys open dyssese drynke mugwort stampyd in wyne & yt shal make þe hole . Another as so*m*me clerkes sayen . þ*at* who so castyth . þ*at* ys to say etyth or drynkyt || þ*ys* herbe no noyous medycen shal mowe hurte hym . & þ*at* f.4r no wylde beste wol {byte} hym gladly . It ys seyde þ*at* yf þow hange a boute thy nek þe root of þ*ys* herbe w*ith* a red threde . no uenemous frosshe shal greue the . The Iuis of mogwort y dro*n*ke w*ith* wyne shall p*ro*fyte also therto . A nother take þ*ys* herbe grene as she growyth . stampe yt & putte yn must & kepe yt tyl yt be wel y fyned & þys wyne shal be medycynal to all þe syknes befor sayd . Thys wyne shal be wel lykynge yn saueur & odour . or smelynge . It co*m*fortyth þe stomak . & helyth þe entrayls þ*at* ben aboute þe herte . yf yt be dronke . And me*n* saye*n* þ*at* yt ys p*ro*fytable to mayny oþ*er* causes .

SOuthernewode as yt ys y radde ys hoot yn þe thyrde degre . & drye yn þe same . hys seed ys moor feruent . yt ys bytwene þe thrydde degre . & þe || fourthe degre . Make þer of a f.4v plaster and yt shal hele synowes þ*at* ben bolle*n* yf yt be leyde þer to . A noþer . Drynke þe cocc*i*on of þ*ys* herbe yt doth good to all þe synowes & to streynesse & to all other causes of þe brest . A nother drynke yt ofte raw w*ith* wyne & yt doth good to þe cowhe & to þe chynke & to ache of þe ludes

89 Southernewode] ii *ext. marg.*

78 byte] byde MS.

& to þe greuance of þe pr*e*ue me*m*ber . And makyth þe to pysse & destroyth þe stone & wormes yn þe bely . It clensyth entrall . & dryueth oute womans floures . It purgyth passyons & dysseses . þ*a*t fallen yn þe whyrlebone of þe hype . It dyssoluyth þe festre & destreth yt . Thys herbe {chasyth} away serpentes thorugh hys odour . Drynke southerwode & yt wol destroue þe uenym of serpentes . If þow haue þe cold feuer . or þan þe dyssese come upon þe drynke þe Ius of *f.5r* southernewod wit*h* wat*er* || medle yt wit*h* comou*n* oyle & wit*h* þ*a*t oyle anoynte þy leymes . Take þe Ius of þ*ys* herbe . & put yt yn þe eere luke warme of hym þ*a*t ys deffe & he shal soon heere . Take southerwode cromes of bred & apples þ*a*t me*n* calle quynsys & sethe hym to gyder yn water & leye yt þan to thyne eyes yt destroyth and helyth þe bocche & þe ache & þe hete of þe eyen . Make of southernewode a playster by yt self . or medle yt wit*h* grece . & yt wol draw oute a shafte or þorne styked yn þe body . Leye þ*ys* herbe only under þy pylowe atte thyne heed & yt wol scure þe hugely to lecherye . Also drynke þe same herbe & yt wol quenche þe lust of lechery . And yt helpyth ayenst þe goute ¶ þ*a*t preuy .

Wermode . ys hoot yn þe fyrst degre & drye yn þe seconde . *f.5v* Thys herbe comfortyth & strengthyth þe sto || mac yn wat wyse euere so ma*n* take yt . but better yt were þer to yf þow sethe yt yn reyne wat*er* . And leet yt be cold thorugh out . And ofte drynke yt yn þ*a*t wyse . It helpyth dyuerse syknesse of þe stomac . In þ*ys* wyse also yt destroyth wormes yn þe bely . & makyth þe laxatyf . & staunchyt þe gret & þe ynmoderat ache of þe wombe . Drynke wermode & makyth ⸤þe⸥ to pysse . Take {narde} of fraunce & wermode stampe hem togyder . & resolue he*m* & temp*re* hem wit*h* mulsa . &

---

118 Wermode] iii *ext. marg.*

---

101 chasyth] chastyth MS. **126** narde] uarde MS.

drynke yt . & so shalt þow purge womens floures souerynly . Thus doth yt also yf þu underput yt w*ith* nesshe wolle . Stampe to gyder wermode . narde & þe tre þ*a*t ys called syler tem*p*re yt w*ith* uenyger & dry*n*ke yt . & so shalt þu wypeaway
þe greua*n*ce || & noyous dysseses of wo*m*mens floures . Take *f.6r*
wermode leues or þe rothe & þe seed of rewe . salte . & pyper & tempre hem w*ith* wyne & sethe hem & drynke hem & so þu shalt purge þe wycked & rawe humorys of þe stomac . Stampe to gedyr wormode & gladen & drynke þ*a*t & yt helpyth þe brest wonderly . Ssho wol stampe wormode w*ith* uynegre & anoy*n*te hym þer w*ith* . hym dare not drede of gnattes flyes . ne flees . Or brenne wormode & þe sauoure of yt dryueth hem away . Ete rawe wormode & smalache to gyder & þ*a*t helpyth þe lyuer . Drynke wermode w*ith* uenygre & yt helpyth þe mylte . Ete or drynke wermode & þ*a*t destroyet þe uenym of padstoles . Drynke wermod w*ith* wyne & yt destroyet þe malyce of uenym of þe hemloke . Drynke
wermod || & yt helpyth ayenst þe bytyng of uenemous *f.6v*
bestes . Stampe wermod & melde yt w*ith* hony & wo*m*mans mylke & anoy*n*te þer w*ith* thyn eyen & þ*a*t makyth hem clere & destroyth þe wannesse & þe bolnyng of þe eyen & þe quytter yf eny þere bee . ffor þe eres þ*a*t ben stopped sethe warmode & lete þe uapur goyn to þe ere & so shalt þow be hoole . Yf þe eres renne of quytter . stampe warmode w*ith* hony & leye to hym & þ*a*t shal esen hem . If þy chekys ben to swolle stampe warmod w*ith* hony & leye yt to þe so or w*ith* ynfurthe . Also stampe yt & leye yt to þe fresshe wondes . for yt helyth he*m* fayre . Stampe wermode & sethe yt yn wyne & make of yt a plast*er* & leye yt to þe wondes & bocches of þe heed & þ*a*t wol hele hem . A bathe of he*m* ||
wol destroye aky*n*ges . Drynke þe yuys of wormode w*ith* as *f.7r*
muche wyne as yt ys . & þan shalt þow not be trauayled w*ith*

---

139 wormode] for fleu*m* *ext. marg. H3* **147** eyen] for eiin *ext. marg. H2*

brakyng of þe see . Leye wermode yn lynnyn clothe . & gyrde yt a boute thyn lyndes & þ*at* wol destroye þe ynmoderate ache of þe grynde . Or stampe wermode w*ith* hony & wyne & make þer of an emplast*er* & leye yt to þe soor grynde . Or wete alynnyn cloute yn þe Ius of wormode & bynde yt aboute þe soor grynde . The smel of wormode wol make þe syke for to slepe . And so yt wol yf yt be leyde under hys heed hym un wyty*n*g . The asshes of wormode blackyth heer yf be medled w*ith* oyle & waxe . yf þu wolt ofte anoynte þyne here w*ith* þ*ys*
f.7v oyneme*n*t . leye wermode yn þy cheste & þere shal || no motthe come þere yn . Stampe wermode w*ith* hony & yt wol hele ache & swellyng þ*at* fallyth under þe tonge . The same medycyne wol hele & destroye þe wa*n*nesse . & dyscoloryng þ*at* ys wont to houe re aboute þe roundenes of þe eyen The Ius of wormode w*ith* þe galle of an oxe helyth þe sownyng of þe yere . A plastre of wermode resoluyth þe hardenesse of þe splene yf þu putte hony þer to Of wormode make a subfumygac*i*on & yt wol drye up þe sky*n*ne þ*at* þe chylde lyeth yn yn hys modrys wombe & makyth þe flores for to renne oute faste Sethe grene wermode yn oyle as yt growyth & a noynte þerw*ith* þe gryndes & þ*at* shal do muche p*ro*fyte to þe stomak . Lete wermode lye & soke yn wyne & w*ith* þ*at*
f.8r wyne temp*re* tyn ynke & þere shal neuer mouse || ne ratte gnawe þe boke þ*at* ys wreto*n* w*ith* þ*at* ynke

Netell ys clepyd yn greke aculiphe she ys hugely hoot & þerefore she ys clepyd urtica yn latyn for so muche þ*at* she wol brenne hys fyngers þ*at* handeleth hyr Drynke nettels & so shal þu hele þe Iayndys Eete & drynke nettels seed w*ith* hony & yt wol destroye þe sykenysse of þe colyke Drynke ofte nettel seed & yt wol hele þe of cowhe . for yt puttyt a way þe colde fro þe longes & þe ache of the wombe &

---

173 eyen] of þe iene *ext. marg. H3* **175** yere] of þe iere *ext. marg. H2*
184 Netell] iiij ext. marg. **189** nettel seed] netyll seed *ext. marg. H3*

swellyng To alle these afore sayd passyons ys þe p⌊o⌋uder of þe netel or of nettel seed good medled w*ith* hony So ys also of þe self grene herbe þe Ius dronken w*ith* wyne . Stampe nettel leues w*ith* salte & make þer of a plastre & yt wol clense foule wondes & do good to bocches Thys plastre ys good ayenst || houndes bytyngge & cancres & þe syknes þ*a*t *f.8v* men callen p*ar*odyda . And þys reformyth & conceyueth þe flesshe . & luxatura þat ys go fro þe boon . and þys dryeth up wicked humours . The netyl root stampyt w*ith* uynegre abatyth þe swellyng of þe splene . Ayenst þe podagre yt ys good & also to alle þe syknesse of þe toon . yf yt be made yn plastre & leyde to . Or y sode*n* yn oyle & þe lymes be anoynted w*ith* þe oynement þerof . Putte yn thyn nose the Iuys of þe nettel leef & yt wol make þy nose to blede . Make of nettel & of myrre a subfumygac*i*on & yt wol dryue oute wo*m*mens floures of þe matryce of ouer muche humo*urs* greued & heuyed sperryd be fore þe pryue me*m*bre . frote yt wel w*ith* nettell leues or w*ith* þe Iuys of nettell . Drynke nettelles or her seed w*ith* wyne & yt wol meue þe to lecherye . But || mor strongly yt meueth to lechyry yf þow *f.9r* stampe yt w*ith* salt . hony & pepyr & dry*n*ke all þuse yn wyne . The foure footed beste þ*a*t wol not suffre hys male . shal be froted wel w*ith* nettell & a noon she wol sto*n*de stylle to hyr male . {Thus} excytyth & scuryth þe nettel þe naturel heet . Drynke nettel seed w*ith* hony & yt wol hele þe syknesse þ*a*t ys called pleuresis . It helyth þe brest & þe lunges . Drynke yt w*ith* mulsa & yt wol make þe wel to pysse . Sethe nettls yn oyle & drynke þe cocc*i*on & yt wol make þe laxatyf . Take nettles seed & rolle yt yn þy mouthe clos & yt wol allaye þe {bolnyng} of þ*a*t parte of þe mouthe þ*a*t ys called uua . ffrote wel abarey*n* bestes cunte w*ith* nettell

---

210 But] mor strongly *bot. marg.*

---

214 Thus] Tus MS. **220** bolnyng] boluyng MS.

leues or w*ith* þe Iuys þer of & þe best shal conceyue . A *f.9v* noynte þe wel w*ith* þe oyle þ*at* nettelles || be soden yn & yt wol make þe to swete. Take þe Iuys of nettell seed & a noynte þer w*ith* þyn heed & yt wol lette & represse þe fluxe of þe heed . Nettel seed shal be gadred yn august & þan shal yt be holsom & p*ro*fytabele to many causes .

Garlyke ys hoot & drye yn þe fourthe degre . Ete garlyke or anoynte þe sore places . & yt wol hele bytynges or styngynges of snakes & of addres . Medle garlyke w*ith* hony þ*at* wol heele hou*n*des bytynge yf þow anoynte þer w*ith* þe bytynge place . The sauor of garlyk stampyd dryueth away noyous wormes . Sethe garlyke yn mulsa & putte to yt alytel uenygre & drynke yt & þ*ys* wol destroye wormes yn þe wombe & þe trenches . Wyth þe same cure þow may heele þe body þ*at* ys *f.10r* borst oute for colde . Sethe garlyke pylees yn || oyle & þ*at* oyle wol hele þe bytynge of dedly & uenemous bestes yf þe bytyn place be anoynted þer w*ith* . Anoynte þy share w*ith* garlyke soden w*ith* mulsa & uenygre & þys wol destroye þe swellyng & þe ache of þe bladdre . The saam wol garlyk pyles do yf þow sethe he*m* yn water & ley hem yn þe manere of a plastre to þe share . Sethe garlyk yn hys pyles & þer yn bathe wel & long a woma*n* & she shal a noon be delyueryd of hyr after byrden . To þe same hylpyth a subfumygac*io*n of garlyk . Sethe garlyk yn gotes mylk & ete yt & yt helpyth aye*n*st many dysseses of þe lunges and so yt dothe also yf þow ete yt rawe . Sethe garlyk w*ith* centory & yeue yt he*m* þat han þe dropesye for þ*at* dryeth up þe watery humours . Sethe *f.10v* garlyk || w*ith* corya*u*ndre & wyne ete yt & drynke þys wyne for þe syknesse þ*at* ys callyd neufresys & for þe ston yn þe reynes & for þe Iaundys & yt makyt nesshe wombes . Sethe garlyk w*ith* benes stampe yt & make þer of aplaster & lay yt

---

228 Garlyke] u̲ *ext. marg.* **246** dysseses] for the breste *ext. marg. H3*

---

252 þer] w*ith* *exp.*

to þe heed or anoynte þer w*ith* þe temples of þe heed & þ*a*t wol destroye þe ache of þe heed. {Stampe} garlyk w*ith* gose grese & handle yt wel atte fyre & put yt yn þyn ere leuke warme & þ*a*t staunchyt þe ache of þe ere & soueraynly yt makyth þe for to here . Sethe garlyk yn water & ete yt ofte & yt destreyth þe cowhe & staunchyt syghynges . Ete garlyk wheþer þu wolt rau or soden & yt wol claryfye þe uoyce . but better helpyth þe soden þerto . Stampe garlyk and mercuryal . sethe hem & ete hem . þat wol destroye þe seknesse þ*a*t ys called tenasmon . Stampe garlyk w*ith* swy ||nes grece . & *f.11r* make þer of aplastre & yt wol destroye bolnynge . yf þow ley ofte þys playstre to þe bolne place . Ete atte morwe fastyng garlyk & drynk wyne þer to & þ*a*t day shall non unknowe water*ys* do þe harme ne chau*n*gyng of places .

Planteyne ys callyd yn greke Arnoglossa she hath leues lyke a lambys tonge . There are tow maner*ys* of playnteyne . þe more & þe lasse . And þe lasse ys cleped lanceolata for hyr leues be shapen sharpe as a spere . Pla*n*teyn ys cold & drye yn þe thrydde degre natheles þe moor þ*a*t ys seyde Arnoglossa hath þe grett*er* myght & uertu . Arnoglossa wol drye moyst wondes & clense hem þ*a*t ben foule yf she be medled w*ith* hony and salte & soden yn uenygre & leyde þerto . Take þys same herbe & a noþer þ*a*t ys brude & dyghte he*m* yn þe same wyse & ete hem & þ*a*t wol || stau*n*che þe fluxe of þe *f.11v* wombe & þe blody menysone & þe flyxe of þe wo*m*be þ*a*t w*ith* ache . The same doth yt leyde yn a plastre & yt restreyneth þe blode . ffrote w*ith* þe same hony a blak spotte & yt wol turne ayen to þe same coloure þ*a*t yt was before . Meldle planteyn w*ith* shepes mylke & yt wol hele brynnynges & sc⌞a⌟ldynges . Stampe only planteyn leues & yt wol hele houndes bytynge & a bate þe bolnyng yf yt ⌞be⌟ leyde þer to .

---

267 Planteyne] uj *ext. marg.*

---

254 Stampe] Sampe MS. **283** Stampe] Sampe MS.

{Stampe} þys herbe w*ith* salte & yt wol destroye þe cornels yf þey be leyde þerto . Sethe playntey*n* as wortes & ete yt for ys good for þe dropesye . And yn þe same wyse yt helpyth hem þ*at* han þe chynke or þe fallyng euel . Holde longe yn þy mouthe þe Iuys of planteyn & rolle yt wel þere yn & yt *f.12r* purgyth þe foule wondes of þe mouthe . Helde þe Iuys || of planteyn yn festres w*ith* a syry*n*ge & þ*at* wol hele hem . The Iuys of planteyn ys for þe ache of þe eres yf yt be helde yn hem . Wyth þe Iuys of planteyn anoynte þe place . where as ys þe maladye þ*at* ys clepyd Ignys sacer & þ*at* wol make yt ho⸤o⸥le . Drynke ofte þe Iuys of planteyn & yt wol hele þe tysyk & hem þ*at* speten blood . Take þe Iuys of planteyn by a clystery & yt wol hele blody menysone . A noynte ofte þyn eyen w*ith* þe Iuys of planteyn & þ*at* wol hele þe bolnyng & þe hete of hem . Chewe wel þe moor & yt wol represse þe bollen gomes & ful of blood . And yn þe same wyse yt staunchyth þe to the ache . Hange þe rote of þ*ys* herbe aboute þy neck & yt wol do away þe heed ache . Wete wolle yn leuke *f.12v* Iuys of planteyn & underputte yt & yt || wol restreyne þe corrupc*io*n or blode þat rennyth out of wo*m*me*n* . leye aplastre of planteyn roote to þe place þ*at* þe scorpyon hath y stong & yt wol make yt hoole . To alle þuse for seyd causes þe cocc*io*n of þ*ys* herbe ys good but yit bett*er* ys þe seed of yt soden yn wyne . Drynke þ*ys* planteyn & yt wol destroye & heele þe ache of þe bladdre & of þe reynes . It ys seyd þ*at* yn hem þ*at* beren þ*ys* herb ys rotes & hange yt aboute hyr neckes þey shal neuer cowhe yf þey bere hem alway . Take thre rotes & stampe hem & medle hem yn iij cuppes of wyne & w*ith* as many of water . & yeue þys to hem þ*at* han þe feuere before þe comyng of þe quakyng uppo*n* hem & so shalt þow putte away þe feuer t*er*cya*n* . Take yn þe same

312 þys] pla*n*tay*n* *ext. marg. H3*

290 festres] wondes *exp.* **305** yt[2]] w *exp.*

manere foure rotes of þe same herbe w*ith* foure cuppes & yt wol putte away þe feuer quarteyn . Here note þ*at* þys cuppe ys clepyd yn latyn Ciatus || Ciatus ys asmuche as an eye shelle *f.13r* my co*n*teyne & holde . Also planteyn þe lasse ys good to þe bocches of þe nostrelles yf þow anoynte hem w*ith* þe Iuys of þys herbe or make of yt aplastre . In þe same wyse yt ys good to þe bocches of þe eyen yf yt be leyd þer upon . ix days w*ith* nesse wolle . ffor þe ache of þe wombe . leye upon þe wombe of þe leuke Iuys of þ*ys* herbe & was she yt . ffor þe wormes yn þe wombe . Drynke ofte þe Iuys of þ*ys* herbe by yt self or melde yt w*ith* olde swynes grece & leye yt þer to . Whan yt ys medled w*ith* þe same grece & þer of ys made a plastre yt ys good to stanche & abate bolnynges . And þe same wyse yt ys good to þat euel þ*at* ys called p*ar*otida & also to fresshe & newe wondes . Drynke of þys herbe Iuys . ij . houres before þe accesse & yt wol hele þe quarteyn . Drynk þe Iuys of þys herbe & yt wol putte oute þe afterbyrdou*n* of þe secu*n*dyne . || Stampe þys herbe w*ith* wyne or uenygre & emplastre yt & *f.13v* so shalt þu hele & a swage þe ache of þe feet goyng . So doth sed of þys herbe ⌞yf⌟ yt be drunke & þe Iuys medled w*ith* resons . Thys herbe ys good to dyuerse syknes of þe bladdre for þ*ys* herbe hath mygth & uertu for to drye þerfor she ys good to bocches & dyslac*io*n of þe body .

REwe . ys hoot & drye yn þe thrydde degre . She doth muche good to þe stomak yf yt be ofte ydronke she openyth þe nosestrelles & dryeth up þe blood . She puttyth oute þe chyld & repressyth lechery yf yt be dronke . And also staunchyt þe cowe & purgyt wo*m*mens floures . Sethe rewe yn water & þe fourthe parte uenygre & drynke þ*at* decoc*io*n . yt wol destroye frety*n*g yn þe bely . It helpyth þe longes & þe brest & þe ache & dessese of þe rybbes þ*at* ys called pleuresys . It destroyth þe passyon þat fallyth yn weher || lebon of þe thye . *f.14r*

338 Rewe] uij *ext. marg.*

And also thylk goute þ*at* ys clepyd arthetica . And eke þe feuers yf þow drynke yt . Yf þow sethe grene rewe yn oyle & þer w*ith* leuke anoynte w*ith* þ*ys* ale þe mothe of þe matryce & yt shal heele yt from bolnynge . Helde yt yn w*ith* a clystery & þ*at* wol hele þe swellyng of þe entrayles . bothe to þe moder & eke to þe ent*ra*les doþe rewe good yf she be dronke w*ith* wyne . Sethe rewe yn oyle & ete yt or drynke yt & so shalt þow destroye þe wormes yn þe wombe . Sethe longe fygges & rewe yn wyne & þe lycoure þer of ys good to hem þat han þe dropse . And so doth þe self co*n*fecc*i*on of yt yn þys wyse . yf yt be emplastred by anyght . Ete rawe rewe & yt wol claryfye þe syght . But bett*er* yt helpyth yf þow make an oynement of þe Iuys of rewe & of þe Iuys of fenel w*ith* þe galle of a kocke & w*ith* hony as muche as ys of þe rewe & w*ith* þys anoynte
f.14v þe eyne ofte . Medle þe Iuys of rewe w*ith* || þe oyle of roses & uenygre & þys onyment wol cesse þe hed ache . Thryst oute þe Iuys of rewe & helde yt yn to þe nostrelles þ*at* bleden & yt wol stanche þe blod . Chawe þe Iuys of rew yn þe pylle of a poune garnet & holde yt yn to þe ere & þ*at* wol hele þe ache of þe ere . Medle þe Iuys of rewe w*ith* oyle roset cense & uenygre & myrre & þ*ys* co*n*fecc*i*on by ofte anoyntyng wol hele þ*at* syknesse þ*at* ys called ignys sacer . Thys oyneme*n*t wol heele bocches of þe heed out of þe wyche rennyth a fatte humour & eke þe stabbe þ*at* ys called darte outher herpeta & eke þe bocches þ*at* rysen yn þe nosstrelles . Metrydates preuyth ofte þ*at* rewe eten or dronkyn rawe wol destre uenym . ffor he þ*at* etyth fastyng rewe mynt leues w*ith* a lytyl salte & too fygges ij akorous & xx nottes þan þar hym not drede of no bestes uenym . Thys also techyth þe wesel . ffor
f.15r whan she shal fyghte w*ith* þe addre she wol fyrst || ete rewe & walowe hyr self þer yn . Sethe rewe yn a lytel boter & oyle & yt wol destroye þe bolnyng of þe matryce yf she be putte under leuke . In suche wyse doth she good to þe dyssese of thylke gutte þ*at* ys clepyd Colon & to all þe maladyes þ*at* ben

w*ith* yn þe body . {Stampe} rewe ⌞w*ith*⌟ lorer leues & make þer of aplastre & þ*at* wol destroye þe swellyng of þe ballok . Take peper comyn & nit*er* yn euene weyght & of rewe as moche as all þuse thre but loke þ*at* þe comyn be wel soked yn sharpe uenygre & ofte dryed uppon an hoot place of yron þan shul all þuse be sta*m*pyd to gydre smal & made up w*ith* hony . Thys wol hele þe ache of þe brest of þe sydes & of þe mawe & eke of þe reynes yf yt be ofte eten . Thys wol an⌞e⌟yntyse colera & make þe nesshe wombed w*ith* oute greuau*n*ce . It co*m*fortyth þe stomak & makyth good degestyon . ||

NEyther þe rose coloure ne þe lylye may ouerpasse þe uiolet *f.15v* nether yn beute ne yn strengthe . or uertu nor yn odour . It ys seyde þ*at* uyolet ys moyst & colde yn þe fourthe degre . There are of uyolet*es* thre maneres þe wyche be knowe by her floures þ*at* ben dyuerse The fyrst ys wythe . The secu*n*de ben blake . The trydde of purpul coloure . And though they ben of dyuerse coloures yit þey han alle oo uertu & myght yn medycyn . Uyolet helpyth & restreynyt places þ*at* ben yn flammat & hoot yf þey be stamped & leyde to hem plast*er* wyse . Uyolet destroyth þe heed ache yf yt be dronken or smelled outher heed ycouerd þer w*ith* . Water þ*at* þe uyolet hath be soden y*n*ne ys good to þe dysseses ⌞of⌟ þe gry*n*de yf yt be ofte bathen & wasshed þe reyn . It ys seyde þ*at* purpul uyolet helpyth & destroyt þe fallyng euel specyaly yn chyldryn . Yf she be dronke yn wat*er* || Stampe uyolet w*ith* *f.16r* myrre & safferon & ley þ*ys* emplastre to þe bolnyng of þe thye & yt wol hele yt . Stampe uyolet & hony & uenygre & þer w*ith* anoynte þe bocches of þe heed . Wyth þe water þ*at* uyolet ys soden yn . Wasshe oft þe moder & yt wol abate þe

---

388 eke…reynes] bon*um* est *ext. marg. H2* **389** colera] rew *ext. marg. H3* **392** uiolet] uiij *ext. marg.*

---

381 Stampe] Sampe MS.

bolnyng of hyr . Medle uyolet w*ith* wax & anoynte ofte þer
w*ith* þe chynes of þe erse þe wyche Grekes clepen Recadyas or
ley yt þerto & þ*at* wol make hem hole . Medle uyolet w*ith*
hony & þer w*ith* anoy*n*te þe whelkes . þ*at* wol destroye &
hele he*m* . or emplastrye yt to hem . The x^{e} uertu uyolet seed
purgyth wo*m*mens floures yf yt be dronke . The ix^{e} uertu þe
rootes of hyr stamped & medled w*ith* uynegre dryeth þe
splene . yf þey be dronke . or leyde þer to . The xij^{e} u*er*tu . It
ys seyde þ*at* yn þe same wyse þow mayst cure þe hot podagre .
The xiij u*er*tu drynke grene uyolet or þe floure . or þe Iuys ||
f.16v of yt & so shalt þow destroye þe red colre yn þe stomak .
The xiiij u*er*tu drynke uyolet w*ith* fresshe water I medled . &
yt wol destroye all sykenesse þ*at* comet of colera rubea or of
blod yn þe tendre & nesshe sydes or yn þe lunges And þe
cowhe of chyldren & þe syghyng yn þe same wyse . The xu
u*er*tu as þow makyst oyle of roses . so shalt þow make oyle of
uyolet & þ*at* ys p*ro*phetable to many causes as men sayen .
for yt wol destroye þe ache of þe erys & þe sownyng þere of
yn also . And to þe heed yt p*ro*phytyth . Wat maner ache
euere holde yt . The xuj u*er*tu helde yn or drynke þe oyle . or
anoynte þer w*ith* þe wombe & þ*at* wol sle all þe wormes þ*at*
ben þere yn . The xuij u*er*tu It acoldyth esely þe body &
resoluyth yt of slomerynge . The xuiij u*er*tu anoynte w*ith*
oyle þe eres of þe heed & þ*at* wol destroye þe scally dust of
yt . The xix u*er*tu If the sculle or brayn pa*n*ne be broke or
bowed so þ*at* þe pacyent may not speke . Stampe uyolet & do
hym for to dry*n*ke yt yn wyne fyrst . After ward yf þe ryght
f.17r syde of þe heed be hurte . Stampe || uyolet & bynde yt to þe
lyfte foot sool . yf yt be þe reue⌊r⌋se . Do þow þe reuerse
anoon þe boon wol {slepe} ayen & yn þe same day shal þe
pacyent speke . as seyth þe leche . The xx u*er*tu þe root of þe

438 Stampe] uyolet *bot. marg.*

440 slepe] sleppe MS.

whyte uyolet wol stau*n*che þe fluxe of þe wombe . be yt olde . beyt newe yf þow holde yt yn þy mouthe swolewe þe Iuys of yt . And yf þow take lyquoryce þ*er* w*ith* & chewe w*ith* yt . hys u*er*tu ys mouche þe spedyer .

SMereworte or Aristologia . hath . iij . maneres . The fyrst ys seyde longe . for hys root ys longe . That other ys seyde yn greke clunatis . Thys ys almost euen of myght to þe secu*n*de þ*at* ys seyde rounde Alle . iij . ben hoote yn þe secunde degre & drye yn þe fyrst degre . The fyrst u*er*tu drynke þe rounde w*ith* wyne & she wol hele alle uenemous bytyng & destroye þe uenym þ*at* me*n* haue eten or dronken & dryueth oute þe afterberden . The sec*u*nde u*er*tu þys herbe drynke w*ith* wyne & peper p*ur*gyth þe moder after þe chyldes byrthe || from all *f.17v* corrupc*i*on & fylthe . And so yt wol do . yf yt be putte oonly undernethe . The thrydde u*er*tu thys herbe doth good to hem þ*at* han þe chynke & to þe dysseses of þe sydes or rybbes . she wol destroye colde þ*at* man hath take yn hys body yf yt be dro*n*ke w*ith* sauored water . or yn eny oþer sauory thynges þ*at* ben p*ro*fytable . The . iiij . u*er*tu stampe þys herbe & ley yt as aplastre yt wol brynge oute nayle or þorne ouþ*er* arowe þ*at* be styked yn manys body . The . u . u*er*tu Medle smere worte w*ith* hony & yt wol clense wondes & hele hem . The uj u*er*tu Medle w*ith* þe for sayd two gladyn & þer w*ith* anoynte þe go*m*mes & þ*at* wol kepe þe tethe fro rotyng & fylthe . The uij u*er*tu dry*n*ke þ*ys* herbe w*ith* uenygre & yt wol dyssolue þe harnes of þe splene . The uiij u*er*tu dry*n*ke her w*ith* hoot water . or wyne & yt wol hele þe ache of þe syde . The ix u*er*tu drynke her w*ith* water & yt wol destroye þe euel feuers . The x u*er*tu drynke her yn þe sa || me & aboue alle þyng*es* yt ys good for þe cra*m*pe . The xi *f.18r* u*er*tu In þe same wyse she wol destroye þe harde podagre . yf yt be dronke ofte . The xij u*er*tu In þe same wyse she wol

---

446 Smereworte] ix *ext. marg.*

destroye & swage þe ache of þe wombe & þe fallyng euel & þe palesy also . The xiij u*er*tu . the smoke of þ*ys* herbe wol chace away alle deuels & gladyth younge chyldryn . The xiiij u*er*tu þe roote of þ*ys* herbe wol sle wel festres yf yt be wel clensed & y put yn to þe hool faste . The xu u*er*tu drynke þ*ys* herbe wi*th* water or wi*th* wyne & yt wol destroye þe yoxe . The longe smere worte may do alle tho þ*a*t I haue seyde . þ*a*t þe rounde may do . but netheles þe longe hath weyker stryngthe þan hath þe rounde werefore so*m*me . whan þey may not haue the rounde . þey take as {muche} weyth of þe longe . as þey wolde of þe rounde yf þey hade yt & halfe so *f.18v* muche more . The decocc*i*on of þe longe || doth good wonderlyche yn bathynge & was shynge . And yf she be dronke wi*th* water she wol heele þe dysseses of þe splene . If she be stamped & leyd to she wol draue oute what þyng euer yt be þ*a*t ys stykyd yn manys body . Also she wol destroye þe wycked humorus of þe matryce & purgyt hyr . Plinius sayth þ*a*t þe woma*n* þ*a*t leyeth þ*ys* herbe to her pryue membre wi*th* beef after þ*a*t she hath co*n*ceyueth . she shal haue a sone . for þys herbe formeth males yn thylke wyse . The xuj u*er*tu Medle þe rounde wi*th* lyme . & stampe hem to gedre & þys quellyth fysshes . & þ*er*for so*m*me me*n* clepen yt uenym of þe erthe .

ACHE ys clepyd Apium yn latyn . for thy þ*a*t þe cappe of uyctours & ouercomeres yn olde tyme were wont to bere hyt whan þey hadde ou*er*come her enemyes . It ys seyde þ*a*t alsydes toke uppon hy*m* fyrst for ⌞to⌟ were suche a croune & *f.19r* oþ*er* me*n* afterwarde used furthe þ*a*t maner || So*m*me supposen þ*a*t þ*ys* herbe ache Smalache was seyd Apium . for thy þ*a*t bees ben wont to sytte uppon þ*ys* herbe & souke oute þe Iuys of hyr floure coueytously . Grekes clepen þ*ys* herbe

---

497 Ache] x *ext. marg.*

---

483 muche] nuche MS.

Selino*n* .or Solumem It ys hoot & drye yn þe trydde degre . The fyrst u*er*tu . Medle þe Iuys of ache wi*th* whyte brede cromes & emplastre yt by anyght to þe eye þ*a*t ys bolle & þ*a*t wol abate þe bollnyng of þe tetes & staunche þe feruour of þe stomake & destroye þe bolnyng & þe uentosyte of yt . The secunde u*er*tu ete or drynke þys herbe rawe & yt wol make þe to pysse . but better doth þe cocc*i*on of þ*ys* herbe root . As also doth þe seed of smalache yf yt be dronke ofte . The iij u*er*tu þys herbe doth profyte to uenemous bytyng . but better ys þe seed þerto or þe decocc*i*on emplastred . yn þe same wyse wol {staunche} þe cowhe . yf yt be dronke ofte . The iiij u*er*tu In þe same wyse she wol harde þe wombe & staunche þe uomyte || yf she be dronke . The u u*er*tu Medle ache wi*th* *f.19v* water & a lytel uenygre & yt wol restore to þe syke colure þ*a*t he hat lost . The uj u*er*tu Ete yche day fastyng smalache rawe & yt wol destroye þe quotydyan . If also þow drynke yt wi*th* water afore þe quakynge of þe feuer . The uij u*er*tu drynke smaleache wi*th* þe Iuys of fenel & yt wol helpe hem þ*a*t han þe dropese . or dyssese of þe splene or bolnyng yn þe mawe . The uiij u*er*tu wi*th* þe Iuys of ache a noynte þe frakelyd face & þ*a*t wol destroye þe frakeles alle The ix u*er*tu þe Iuys of smalache medled wi*th* mele . or floure of whete & þe whyte of an eye & emplastred . wol clense wondes & bocches yf yt be leyde ofte*n* tymes þer to .

SAueyne . ys drye & hoot yn þe thryd degre . The fyrst u*er*tu Medle sauyen wi*th* hony & yt wol drye faste abocche or wonde & clense yt wel . The ij u*er*tu þys emplastre wol hele a feloun . þe wyche þe comou*n* peple clepen þe goute bocches The iij u*er*tu saueyn wol delyuer wel || wome*n* of her floures *f.20r* & to þe deed chylde to be boor . yf yt be dronke ofte wi*th*

---

509 stomake] for the stomac *ext. marg. H3 marg.* **529** Saueyne] xj *ext. marg.*

---

515 staunche] stauche MS.

wyne or stamped . other be leyde to þe matryces mouthe . The ⌞iiij⌟ u*er*tu saueyn medled w*ith* ache rootes . wol make þe skyn to glytere & shyne . Sauyn wol do good to alle sykenesses þ*at* ben take of colde yf hyr decocc*i*on be dro*n*ke w*ith* wyne or wat*er* .

LEeke as ys yt y seyde . Ipocras used leeke yn many of hys medycyns . The fyrst u*er*tu ypocras þ*at* gret leche . yaf þe Iuys of leeke for to drynke to hym þat casted oute bloode þe wyche me*n* ben cleped {Emoptoycy} . The . ij u*er*tu w*ith* ij *dragmes* of dust of encense . or of galle *dragme* . i . of leeke seed & a lytel of myrre . Whan alle þuse be wel stampyd to gedyr & soden yn wyne It wol be a good drynke for hem þ*at* speten bloode & to hem þ*at* bleden at nose . The iij u*er*tu þe Iuys of leeke wol staunche þe blood of þe nose yf þe nostrelles *f.20v* {furthw*ith*} be anoynted || w*ith* yt w*ith* ynne . The iiij u*er*tu þe same ys good for rennyng or flowyng of broken bocches . The u u*er*tu þe woma*n* þ*at* etyth leeke often tymes shal conceyue lyghtly . The uj u*er*tu stampe leke w*ith* hony & leye yt to a bocche or wonde & yt wol do good þerto & hele yt . The uij u*er*tu Medle þe Iuys of leeke w*ith* ptisane . & yt wol do good to dystillac*i*on of humors of þe heed to þe lunges & to þe dysseses of þe brest . & makyth a shylle uoyce & destroyt þe cowhe þ*at* harmeth þe entrayles & to alle causes þ*at* ben seyd tofore . ys þe Iuys of leeke good allone . The uiij u*er*tu Ete leke & drynke wyne to or drynke þe Iuys of leke w*ith* wyne & þys wol make þe harde wombed . Sethe þe whyte of lekes yn wyne . & after þe fyrst boylyng take yt oute of þe wyne & boyle yt yn water & yeue yt to drynke . & þ*at* wol staunche þe flyxe & make þe hard wo*m*bed . So yt doth also yf yt be soden yn wyne & y dronke . And þ*at* same *f.21r* ys good to dystroy || uenym of addres . or eny uenemous

---

540 Leeke] xij *ext. marg.* **563** flyxe] for the flyx *ext. marg. H3*

---

543 Emoptoycy] Euotoycy MS. **549** furthwith] furw*ith* MS.

best . The ix u*er*tu Medle þe Iuys of leeke w*ith* gotes gal or w*ith* mulsa . & helde yt luke yn to þe ere þ*at* akyth & yt wol abate þe workyng of þe ere . The x u*er*tu Medle þe Iuys of leeke w*ith* woma*n*s mylke & yt wol destroye an olde cowhe . & do muche good to dyuerse syknesse of þe lunges . The xi u*er*tu the leke destryth the uenym of þe padstoles yf yt be eten . The xij u*er*tu . Medle to gyder . ij . partes of þe Iuys of þe leke . & þe trydde parte of hony . helde yt yn atte nosestrelles . or atte eres & yt wol abate þe heed ache . The xiij u*er*tu as leches sayen þere ys no þyng so profytable to þe ache of þe lendes . as ys þe Iuys of lekes y dronke w*ith* wyne . The xiiij u*er*tu leke or þe Iuys of leke ys good for to consounde & hele bocches . & for to allente & mollyfye þe hardnes of a postome ⌊or⌋ of a bocche The . xu u*er*tu stampe leke & salte & leye hem to a newe fresshe wonde & þat wol close yt a noon . The xuj u*er*tu Ete rawe || leke & yt wol *f.21v* putte away dronkenesse . & scure to lechyre & make þe wo*n*de nesshe þ*at* ys harde .

NEpte ys called yn greke . Calamentu*m* & yt ys drye & hoot yn þe myddel of þe thrydde degre . The fyrst u*er*tu drynke þys herbe w*ith* methe & yt wol turne all þe body yn to a swoot . The ij u*er*tu Oyle of þe decocc*i*on of þ*ys* herbe . wol destroye þe feuers yf all þe body be anoynted of yt before or þe colde take þe pacyent & yt wol put away þe cold also . The iij u*er*tu stampe þys herbe grene & ley yt to þe thye of hym þ*at* hath dyssese yn hys whyrlebon*e* þus yt brennet up þe skyn as yt ys seyd . & so dryet up þe humours . & so putte away þe dyssese & ache of þe whyr⌊le⌋bon*e* . The iiij u*er*tu Medle þe Iuys of þys herbe yn drynke & yt wol purge wo*m*mans floures . The u u*er*tu . Elephancya ys amaner of lepre & yt ys cleped þys name . for ryght as an olyfaunt ys hugest of alle bestes . so ys þys || maladye gretyst of alle maladyes & lepres . *f.22r*

---

584 Nepte] xiij *ext. marg.* **588** feuers] for the ackes *ext. marg. H3*

Drynke Calamynte y*n* þe begynnyng of þys maladye w*ith* wyne for yt wol waste & co*n*sume þe humours þ*at* þys maladye ys norysshed by . & so cure þe man . The uj u*er*tu S⌞t⌟ampe þys herbe & leye yt to þe place þ*at* ys y stunge w*ith* eny serpent & so shalt þow heele þ*at* place . The uij u*er*tu drynke Calamynte yn wyne & þ*at* wol putte away uenym . The uiij u*er*tu Calamynte y dronke wol sle wormes yn þe bely . The ix u*er*tu Medle þe Iuys of calamynt w*ith* salte & hony & þ*at* wol sle þe wormes þ*at* rennen yn eny place of þe body . The x u*er*tu yf a woman þ*at* ys w*ith* chyld drynke Calamynte yt wol delyuer hyr of hyr warpelyng þus wol þys herbe do yf she be grounde & y putte unther þe woman . The xi u*er*tu þys herbe y dronke w*ith* wyne wol clense & hele þe Iaundys & þe streyghtnesse of þe brest & þe chynke . The *f.22v* xij u*er*tu . || on þe same wyse It wol hele þe olde ache & þe greua*u*nce yn þe syde . The xiij u*er*tu stampe þys herbe & ley yt to þe blak cicatrices . & þ*at* wol brynge hem to þe coloure þ*at* þey hadden fyrst . But better helpyth þys herbe . yf she be soden yn wyne & þan emplastred . The xiiij u*er*tu drynke þe Iuys of þ*ys* herbe yn wyne & yt wol destroye þe greuau*n*ce of þe stomak & þe ache . The xu u*er*tu þe smoke of þys herbe chasyth serpentes oute of þe house þ*at* þ*ys* herbe ys brent yn . The xuj u*er*tu It ys seyde þ*at* þys herbe y dronke w*ith* wythe wyne wol put away þe yoxe & yn þe same wyse she wol make a body costyf yf yt be dronke ofte . There ben iij maneres of Calamentes . One ys lyke to The seconde ys lyke pulyol þ*at* ys brother worte . The iij ys lyke u*n*to mynte .

FEnell ys called yn greke Maratrum . It ys hoot & drye yn þe *f.23r* secunde degre . The fyrst u*er*tu þys dronke || w*ith* wyne wol destroye alle maner uenym . & hele all maner uenemous bytynges . The ij u*er*tu In þe same wyse she wol scure & prycke to lechery . The iij u*er*tu the addre wol ete fenel whan

625 Fenell] xiiij ext. marg.

hyr eyen dasewen . & so she getyth ayen clere syght & þerby yt ys preueyt þ*a*t fenel doth p*ro*fyt to ma*n*nys eyen . The eyen þ*a*t ben duske & dasewed shul be anoynted w*ith* þe Iuys of fenyl rootes & medled w*ith* hony & þys onyment shal putte away all þe dasewenesse of hem & make hem bryght . The iiij u*er*tu wrynge oute þe Iuys of grene fenel seed & drye þ*a*t ayen þe sonne & þ*a*t ys a gret & myghty medycyne to þe sores of þe yen of what so euer cause yt come . The u u*er*tu putte yn at ere þe Iuys of fenell & yt wol sle alle þe wormes yn þe ere . The uj u*er*tu sethe fenel yn wyne & drynke yt for þ*a*t wol abate þe swellyng of þe dropese . And yn þe same wyse yt wol hele uenemouse bytynges . & þe longes . || & þe *f.23v* mawe also . The uij u*er*tu the noryce . þ*a*t hat defaute of mylke shal ete ofte or dry*n*ke fenel . or þe Iuys & so shal she haue mylke ynow . The uiij u*er*tu sethe yn wyne or yn wat*er* þe rotes of fenel . & þ*a*t decocc*i*on wol hele þe ache of þe reynes . & þe passyons . & greuau*n*ces of þe {bladder} . The ix u*er*tu ete fenel or drynke þe Iuys of yt . & þ*a*t wol make þe to pysse wel . And dyssolue womans floures . Or stampe fenel & bynde yt to þe share & yt wol do þe same . The x u*er*tu the roote of fenel soden yn ptysan ys medycynable for þe reynes . The xj u*er*tu drynke þe Iuys ˪of˩ fenel yn wyne & þ*a*t wol staunche brakynge . The xij u*er*tu þe Iuys of fenel dronke w*ith* wyne asswagyth also þe hete of þe stomak . The xiij u*er*tu þe root of fenel soden yn wyne & emplastred to þe yerde of ama*n* abatyth lyghtly þe ache þ*a*t fallyth þe reyn The same doth þe decocc*i*on of yt yf yt be dronke or used as a bath to þe yerde . And þe same doth yt . yf þow putte to yt oyle || & anoynte þer w*ith* þe place . The xiiij u*er*tu . stampe *f.24r* & melde þe Iuys of fenel w*ith* oyle & þer w*ith* anoynte þe place þ*a*t ys swollen thorugh a buffet or eny oþer cause . for þ*a*t wol abate & staunche þe swellyng . Also yt wol do þe same yf þow stampe fenel w*ith* uenygre & make þer of a

646 bladder] badder MS.

plaster & ley þ*er* to . The xu u*er*tu fenel seed drunke w*ith* wyne . scoryth to lechery & a batyth þe ache of þe sydes . The xuj u*er*tu þe decocc*io*n of fenel drunke ofte wol make olde me*n* to seme longe yong . Thys preueth autours & phylosophers . for serpentes whan þey ben olde & wylnen to waxe myghty & stronge & yonge ayen þey gon & ete of fenel . & so þey be come yongly & myghty .

LEtuse ys colde & ryght moyst & þer for þys herbe puttyth away many dysseses . yf she be eten . And she doth þe same yf she be stamped & leyde to as a plastre . The ij u*er*tu letuse ys *f.24v* p*ro*phytable to þe stomak she makyth a body to slepe || wel & she makyth a body laxatyf . To all þuse causes þys herbe ys better soden þan rawe & y eten . The iij u*er*tu the seed of letuse y dronke w*ith* wyne . destryeth & puttyth away ueyne dremes & allso yt stau*n*chyt þe flyxe of þe wombe . The iiij u*er*tu who so ys yn slepe ofte pollute thorugh hys sperme . Ete he þys herbe & drynke þe Iuys of yt & he shal sone be staunchyd of suche pollucyouns . The u u*er*tu to þe stomak ys letuse best for to ete rawe & unwasse . The uj u*er*tu þe noryce þ*a*t wol often tyme eten letuse shal haue mylke ynow . But so*m*me me*n* sayn who so usyth muche for to eten þys herbe he schal be blynde þere thorugh .

THe Rose as us semeth may ⌞be⌟ clepyd floure of all floures syth she passyth all oþer floures by dyuerse maneres yn sauorre & yn kynde or maner . Of roses þer ben dyuerse maneres . ffor som rose ys y cleped Rosa emoroda . And þys I *f.25r* || trow be þe red rose . Thys ys allso cleped {Rosa canina} . Another ys seyd þe wylde rose & atte rome she ys called Salimica . The fyrst u*er*tu þe Rose staunchyth þe blody

670 Letuse] xu *ext. marg.* **685** Rose] xuj *ext. marg.* **688** I] trowe be *bot. marg.*

689 Rosa canina] Rosa camina MS.

me*n*son of wo*m*ma*n* ynceste . The ij u*er*tu drynke þe Iuys of Roses & þ*at* wol staunche thylke flyxe þ*at* ys cleped diarria . The iij u*er*tu anemplastre of Roses wol drye up roten wondes . The iiij u*er*tu as sayth Constantinus þe Rose ys hoot & drye . thys ys sayd of þe wyld Rose as I trowe . Of þ*at* oþer þ*at* ys to say . of þe garden Rose folowyth here aft*er* . The Rose natheles may not {hepe} us thorugh hyr sauor . ne thorugh hyr bute . but she ys good yn many dyuerse medycynys . She ys drye & colde yn þe fyrste degre . The fyrst u*er*tu Rose wol abate þe holy fyre yf she be stamped & leyde þere to . An yn þe same wyse yf þe stomak be to hoot or þe entrayles ouer muche . þe wyche ben cleped precordya || {Stampe} þe Rose . & emplastre hyr þere to & she wol abate *f.25v* þe hete . The ij u*er*tu abathe of þe Roses sode*n* yn wyne . or a drynke wol staunche þe fluxe of þe matryce The iij u*er*tu In þe same wyse þ*at* þe Rose staunchyth þe fluxe of þe matryce she wol staunche þe fluxe of þe wombe . The u u*er*tu þe pouder of þe drye Roses helpyth to many sores of þe mothe . The uj u*er*tu þe pouder of þe Rose floure froted upon þe lyppes or medled wi*th* hony . ys good for brekyng of þe lyppes or of þe go*m*mes . The uij u*er*tu alle maner unkynde hetes wol þe Rose destroy yf she be stamped all grene & plastred þer to or yf she be stamped & drunke wi*th* mulsa . The uiij u*er*tu of þ*ys* Rose ys made oleu*m* rosaceu*m* þe wyche ys p*ro*phytable to many causes . And specyaly yf yt be dronke yt wol nesshe þe wombe & quenche þe yn moderat het of þe stomak . The ix u*er*tu wi*th* || þys oyle wasshe or bathe or a *f.26r* noynte wel þe heed so mayst þow staunche þe ache & þe heet of þe heed þ*at* ys ou*er*muche The x u*er*tu þys oyle wol haue oute also & clenly þe felthe of wondes & fylle wi*th* good flesshe þe depe wondes yf yt be medled wel wi*th* stronge

---

704 Stampe … &[1]] Sampe þe Rose & *top marg.*

---

698 hepe] hepe MS. **704** Stampe] Sampe MS.

uenygre . And yn þe same wyse yt ys good for brennynges of fyre . or scaldyng of wateres . The xi u*er*tu þys oyle y holdyn longe yn þe mothe wol sone staunche þe tothe ache as yt ys seyd . The xij u*er*tu þ*ys* oyle wol make harde browes nesshe . yf þey be anoynted þerwi*th* . The xiij u*er*tu þ*ys* oyle wol do away þe ache of þe membres wi*th* ynne yf yt be under putte . And þys oyle ys good for many causes of þe matryce . Dyuerse me*n* makyn dyuersly þ*ys* oyle . but þe greet clerke palladius wrytyth of yt yn þ*ys* wyse . Take of þ*a*t þat ys reed of þe *f.26v* Roses floure an unce || & þer to a pounde of oyle . & putte alle þuse yn a glas . & stoppe yt faste & uij dayes allone hange yt yn þe soune . So*mm*e sayn þ*a*t yt shulde be honged atte fyre . or atte sonne fourty dayes & afterwarde {eek} streyneyt thorugh a clene clothe & kepyt yt wel for dyuerse medycyns

Affter þys gentel & golden Rose ryghtfully shal folewe nex after þe seluerne lylye . þe wyche yf þey be lykned to þe Rose yeuyth not stede ne sauore nether fayrnesse yit yn many causes þe lylye ys as p*ro*fytable to me*n* as ys þe Roses for medycynes . The fyrst u*er*tu þe lylye rote rosted under þe coles & after stamped smal wi*th* comune oyle wol hele wonderly brynnyng or scaldynge yf yt be a noy*n*ted þer wi*th* . But better yt wol do yf oyle of Roses be Ioyned þer to . The ij u*er*tu þe lylye root dyghte yn þe saam wyse & unther put *f.27r* makyth nesse þe harde || matryce . The iij u*er*tu A plast*er* made of lylye leues soden . helyth þe synowes þ*a*t be drawen to gydres & nesshyt hem & yn þe same wyse yt helpyth þe ly*mm*es þ*a*t ben brent . Also yt helpyth addres bytynges . The iiij u*er*tu þe lylye root soden yn wyne . destroyth þe uenym of padstoles . The u u*er*tu stampe þe lylye root & sethe yt yn wyne & þ*er* of a plast*er* wol drawe oute nayle or thorne styk .

---

739 lylye] xuij *ext. marg.*

---

735 eek] ee MS. **752** sethe] yt yn ou *exp.*

outher arowe stykyd yn yn þe flesshe but þ*ys* plastre schal not be meued tyl after iij dayes . The uj u*er*tu It ys seyd þ*at* þe lylye soden yn swynes grece or shepes talowe wol make heer to growe yn þe lymes þ*at* ben brent . The uij u*er*tu Men say þ*at* lylye rotes soden yn wyne . & drunke purgyth euel bloed by þe wombe . & so yt doth good & p*ro*fyt to þe splene . And so yt helpyth þe kunte & purgyth wommens floures . Al þys wol yt do yf yt || be soden yn olde wyne & leyde to as a *f.27v* plast*er* . The uiij u*er*tu the lyly rotes stamped wel & {medled} w*ith* hony ys medycyne for broken . or kutte . outher y hurte synowes . The ix u*er*tu þere ys no þyng better to drye up wondes þan ys þe Iuys y thurst oute of þe lyly leues medled w*ith* uenygre & soden yn hony . Of þys Iuys shal be fyue partyes . & of hony & uenygre shal be foure partes & of yuy*s* þe u parte . þ*ys* wol drye up bocches . olde wondes & newe & close hem fayre . The x u*er*tu lyly rotes soden & stamped & medled w*ith* cerotes or w*ith* wax & bouter wol strecche oute alle þe ryuelynges of þe face & do away alle þe frakles of þe skyn yf yt be a noynted þer w*ith* The xi u*er*tu þe same oynement wol purge & destroye þe meseles þe wyche ben cleped yn latyn lichene or uariole . The xij u*er*tu stampe lyly leues & þe Iuys þer of under putt to kuntes makyth nesshe . And þys Iuys as yt || ys seyd may make abody to *f.28r* swete þ*at* ys anoynted þer w*ith* . The xiij u*er*tu thys same Iuys ys good to maturyng of bocches & yt clensyt hem .

SAuerey ys seyde yn latyn Saturya & yn greke Tymbrya . The fyrst u*er*tu sauerey ys hoot & drye yn þe fourthe degre . Drynke þys herbe w*ith* wyne & yt wol make þe to pysse . And also yt purgyth wo*m*mens floures . The ij u*er*tu . In þe same wyse she wol putte oute a chylde of wo*m*ma*n*s wombe though yt be deed þereyn & clense alle þe guttes of

779 Sauerey] xuiij *ext. marg.* **782** floures] menstrua *ext. marg. H3*

763 medled] meldled MS.

wo*m*ma*n* . The iij u*er*tu þe pouder of sauerey wit*h* soden hony under putte . or eten or soden wit*h* wyne or mulsa wol make a body spette away þe glatte abowte þe brest . The iiij u*er*tu þys pouder largely drynke wit*h* leuke wyne wol abate þe fretynge of þe wombe . And þys preued macer ofte . as he *f.28v* wrytyth yn hys boke . || The u uertu þere ys a syknesse þ*a*t ys called litargia . þe wyche as leches sayn ys co*n*trary to frenesy . The litargius ys eu*er* slepyng yn hys syknesse . but þe frentyke ma*n* may not slepe : To hym þ*a*t ys takyn wit*h* so dedly a slepe medle sauerey wel wit*h* uenygre & þere yn wasshe hy*s* heed of tyme . & so shal he be hoole of þe heue slepe . The uj u*er*tu Euery wo*m*ma*n* þ*a*t ys wit*h* chylde . fle she euer þys herbe . þat she not touche yt . for not only puttyth oute sauerey hyr chylde whether yt be quyk or deed yf she ete sauerey . but also yf sauorey be under put to þe woma*n* þ*a*t ys wit*h* chylde . The uij sauorey stamped wel & dronke yn a lytel wyne or eten wit*h* aneye . wol staunche brakyng . An yn þe same wyse she wol scure to lechery . & wonderly . yf she be dronke largely drye or grene . as leches sayn . Sauerey & tyme ben euene yn myght yn þys . And *f.29r* þerfor þey || co*m*maunde for to take sauorey yn þe stede of tyme . Where þ*a*t ys no tyme . & stampe yt & drynke yt wit*h* wyne hony & peper & þys wol scure unto lechery hugely as yt ys seyden .

SAuge ys cleped yn latyn . Salgia & saluia & yn greke lilifagus . The fyrst u*er*tu sauge dronke wit*h* mulsa doth good to alle þe dysseses of þe mawe . In þe same wyse she wol delyuere a woma*n* of þe chylde þ*a*t ys ded yn her body . And purgyth wo*m*mans floures . & makyt a body to pysse faste . The ij u*er*tu sauge stampyd wit*h* salt & emplastred . curyt uenemous bytynges & staunchyt þe blod of newe wondes . The iij u*er*tu þe Iuys of sauge y dronke wit*h* wyne wol

---

809 Sauge] xix *ext. marg.*

staunche þe olde cowhe & þe ache yn þe syde . The iiij u*er*tu þe wyne þat sauge ys soden ynne wol destroye þe ycche of þe kunte & of a manys yerde yf yt be wasse þer w*ith* . The u u*er*tu þe Iuys of sauge wol make heres blak yf þey be || ofte *f.29v* noynted þer w*ith* yn þe hoot sonne .

HOrsehelne ys cleped . Enula comounly Elena & leches clepen yt Elenum Alme*n* knowe wel þe shappe of þys herbe . ffyrst þys herbe ys moyst yn þe fyrst degre & hoot yn þe secunde degre . The decocc*io*n of þys herbe dronke . purgyth wo*m*mans floures . The ij u*er*tu In þe same wyse she makyth a body to pysse fast . And also she wol delyuer þe chylde þ*a*t ys ded yn þe moders wombe . And also she makyth hym nysshe wo*m*bed þ*a*t ys costyf . The iij u*er*tu þe root of þys herbe stamped & emplastred to þe thye wol hele & destrye þe passyo*u*n & þe ache of þe wyrlebon þe wyche ys seyd Ciat*ica* . The iiij u*er*tu þe leues of þys herbe soden yn pyement & lapped aboute þe reynes wol hele þe ache & þe dyssese of þe reynes . þe wyche ys seyde Nefresis The u u*er*tu þe pouder of þe root of þys herbe eten w*ith* hony . wol destroye þe cowhe . And yn þe same wyse doth || yt helpe & *f.30r* medycyne hem . þ*a*t han þe chynke cowhe . i . Ortho⌞no⌟nicus . Ortononicus ys he þ*a*t drawyth yn as . muche eyre . as he puttyth oute Asmathic*us* ys he þ*a*t putyth out moor of þe eyre þan he resceyueth Disnoicus ys he þ*a*t takyth yn moor þan he puttyth oute . In al þese thre ben knowhers but dyue⌞r⌟sly . as yt ys before seyde . The uj u*er*tu . As so*m*me me*n* sayn & afferme . The Iuys of þys herbe w*ith* þe Iuys of rawe yn euen mesure soden to gydre doth muche good & p*ro*fyt to hem þat ben broke . yf þys decoccyon be y dronken .

---

822 Horsehelne] xx *ext. marg.* **826** floures] menstrua *ext. marg. H3* **832** Ciatica] ciatica *ext. marg. H3* **836** cowhe] for the breste *ext. marg. H3*

YSope ys drye & hoot y*n* þe thrydde degre . The decocc*i*on of ysope w*ith* hony & drye fygges eten or dronke wol helpe hem þ*at* han þe cowe ou*þer* þe pose . The ij u*er*tu þys same decocc*i*on helpyth hem þ*at* are hors or haue dyssese yn þe lunges . The iij u*er*tu þys decocc*i*on destroyt wormes yn þe þe *f.30v* bely . The iiij || u*er*tu If þer be eny dystyllac*i*on or fallyng of þe humours from þe heed to þe brest þe wyche ys wont to gender þe kowhe & þe tysyk . þys same decocc*i*on wol hele yt yf yt be dronke ofte . To all þe dysseses afore seyd . þe poudre of ysope meled or confecte w*ith* hony ys good & medycynable . The u u*er*tu grene ysope stamped & melde w*ith* oxiniel . þ*at* ys to say w*ith* amaner of drynke þ*at* ys made w*ith* uenygre & hony . & þe tweynte partes uenygre . & þe thrydede of hony & y dronke . þys wol make nesshe wombed þ*at* ys costyf . The uj u*er*tu In þe same wyse yt puttyth away þe noyous wynde & uyscouse & glatty fleume . But better doth þys . yf þow take þer to Cardama . The uij u*er*tu A porc*i*on of ysope grene or drye y dronke w*ith* wyne wol make abodyes face wel coloured . The uiij u*er*tu stampe ysope w*ith* drye fygges & w*ith* nitru*m* & þys emplastred wel to þe splene *f.31r* || þ*at* ys ybolle wol hele yt . And also yt ys wo*n*t to destroye þe dropsye yn dryenge . The ix u*er*tu ysope drunke w*ith* wyne relessyth þe entrayles þ*at* ben streyght out ouermuche . And also yt puttyth away amaner swellynge w*ith* yn furth . The x u*er*tu ofte wasshe þe tethe þ*at* akyn yn þe uynegre þ*at* ysope ys soden yn & þ*at* wol do away þe yn moderat ache . The xi u*er*tu thorugh þe smellyng of brent ysope ys destroyed þe sownyng & þe ryugyng yn þe ere . The xij u*er*tu soden ysope & leyde to þe face wol make bryght & clere þe wannesse . The xiij u*er*tu In þe same wyse . yf yt be cast yn atte nesestrelles yt wol hele þe Iaundyse . The xiiij u*er*tu yt ys

---

847 Ysope] xxj *ext. marg.* **849** cowe…pose] for the brest *ext. marg. H3*

seyd þ*at* a co*n*fecc*i*on of soden ysope & oyle of roses to gedre y helde yn atte ere wol hele þe ache of the ere .

Gladen yn englysse ys clepyd Iris yn latyn for hys floures ben lyke to þe reynbowe . She ys clepyd also || *f.31v* Illirica . for as yt ys seyd yn þe cuntre þ*at* me*n* clepen Illirica growith gret plente of þys herbe . Thys herbe ys hoot & drye yn þe secunde degre . but yn þe root of þys herbe ys hys moost u*er*tu . The fyrst u*er*tu of *þys* herbe . take þe rootes of yt & kutte hem to rounde gobettes ryue hem on threde . so þ*at* noon of hem touche other . If þow wolt drye hem . hange hem yn adrye place yn þe shadowe . for elles shalt þow not drye hem unnethe yn an hool yere . Drynke poudre þer of yn wyne & so shalt þow staunche þe cowhe & gete a wel sauored mothe . Thus also {mayst} þow putte away þe attere & þe rotynesse yf eny þere be wi*th* yn lurkyng & hurtyng or greuyng þe entraylles The ij u*er*tu þys pouder drynke wi*th* mulsa . destroyt þe colre Mulsa ys a drynke maad wi*th* hony & of water . The uiij parte water & þe ix hony . The iij u*er*tu melde þys pouder wi*th* uenygre & þ*at* wol stanche || *f.32r* {gry*n*dyng} of þe wombe . And yn þe same wyse as me*n* saye . yt wol do good to þe ueynes . The iiij u*er*tu thes pouder ys medycynable to hem þ*at* han dyssese yn þe splene . & to hem eke þ*at* ben drawe to gedyr or shortes eyther hurte wi*th* colde . yf yt be dronke wi*th* wyne . The u u*er*tu In þe same wyse It wol soune purge wo*m*mens floures þ*at* taryn & come*n* furthe slowly . The uj u*er*tu a decocc*i*on of gladen rotes wol make nesshe þe hardnesse of þe matryce yf she be ofte tymes wasshe wi*th* *þys* decocc*i*on a lytel chafed before And yeue also þe pacyent to drynke þys decocc*i*on luke . The

---

880 Gladen] xxij *ext. marg. H3* **894** colre] purge coler *ext. marg. H3* Mulsa] mulsa mak cu*m* aqua celidon? *bot. marg. H3* **902** floures] menstrua *ext. marg. H3*

---

891 mayst] myast MS. **897**] grydyng MS.

uij u*er*tu me*n* say*n* þ*a*t þys decocc*i*on caste ynne atte erse wi*th* a clyster wol doo muche good to thylke passyo*un* . þ*a*t ys clepyd Scietica . The uiij u*er*tu of gladen rotes & hony *f.32v* {medled} to geder ben made colluryes or medy || cynes þe wyche under put to þe cunte puttyth oute after byrden . The ix u*er*tu In alle holowe places . These colluryes helyth þe syrynges þ*a*t ben styked yn . The x u*er*tu þe pouder of gladen rotes medled wi*th* hony drye up þe wondes & fylle hem up ayen wi*th* good & clene flesshe . yf yt be leyde þer to . And allso þ*a*t wol regendre flesshe uppon þe bon þ*a*t ys maad bare . yf yt be leyde þerto . The xj u*er*tu take too partyes of þe pouder of gladen rootes & þe thryde parte of þe pouder of olebur þat so*m*me me*n* clepe {clof thunge} & medle þuse too poudres to gyder wi*th* hony a plastre of þys purgeyt & clensyt þe face of frekles & resolue þe pockes And þe welkes of þe face .

WYlde malowe ys clepyd holy hocke & yn latyn we cleped hyr Alltea for she waxyth yn to heyght . And so*m*me me*n* *f.33r* clepen hyr Euisca . for hyr root handled semyth || to be moyst as amaner of slyme so*m*me clepen þys þe wyld malowe . The fyrst u*er*tu þe floure of þys herbe soden yn mulsa purgyt wel wondes . yf þow stampe þys floure & drynke yt wi*th* wyne & make þer of aplaster . The ij u*er*tu In þe same wyse yt wol sprede or sparcle a brood ue*n*nes . & helpe þe akynge eres . The iij u*er*tu In þe same wyse as yt ys seyd . yt ys also good for brusynges . The iiij u*er*tu þ*ys* roose soden . & after warde stamped . & medled wel wi*th* swynes grece & terrebe*n*tine. ys seyde to hele swellynges of þe matryce & all other aches & dysseses of hyr . And so eke she

---

923 Wylde malowe] xxiij *ext. marg.* Wylde ... cleped] Wyld malow ys cleped holy hocke & in latyn we d *ext. marg. H2* **925** semyth] xxiij And *bot. marg.* | to be moyst *bot. marg.*

---

910 medled] nedled MS. **919** clof thunge] clofunge MS.

relaxyth þe synowes of þe matryce . The u u*er*tu In þe same wyse yt wol breke & sparcle abrode harde postomes . The uj u*er*tu all þuse causes þe decocc*io*n of þ*ys* herbe wol helpe . yf þe place þ*at* þe greef ys ynne . be oftymes anoynted or bathed þeryn . Whan yt ys chafed & made || *f.33v* mylke warme . The uij u*er*tu þe decocc*ion* of þe root y dronke yn wyne wol staunche the blody menyson . And putte oute hastely þe aft*er*byrden of wo*m*men . The uiij u*er*tu þys same ys good to hem þ*at* speten blod . Thys wol also destroye þe stoon of þe bladdre . The ix u*er*tu stampe þe seed of þys herbe & putte þerto oyly of olyf & þys onyment wol do away þe foule spottes . The x u*er*tu þys herbe wol destroye eny uenym yf she or hyr decocc*ion* be drunke w*ith* mulsa . The xi u*er*tu þys herbe soden & after warde stamped w*ith* hony wol heele holowe wondes & fylle hem w*ith* good flesshe yf yt be ofte y leyde þerto . The xij u*er*tu A plast*er* made of þys leues of þys herbe soden yn oyle wol make nesshe all hardnesse . & a swage all styfnesse . The xiij u*er*tu þe asshen of þys herbe wol hele uenemous bytyn*g*es yf þey be*n* ofte yleyde þ*er*to .

ANyse as leches sayn ys hoot & drye yn þe secunde degre . The fyrst u*er*tu þe floure of annyse soden wel yn || *f.34r* oyle & bounde unto þe heede . wol staunche þe heed ache . The ij u*er*tu þe decocc*io*n of anyse drunke ofte makyth anoryce to haue mylke ynow . And þys same wol destroye þe dysseses of þe stomak He þ*at* ys syke yn hys stomake . shal cake thre Ciates of þys decocc*io*n Whan yt ys mylke warme & drynke hem of And þys wol opene þe stomake ys mouthe as shal wel shewe gret bolkynge & so shal þe noyous wynde passe oute of þe stomak & w*ith* suche a drynke ys staunched þe gret brakynge . Ciatis ys þe haluendele of Emina . & emina ys ys haluendele of a sextarye . The iij u*er*tu þys same drynk wol

---

950 wondes] for the synew*es* *ext. marg. H3* **955** Anyse] xxiiij *ext. marg.*

make abody to pysse faste & destroye þe same thynges þat letten hym to pysse . The iiij u*er*tu þys drynke wol helpe wel þe matryce . & also þe bathe . or wasshynge yn þys decocc*i*on whan yt ys leuke . The u u*er*tu aneys stamped & dronke yn *f.34v* leuke water wol hele þe ache of þe || entrayles & of þe wombe & yt helpyth þe dygesty*ou*n . & yt helpyth a body sone to goo to sege . The uj u*er*tu Aneys drunke ofte noyeth þe syght & sperryth þe way of chylde getynge . & dryeth up þe humours of þe seed w*ith* yn þe body . The uij u*er*tu þe asshes of Anneys wol frete away þe euel flesshe þ*a*t waxyth yn wondes & yt clensyth wel þe bocches þ*a*t crepen from o place to a noþer . And also yt purgyth foule woundes . The uiij u*er*tu yf þe lytel gobet yn þe mouthe þ*a*t ys cleped uua . be greued w*ith* ouer muche humours & to swolle . þe asshes of anneys seed putt yn w*ith* a fynger . or helde yn w*ith* a clyst*er* wol haue yt up ayen . Wel yt ys seyd þ*a*t þe asshes of þe rotes of aneys be moor sharpe yn wyrchynge þan ben þe asshes of þe self herbe . The ix u*er*tu þese asshes wol helle bocches . & specyaly of a man ys yerde yf þey be leyde ofte þer yn . The x *f.35r* u*er*tu anys seed rosted & smellyd || to all hoot ofte . wol reprysse þe yoxe . The xj u*er*tu sethe aneys floures yn oyle & yt wol be medycynable sp*eci*aly to sores þ*a*t come*n* of colde . And yt wol ofte tymes staunche þe heed ache & yt wol relesse þe bolnynges of þe ueynes And yt destroyt þe colde þ*a*t greueth hem . The xij u*er*tu aneys rotes stamped & leyde to wol take away þe feruent hete of a ma*n*neys eyen . The xiij u*er*tu Aneys seed rosted & leyde to þe Emoroydes wol hele hem & dyssolue þe kernel yn þe erse & eke elles where .

BEteyne ys cleped yn greke Castreon . The fyrst u*er*tu Beteyne drunke makyth a body wel for to pysse & puttyth oute þe stone . The ij u*er*tu Beteyne drunke w*ith* wyne wol helpe hem wel þat han þe dropesye The iij u*er*tu aplast*er*

995 Beteyne] xxu *ext. marg.*

made of beteyne leues wel stamped wol hele þe eyen þ*a*t ben hurte thorugh a stroke & lete þys plaster leye styll to þe eye all nyght || The iiij u*er*tu þe beteyne stamped & leyde to yn a *f.35v* plast*er* wyse wol hele þe ache of þe throte & of þe nek . The u u*er*tu þe Iuys of beteyne medled w*ith* oyle of roses & helde yn to þe eres wol hele hem of many dyu*er*se syknesse . The uj u*er*tu þys herbe brosed wel & put yn to þe nostrellys wol staunche þ*a*t rennyth atte nosse . The uij u*er*tu þe pouder of beteyne seed yn hony wol helpe þe syknes þ*a*t leches clepen Empices . It wol staunche þe cowhe & syghynges . And yt wol also helpe þe stomak of many dysseses . The uiij u*er*tu þys pouder drunke wol meue þe wombe . The ix u*er*tu þe leues of beteyne stamped w*ith* salte & þere of maad a plast*er* wol hele all maner of newe wondes . The x u*er*tu þys pouder drunke w*ith* wyne wol destroye þe feuere þ*a*t ys hoot . The xj u*er*tu beteyne allone stamped & emplastred wol hele þe brekyng of þe heed . The xij u*er*tu beteyne leues soden & emplastred wol do muche good to || dyu*er*se sores of þe eyen *f.36r* whether þey be eten or dronke . The xiij u*er*tu In þe same wyse It wol hele addres bytyngges & smytynges . The xiiij u*er*tu Beteyne eten or dronken wol restreyne þe {renny*ng*} of þe eyen . The xu u*er*tu take Beteyne & as muche of rewe & ete or drynke hem & þ*a*t wol put away þe dyrknes of þe eyen . The xuj u*er*tu þe Iuys of beteyne drunke yn leuke water wol put oute þe blood þ*a*t noyeth þe eyen doun by þe eres . þus sayn leches & þus yt makyth þe eyen hool & clene . The xuij u*er*tu þe Iuys of beteyne drunke yn l⌊e⌋uke water wol purge & delyuer þe greuonce uomyte & colre . And w*ith* þe same drynke ben heled þe sores of þe brest . The xuiij u*er*tu þe decocc*io*n of beteyne drunke helpyth bothe þe splene & þe maw . The xix u*er*tu take iiij unces of beteyne & iij Ciates of || olde wyne & xxuij pepyr cornes wel brayde yn *f.36v* a morter . Caste all þuse to gydre & drynke yt ofte & þys wol

---

1019 rennyng] remy*ng* MS.

hele þe reynes of all hys doloures . The xx u*er*tu An unce of beteyne drunke w*ith* tweyne Ciates of chaued water or wyne wol staunche þe ache of þe wombe . The xxj u*er*tu beteyne etyn w*ith* hony wol destroye þe cowhe & laxe þe costyf wombe . The xxij u*er*tu þe Iuys of beteyne y holden longe yn þe mothe staunchyt þe tothe ache . The xxiij u*er*tu ij unces of playntyne w*ith* one unce of beteyne stamped togydyr & dronke yn leuke water or þ*at* þe colde come wol destroye þe quotydyan feuer . The xxiiij u*er*tu An unce of beteyne resolued yn a Ciate of hoot water doth gret p*ro*fyth to hem þ*at* han þe dropesye . yf yt be ofte ydronke . The xxu u*er*tu Beteyne rotes dronkyn yn mulsa purgyth sone þe noyous *f.37r* humer || rus ryght as doth Elebur . The xxuj u*er*tu Plinius comaundyth to take iiij dra*m*mes of beteyne rotes & yeue hym to drynke yn mulsa or yn uyno passo . for þys wol souereynly purge þe flume by a uomyte uinu*m* passu*m* ys þ*at* . þat ys ythurst oute of drye grapes . leyde yn þe so*n*ne for to drye somwhat & storcle as doth hey . The xxuij u*er*tu þe pouder of beteyne leues drunke yn mulsa doth hem good þ*at* ben y broke . And yt wol also reyse up þe moder to hyr place . yf she be fallen doun . The xxuiij u*er*tu Beteyn drunk w*ith* wyne & namely beteyn seed wol destroye all maner uenyms . The xxix u*er*tu who so etyth beteyn fastynge he shal not þ*at* day be dronke . The xxx u*er*tu An unce of beteyn y dronke yn wyne destroyt þe Iaundese . And yn mulsa she dessolueth wo*m*mans floures . The xxxj u*er*tu A *f.37v* been || weyght of þe pouder of beteyn eten w*ith* hony aft*er* soper . helpyth þe stomak gretly to defye . The xxij u*er*tu Plinius seyth . yf þer be made aboute serpentes a sercle of grene beteyn þey dare not goo ouer ne under þe sercle ne passe oute þer of but þere ryght þey shul by p*ro*cesse of tyme byte & bete w*ith* her tayles hemself to deth . The xxxiij u*er*tu

---

1035 cowhe] for the cuw *ext. marg. H3* **1040** quotydyan feuer] cuartiam feuer *ext. marg. H3*

Menacus sayth & comau*n*dyth to put þys herbe yn alle medycynes for þe stomak as þe most co*n*uenyent & p*ro*fytable herbe to þe stomak amonge alle herbes . The xxxiiij u*er*tu Plinius sayth þ*at* hoo so beryt abowte hym þys herbe þere shal noon euel drynke harme hym . The xxxu u*er*tu And he also sayth þ*at* þe same herbe oftentymes drunke w*ith* wyne wol make a body wel colured & destroye þe wa*n*ne & ledyrcolor .

CAule ys clepyd yn greke brassica yt ys a comou*n* herbe . Natheles yt ys a p*ro*fytable herbe & ryght holsom to many causes . Caton sayth uj hundred || *f.38r* yere before þe tyme þ*at* leches wroot eny medycynes or leche crafte att rome þe Romaynes used caules for her medycynes . And so þ*at* tyme þey fette bothe her methe & hyr medycynes yn þe gardeyn of þe caules . The fyrst u*er*tu caule ys colde ⌊&⌋ drye yn þe fyrst degre as þe same caton sayth caule stamped & emplastred wolle hele wondes not oonly newe but also {oolde} . The ij u*er*tu þe same Caton sayth þ*at* caule wol hele cancres but he co*m*maundyth þ*at* þe place be fyrst wasshe w*ith* leuke wyne or wat*er* And to take þe rawe caule & stampe hem & leye yt to hym yche day twyes fresshe . The iij u*er*tu þe same Caton co*m*maundyth to cake barly mele caule & rewe & coryaundre w*ith* ryght alytel salte & stampe all þese to gydre & make of hem a plastre & þan ley yt to þe wycked podagre . The iiij u*er*tu þys same plastre wol do medycyne || *f.38v* to þe sores of þe toon & of þe Ioyntes þe wyche ys clepyd Arthetica . The u u*er*tu þe same plast*er* wol hele þe festre þ*at* ys clepyd Siringa . And þ*at* dyssese also þ*at* ys clepyd luxatura & many other maner sores . The uj u*er*tu þys same Caton sayth þ*at* hys pysse þ*at* etyth of caule ys ryght good & medycynal to þe

---

1072 Caule] xxuj *ext. marg.* **1087** podagre] for the podagre gowt *ext. marg. H3*

1080 oolde] oode MS.

dysseses of þe synowes yf yt be chaued & therw*ith* þe place y wasshe . The uij u*er*tu þ*ys* same Caton also sayth þ*at* þys uryne wol do muche good to chyldryn helys . yf þey ben oft washe þer w*ith* . The uiij u*er*tu Crisippus sayth of þe uertues of þ*ys* herbe . All leches confyrme*n* þ*at* caule clensyth & makyth clene her eyen . þ*at* eten þere of often grene . And yn þe same wyse yt fyllyth þe noryce tetys w*ith* mylke & purgyth wo*m*mens floures . & yt helpyth þe stomak to defye . The ix *f.39r* u*er*tu It is sayde þ*at* caule muche soden & ete || byndyth & makyth costyf . And half ysoden makyth a body laxatyf . The x u*er*tu dyppe caule yn uenygre & etet so all rawe & yt wol represse & a bate þe swellyng of þe splene . The xj u*er*tu þe seed of caule wol delyuere a woma*n* of þe ded chylde yn hyr wombe . The xij u*er*tu take uenygre & olde swynes grece & caules & stampe hem wel . þan sethe all these to gydre & cast þer to oyle of roses as muche as þow seest good Thys decocc*i*on destroyth þe gret heet of þe feuers . yf þow anoynte þerw*ith* þe stomak . & þe other me*m*bres wyche ben hoot . The xiij u*er*tu take hool alym & sharpe uynegre & caules & stampe þuse to gydre & þ*at* þey be wel yncorporat to gydre . w*ith* þ*ys* {oynemen*t*} þow mayst abate þe lepre & oþer many spottes yf þow a noynte þe place þerw*ith* . And þys same o*n*yment wol kepe þe heres þat þey shal not falle away . The *f.39v* xiiij u*er*tu leches sayn || þ*at* þys oyneme*n*t helpyth muche to swollen ballokes . & oþer dyuerse sores þ*at* fallen yn þe genytrall . And better wol þys do þuse cures yf þow take to þe forseyd thynges soden benes . The xu u*er*tu stampe caule w*ith* femygreke & uenygre & leye þu se upon þe toon þat aken & þ*at* wol helpe þe passyo*un* þ*at* ys cleped artetica passyo So shalt þow also helpe muche þe podagre . The xuj u*er*tu þe asshes of caules wel grounde w*ith* olde swynes grece

---

1122 artetica...1123 passyo] arthetica passio gowte *ext. marg. H3*

1114 oynement] ynemen*t* MS.

& emplastred wol helpe hugely þe olde ache . bothe of þe syde & of þe thye . though þys be a foule medycyne natheles yt ys holsom . The xuij u*er*tu þe seed of caules drunke yn uenygre ys wonte to destroye wormes yn þe wombe . The xuiij u*er*tu of drye caule rotes & brent to pouder or asshen . putte yn þat parte of þe mouþe þat ys clepyd uua . wol drye yt up & so rere yf she be bolne . The xix u*er*tu leches sayen þ*a*t yt ys good || to hym þ*a*t hys hoos forto chewe wel caules & *f.40r*
souke yn þe Iuys . The xx u*er*tu þe Iuys of caules helde yn atte nosestrelles purgyth wel þe heed . The xxj u*er*tu to hem þ*a*t ben malencolyke caule wol gendre groos & gret blod . The xxij u*er*tu he þ*a*t ethet caule fyrst at morwe unneþe shal he fele eny drunkenesse all þ*a*t day . The xxiij u*er*tu Mellitus sayth þ*a*t a caule roote þ*a*t neuer touched þe erthe . aft*er* þ*a*t she were pulled up of þe gro*u*nde . honged aboute þe nek shuld kepe & hele þe uua of þe mouþe from all sores þat are wont to falle þeryn .

Oynouns ben ryght good but of hem semeth not leches for to assente ne acorde to gydre for Diascorides sayth þ*a*t þey bollen þe heed & greuen yt & to make hym {thyrsty} þat etyt hem rawe . Galyen sayt þat oynouns be not good to malencolyous folke but to flumatteke folkes he trowyth þ*a*t þey || ben ryght good . Asclepius sayth þ*a*t þey ben good & *f.40v*
namely to þe stomak . The fyrst u*er*tu oynouns ben hoot & moyst yn þe fourthe degre . The ij u*er*tu þys Asclepius sayth þ*a*t oynouns makyt hym fayre coloured þ*a*t lokyth uppon hem . The iij uertu þ*ys* man sayth also he þ*a*t wol euere daye ete a oynouns fyrst he schal lyue longe w*ith* outen eny syknesse . The iiij u*er*tu leches sayn þ*a*t oynouns wol hele houndes byty*n*ges yf þey be leyde þerto . but fyrst þey must be wel grounde w*ith* uenygre & hony . So*m*me oþer men sayn

1142 Oynouns] xxuij *ext. marg.*

1144 thyrsty] syrsty MS.

oynouns wyne & hony & so leye hem to . & so atte thre dayes ende remeue þe plast*er* . The u u*er*tu Diascorides sayth þ*at* oynouns . salte & rewe shal be leyde to serpentes bytynge & so he sayth yt shal be heled . The uj u*er*tu þe Iuys of oynouns wit*h* womans mylke y helde yn atte ere wol destroye þe ache of þe eres . The uij u*er*tu all leches afferme wel þ*at* f.41r oynouns wol yeue sauour to hym þ*at* etyt hem & || þ*at* þey wol holsomlyche make a body laxatyf . The uiij u*er*tu þe Iuys of oynouns meled wit*h* water & y dronke wol helpe hem whom eny sodeyn soor makyth for to be dombe . The ix u*er*tu þe Iuys of oynouns only drawen yn atte nostrelles . doth away þe noyous humour*s* of þe heed . The x u*er*tu oynouns eten or dronke*n* purgen wo*m*mens floures wha*n* þey taryen . The xj u*er*tu þe Iuys of oynouns wol hele þe brekynges of þe feet or of þe soles . þe wyche þe hardenesse of hosen eyther of shone hath made . yf þow wolt medle þer to hennes grece & wit*h* þ*at* anoynte wel þe place . The xij u*er*tu leches sayn he þ*at* eueryday a morwe frotyth & wasshyth wel hys teth wit*h* þe Iuys of oynouns he schal neuere fele þe tothe ache . The xiij u*er*tu oynouns eten wit*h* bred wol a bate þe welkes & þe bocches þ*at* waxen yn þe mothe . The xiiij u*er*tu f.41v soden || oynouns dypped yn oyle & so ete . staunchyt þe bytynges wit*h* ynfurthe & þe gnawyng of þe blody menyson . The xu u*er*tu oynouns seed drunken helpen he*m* wonderly þ*at* han þe tysyk . The xuj u*er*tu wit*h* oynouns y grounden small . þow mayst restore þe heer of þe heed . yf þow wolt ofte anoynte þerewit*h* þe place . were heres ben fallen away . The xuij u*er*tu oynouns destroyen þe stenche & þe heuy or euel sauour of þe mouthe . The xuiij u*er*tu oynouns y gronde small & plastred doth good ayenst þe Emoroydes . The xix u*er*tu þe Iuys of oynouns y meled wit*h* hony clensyth þe eyen & makyth hem bryght yf þey ben ofte wasshen þer wit*h* .

1162 &] þat þey wol *bot. marg.*

The xx u*er*tu oynouns Iuys meled w*ith* uenygre . ys wont to amende þe spotte*s* of frakles yf þey be wel anoynted þ*er* w*ith* .

AMonge þe herbes þat pictagoras presyd as yt ys sayd . he yaf þ*e* || fyrst & gretyst preysynge unto Synueye Synuey ys bothe *f.42r* hoot & drye yn þe fyrst degre . The fyrst u*er*tu synuey drawyth oute & thynnyth þe uyscouse humours & brennyth þe skyn . so gret ys hys myght . but yn þe seed ys moor uertu þan yn self herbe . The ij u*er*tu synuey seed eten sharpyth þe wytte & scuryth þe wombe . It brekyth þe ston . & makyth þe to pysse & yt purgyth wo*m*mens floures . The iij u*er*tu þe seed grounden smal . & w*ith* leuke water holde & rolled aboute þe palat of þe mothe ayenst þe soune wol clense þe noyous flume of þe heed . The iiij u*er*tu It ys good to ete or drynke þe seed yn fnesynge . for with yt ys resolued yche stryghtnesse of þe heed Thys eten co*m*fortyth þe stomak & stau*n*chyt syghynges . The u u*er*tu þys seed grounden smal w*ith* uenygre & leyde || upon þe addres bytynge wol hele yt . *f.42v* The uj u*er*tu þys seed eten destroyth þe uenym of padstoles & kepyt þ*a*t þe uenym shal not greue þe entrales . The uij u*er*tu It ys sayd afore þ*a*t senuey . & hyr seed bothe for þe gret hete þ*a*t ys yn hem wol brenne & brest þe skyn But w*ith* oute eny doute . seche an adustyoun ys rygth noteful yn many causes for þorfe suche adustyon be draw oute noyous humours of þe heed & dryed up And also þe humoure þ*a*t fallyt fro þe heed to þe lunges & hurtyth hem . The uiij u*er*tu þys adustyoun wol destroy many sykenesse of þe stomak & þe kowhe & þe tysyk . The ix u*er*tu þys adustyoun wol drawe oute þe olde ache & dessese of þe thye by a bladder þe wyche greef ys clepyd yn greke Siasis . The x u*er*tu þys adustyo*un* wol also dryue away þe harde bolnyng of þe splene & of þe mawe & to many oþer olde || causes . ys þys *f.43r*

1190 Amonge] xxuiij *ext. marg.* **1197** floures] menstrua *ext. marg. H3* **1213** stomak] for the stomacke *ext. marg. H3*

adustyo*u*n good & p*ro*fytable . syth þat aplast*er* of þys herbe or of þys seed ys þus p*ro*fytabyle . for by cause leches maken þys plast*er* dyu*er*sely . I wol say shortly how þ*at* mene leches comau*n*dyth for to make yt Take senuey seed & stampe yt wel yn a morter . take þer to iij parte of cromes of wythe bred & cast þer to drye fygges . hony & uenygre . after þ*at* þe age askyth þe quantyte of þe soor suffycyth . for þe moor þ*at* þow castyth yn of drye fygges & hony þe sharper ys þe synuey . but þe moor bred þow castyst yn & uenygre þe moor feble & weker ys þys plaster I counseyle þe þ*at* þow sette not a lytel by þys co*n*fecc*io*n . for y haue preued yt ful notable yn many causes but natheles I wol not þ*at* þow laye yt to many sores but late & selde to gret & olde sores . The xj u*er*tu {Plinius} *f.43v* comau*n*dyt for to take & ley senuey seed w*ith* || senuey rotes yn must & lete hem lye & soke styl . for as he sayth þ*at* wyne ys full p*ro*fytable . & holsom to many sores . after þ*at* yt haue drawe oute þe strengthe of þe seed . þ*at* ys to say . bothe to þe chekys & to þe stomak & to þe ⌞e⌟yen & to many dyuerse dysseses of þe heed . The xij u*er*tu So*m*me maken oyle of þys seed þ*at* ys fyrst steped & þ*ys* oyle ys medycynall to þe lendes & to þe synowes þ*at* ben astonyed . The xiij u*er*tu þe Iuys of senueys tendre stalke wol destroye þe tothe ache yf yt be rolled wel yn þe mouthe & ofte y swolewed ynne . The xiiij u*er*tu synuey seed eten wol helpe þe uoyce & amende yt . for yt wol make {lygthe} & souple þe ueynys þ*at* þe uoyce ys gendryd by . The xu u*er*tu þys seed stamped & medled w*ith* olde swynes grece & emplastred wol destroye wennes & *f.44r* dyssolue hem . The xuj u*er*tu It || ys sayd þ*at* senuey seed also ys good & helpyng to hem þ*at* han þe fallyng euel . The xuij u*er*tu þys also wol drye þe matryce & so helpe many causes of hyr dyssese . The xuiij u*er*tu It ys a gret medycyne

---

1222 seed] No*ta* hi[c] *ext. marg.* **1224** hony] cietica *ext. marg. H3*

1231 Plinius] Pliuius MS. **1243** lygthe] lythe MS.

for to take & stampe þys seed w*ith* drye fygges & so to leye yt to hys heed þ*at* ys lytargicus . þ*at* ys to say Whan hys hedys newe shaue . or stampe & grynde þys seed w*ith* hony . or swynes grece & noy*n*te þe feet of þe lytarge . The xix u*er*tu In þe same wyse ys þys seed helpyng to destroye Allopiciam yf yt be ofte anoynted yn de grynde Allopes yn greke ys seyde uulpes yn latyn þ*at* ys a foxe yn englysshe & þer of ys seyd Allopicia a maner of lepre þe wyche makyt men to lese þe heer of her heed & of her browes . The xx u*er*tu þys seed stamped w*ith* uynegre & anoynted woll destroye certeyn lepres . The xxj u*er*tu þys seed eten a fore ⌞þe⌟ axses || *f.44v* co*m*me*n*ly wol cure & hele þe accesse . or feuere þ*at* ys clepyd {p*er*yodica} febrys þat ys the quotydyan .

Whyte pepyr or whyte synuey ys clepyd yn latyn Eruca þ*at* ys hote & drye yn þe myddel degre . but she ys not so drye as she ys hote . The fyrst u*er*tu þys herbe eten helpyth for to defye . The ij u*er*tu þys herbe eten & drunke wol make þe eter wel for to pysse . The iij u*er*tu þys herbe eten wol destroye þe chyldryns kowhe . The iiij u*er*tu þys herbe grounden small w*ith* hony & bounden to wol clense þe sken of spottes & þe face of frakles . The u u*er*tu þe root of þys herbe fyrst sode & afterwarde grounde small & þan emplastred to þe place wol hele þe boon breche . The uj u*er*tu þe seed of þys herbe grounden & drunke w*ith* wyne wol hele alle deedly strokes . The uij u*er*tu þys herbe grounde small w*ith* oxe galle & anoynted upon þe place ory plastred wol destroye þe blake spottes . The uiij u*er*tu þys herbe grunde || *f.45r* small & drunke w*ith* wyne & a gret qua*n*tyte wol harde þe felynge ayenst betyng as men sayen . The ix u*er*tu þys herbe or hyr seed putten yn metes makyth hem wel sauoured . And þe Grekes clepen þys herbe Euȝimu*m* . for þy

---

1263 Whyte pepyr] xxix *ext. marg.*

1262 peryodica] pyodica MS.

þ*at* hys Iuys ys good & sauoured . The x u*er*tu þys seed eten or drunke scuryth gretly to lechyry . as leches conferme & also many poetes . The xj u*er*tu þys herbe ys ryght holsom for ete wit*h* letuse for hyr heete makyth a tempernesse to {letuse} colde .

KErso*u*n ys sayde {Saturi*u*m} & eke a noþer name Cardamomum þys herbe ys hoot & drye yn þe meddel of þe thrydde degre . The fyrst u*er*tu of þys herbe yf yt be often ete yt woll destroye lecherye dryeng up þe seed of þe eter And so wol also rewe . The ij u*er*tu þys herbe grounden small & medled wel wit*h* wyth soure dowe wol destroye a felou*n* yf *f.45v* þys be wel || plastred to þe place . And þys same medycyn wol hele thylke sore þat ys cleped furniculus . for þys plastre wol make yt for to rote & to quytre & so passyth away þe ache & þe gref of yt . The iij u*er*tu þys same plast*er* wol do away wertes . The iiij u*er*tu wasshe þyn heed wit*h* þe Iuys of þys herbe & þyn heere shal not fall as yt ys seyd . The u u*er*tu helde þe Iuys yn to þe eere of þ*at* syde þ*at* þe tothe akyth & yt wol staunche þe totheache . But þe seed of þ*ys* herbe ys more myghty þan þe herbe . The uj u*er*tu þys seed drunk wit*h* wyne wol delyuere a wo*m*ma*n* of hyr chylde . yf yt be deed yn hyr wombe And yt sleeth wormes of þe wombe And þe same wyse as men sayn yt wol destroye all ueny*m*ys ffor as yt ys sayd þe self odour of þys herbe or seed cast ynto coles dryuyt away serpentes . The uij u*er*tu þys seed drunken ofte ⌊yn⌋ uynegre wol represse þe splene . The uiij u*er*tu þys seed *f.46r* drunke || ofte wit*h* uynegre & þan plastred . wol hele sc⌊i⌋atica pasio . as leches sayn þys medycyn ys {ryght} good & p*ro*fytable . The ix u*er*tu þe Iuys of þys herbe anoynted

---

1286 Kersoun] xxx *ext. marg.* **1291** feloun] for the felon *ext. marg. H3* **1296** wertes] for w*erte*s *ext. marg. H3*

1285 letuse] leuse MS. **1286** Saturium] Naturi*u*m MS. **1308** ryght] rytgh MS.

w*ith* hony wol hele þe mesels . The x u*er*tu yf þyn heed ycche . or be ful of bocches take kersen & medle hem w*ith* gose grece & þer w*ith* a noynte ofte þyn heed & so shal þow destroye eyþer of hem . The xj u*er*tu þys herbe or hyr seed soden yn fresse gotes mylke & y dronke leuke wol destroye þe ache & greef of þe brest . The xij u*er*tu kerso*un* seed gronden small a dragme weyght . & dro*n*ke w*ith* leuke water . wol make þe nesshe wombe as many men yt sayn . Thys seed eten w*ith* hony wol staunche þe cowe & do muche good to þe streytnes ¶ of þe brest .

POpye ys colde & drye & as yt ys seyde þer ben iij maneres of yt ffor þe floure of one ys wythe . of a noþer yt ys reed as ys þe || roos & of þe iij somdele redde & pale And þys ys of *f.46v* lasse shappe þan ben þe toþyr Thys ys cleped comou*n*ly whyte popye but he ys best whos floure ys whyte Of þe tender bolles of þys men maken opium þus . They kutten a lytel þe utmyst sken of þe popyes bolle & þe mylke þat comet oute þere of þey take & reserue yt drye . And þys opium ys good for many syknesse or medycynes So*m*me taken þe selfe bolles as þey growen w*ith* her mylke þey grynden hem & thursten oute of hem þe lecour & drye yt at so*n*ne . Thys ys not so myghty as ys þe fyrst . The fyrst ys sayd opium & þe secunde ys Capitellum . The iij whyte floure of popy þ*at* beryth floures of þys coloure . men maken oyle of þe seed whan yt ys stamped & grou*n*de small . Thys oyle ys good yn tast & wol make a body to slepe fast . The iij maner of popy þ*at* is to say þ*at* beryth || þe wythe floure & blak seed . wol *f.47r* yeue good sauore yf she be dronke . as þe toþ*er* tweyn . The fyrst u*er*tu þe decocc*i*on of yche of þuse drunke leuke wol yeue to þe syke an esy slepe but yf he shal dye sone . And so yt wol do yf þe syke bodyes face be wel wasse þer w*ith* . The ij u*er*tu þe blak seed drunke w*ith* wyne wol make a body

---

1320 Popye] xxxj *ext. marg.*

costyf as yt ys seyde . The iij u*er*tu In þe same wyse she wol staunche þe fluxe of þe matryce . The iiij u*er*tu þys seed y dronke makyth a body to slepe . And yt staunchyt þe wycked kowhe . But loke wel þ*at* þow neyþer ete ne drynke neu*er* attones a peny weght of þe seedes at most . ffor why who so takyt of hem moor . he shal of tyme take þer of hys dethe or at lest fal yn to a lytargie . The u u*er*tu a plaster of popy leues wol abate þe bolny*n*ge of þe chekes . The uj u*er*tu þ*ys* plastre *f.47v* wol destroye þe sykenesse þ*at* ys || clepyd þe holy fyre & yn latin sacer ignis The uij u*er*tu yf þe ueyne þ*at* þe uoyce {comyth} oute by . be sharpe . or harre eyther by colde or by syngynge or by etyng . or drynkyng or by eny mete . leye þys medycy*n* þer to & yt wol make þe ueyn softe & lyght . The uiij u*er*tu It ys seyde þat grekes clepen all maner popye miconiu*m* þe whyte popye ys nobler & moor p*ro*fytable þan þe toþer twyne . Whan þe bolles of þys popy ben ful of mylke gadre hym sethe hem yn two partes of water & þe iij of hony tyll all þuse be so thycke as yt were fyne hony And kepe wel þys decocc*io*n for yt ys ryght good to many causes . Thys decocc*io*n eten or drunken ⌞makyth⌟ þe for to slepe . The ix u*er*tu þys decocc*io*n wol yn þe same wyse destroye þe cowhe & make a body costyf & purge þe rewmes þ*at* fallen doun fro þe heed & of þe uocale ueyne . The x u*er*tu as I haue seyd to *f.48r* fore The opiu*m* made of þe tendre bolles of þys || whyte popy . þow shalt take yt & medle yt w*ith* oyle of Roses & þer w*ith* anoynte þyn heed þys oynement wol staunche all þe ache of þe heed & make þe to slepe esely . The xj u*er*tu þow shalt cast þe safrom {chyres} þ*at* smellen swete yn to þys oynement helde yn atte ere & þ*at* wol staunche þe ache of þe ere . The xij u*er*tu grynde wel þys oynement w*ith* wo*m*mans mylke & safron & thus þan ofte anoynted wol hele þe hoot podagre .

1372 podagre] podagre *ext. marg. H3*

1352 comyth] cornyth MS. **1369** chyres] chyses MS.

The xiij u*er*tu ley þys oynement under þyn erse & yt wol make þe to slepe . And as yt ys trowed yt wol do þe same by hys sauor oonly .

COriaundre ys colde ypocras sayt þat coryandre ys hoot for yt ys bytter yn tast Galion sayth þ*at* coryau*n*dre hath somdele a sterne & styffe u*er*tu for yt wol sle þe wormes of þe wombe & þe trenches yf she be dronke w*ith* wyne or uenygre medled þere a || mo*u*nke . The u*er*tu Coryaundre co*n*fecte w*ith* *f.48v* resouns & hony & emplasterd wol a bate dyuerse swellynges & namely of þe ballockes . The iij u*er*tu coryaundre seed drunke ofte w*ith* water wol staunche þe fluxe & make hym costyf þ*at* ys laxe . The iiij u*er*tu take Ceruse & þe froth of seluer caste hem to gyder & grynde hem smal . þan cast to þuse þe Iuys of coryaundre & uenygre to þuse foure medle þe oyle of roses & grynde to gydre all þuse . Thys precyouse oynement wol destroye þe holy fyre & put away þe hoot bolny*n*ges . And yf þys confecc*i*on semyth þe to heue costlewe . The self Iuys of coryaundre medle w*ith* fyne uenygre ys good to þys malady . The u u*er*tu þe Iuys of coryaundre medled w*ith* cromes of whyte bred of clene whete . staunchyt all maner of hetes þ*at* ben ouer muche . The uj u*er*tu þys Iuys medled w*ith* ben mele & emplastred wol destroye wennes . or || kerneles & þe feruent whelkes . *f.49r* The uij u*er*tu many men han wrete þ*at* þe cornes of coryawndre seed eten before þe accesse or tremlynge of þe feuer wol destroye þe tercyam . And þe same wol þys seed do yf be gadred atte morwe be fore þe so*n*n rysynge & leyde under þe pacyentys heed . The uiij u*er*tu Zenocates seyde þat a wommans floures shulde sayle hyr as many dayes as she ete Coryaundre seed cornes . The ix u*er*tu so*m*me me*n* co*n*dempne*n* þe co*n*tynuall & custumable etynge of Coryau*n*dre . ffor þey holde þ*at* whoso etyth yt costumably he

---

1376 Coriaundre] xxxij *ext. marg.* **1395** or] kerneles *bot. marg.*

shal take hys deth þer by or som oþer gret meschyf . or syknesse . The x u*er*tu who so dare not ete pyper for hys heete yn sauce caste he to yt coryaundre . for yt ys colde & wol alay þe gret hete & uyolence of þe pyper .

ARage ys cold yn þe fyrst degre & moyst yn þe secunde . The fyrst u*er*tu Arage eten wol make þe laxe . The ij u*er*tu aplastre of arage soden or rawe || *f.49v* wol solue dyuerse hardenesse & also drawe oute nayles . The iij u*er*tu þys emplastre wol drawe away sone þe nayles or spere of þe flye þ*at* ys cleped scrabro And yt destroyth also þe holy fyre The iiij u*er*tu arage y grounde small wi*th* nytrum . hony & uenygre wol abate þe podagre . The u u*er*tu arage seed as Galien sayth y dronke ofte wi*th* wyne wol destroye the Iaundyse .

MYnte ys hoote & drye yn þe secunde degre . The fyrst u*er*tu mynte y drunke helpyth þe dygesty*ou*n . comfortyth þe stomake & staunchyth þe uomyte & sleeth wormes yn þe bely . The ij u*er*tu wasse þy ballokes yn þe water þ*at* mynte was soden yn & þ*at* wol hele many dyuerse syknes & greuans of hym . The iij u*er*tu mynte Iuys maad leuke . & drunke wol wonderly claryfye þe uoyce . The iiij u*er*tu mynte sta*m*ped & leyde to þe tete . makyth yt ful of mylke . The u u*er*tu helde yn || *f.50r* atte ere þe Iuys of mynte wi*th* hony . so shalt þow abate þe ache of þe ere . The uj u*er*tu frote ofte þy tung wi*th* mynte & þ*at* wol hele þe rownesse of þe tung . The uij u*er*tu Mynte Iuys drunke wi*th* sapa wol delyuer sone a woman & allaye hyr throwes . Sapa ys wyte & small wyne . or þe wyne medled wi*th* þe Iuys of som herbe . The uiij u*er*tu Mynte stamped wi*th* salte & leyde upon wol hele þe bytyng of an hounde . The ix u*er*tu þe Iuys of myntes medled wi*th* uenygre . helpyt hem þ*at* speten or spewen blode . The x

---

1409 Arage] xxxiij *ext. marg.* **1419** Mynte] xxxiiij *ext. marg.*
1421 stomake] for the stomack *ext. marg. H3*

u*er*tu My*n*te Iuys putte under þe matryce a fore þe kunte makyth þ*a*t þe woman shal not co*n*ceyue atte þ*a*t tyme . The xj u*er*tu Myntes Iuys dryeth bocches . The xij u*er*tu Myntes stamped & leyde to wol hele þe wondes of þe heed . The xiij u*er*tu Mynte Iuys medled wi*th* þe {rennynges} . wol not suffre chese for to roote þ*a*t ys made wi*th* tho rennynges . Leye grene mynte aboue þe chese & þ*a*t wol do þe same . ||

SKyrwyt hath no u*er*tu but yn hys seed only & yn hys root . *f.50v* The fyrst u*er*tu a decocc*i*on of þuse rotes yn mulsa wol hele þe greuaunce of þe splene & of þe mawe & þe ache of þe lendes . yf she be dronke . The ij u*er*tu þe rotes soden yn mylke & drunke . wol hele þe chynke though she be olde & also staunche þe fluxe . The iij u*er*tu þys rote as so*m*me me*n* sayn hanged a boute þe nek . wol abate þe swallyng of þe ballokes . The iiij u*er*tu þys rote as so*m*me me*n* sayn he þ*a*t beryt aboute hym skyrwyt or etyth yt no serpent shal mowe hurte hym The u u*er*tu who so etyth muche skyrwyt yt wol scure hyn to lechery . The uj u*er*tu scrape þy tethe aboute wi*th* þys root & yt wol destroye þe gret to the ache . The uij u*er*tu þe seed of þys herbe dronke wi*th* wyne wol abate þe swellynge of womans wombe thorugh þe wyche she semyth of þ*a*t she ys wi*th* chylde & yt ys nat so . The uiij u*er*tu || þys *f.51r* seed grounden smal wi*th* hony & leyde to cancres . yt helyt hem . The ix u*er*tu þys herbe ys clepyd pastinaca . for þy þ*a*t she ys good to ete þ*a*t ys to say hyr rootes . for þere ys no root bett*er* for to ete þan ys þe skyrwyt root .

CErfoyle ys ryght hoot & sharpe The fyrst u*er*tu cerfoyle ground wi*th* hony & leyde unto cancres helpyth hem . The ij

---

1443 Skyrwyt] xxxu *ext. marg.* **1452** The ... uertu] to restore *ext. marg. H3* **1453** tethe] for the tothe *ext. marg. H3* **1462** Cerfoyle] xxxuj *ext. marg.*

1440 rennynges] renmynges MS.

u*er*tu cerfoyle drunke w*ith* wyne wol hele þe ache of þe syde . The iij u*er*tu cerfoyle dronke w*ith* mulsa wol destroye þe pyppe . The iiij u*er*tu Also w*ith* þe oyle þat cerfoyle ys soden ynne anoy*n*te þe body & yt puttyt away þe colde . The u u*er*tu solue also cerfoyle w*ith* uyolet & uenygre & þys drynke wol sle þe wormes of þe bely & þe tre*n*ches . The uj u*er*tu Also cerfoyle drunke w*ith* wyne wol make a body for to pysse & yt purgyth wo*m*mens floures . The uij u*er*tu aplastre of olde cerfoyle & of olde swynes grece & of uyrgyne waxe to gydre wol hele || *f.51v* and represse not oonly þe parodycas knobbes þ*a*t waxen yn þe feuers but also all maner swellynges yf yt be ofte yleyde un to þe place . The uiij u*er*tu {Cerfoyle} eten w*ith* fyne uynegre wol staunche þe fluxe & staunche also þe spuynge . The ix u*er*tu ley uppon þe share powned cerfoyle & drynke & þe Iuys of cerfoyle & wol opene al þe ueynes of þe uryn yf þey be sperred . The x u*er*tu who so hath þe syknesse þ*a*t ys clepyd uertylago sethe þys herbe & bynde yt to hys temples & to hys front But fyrst wasshe hys hed yn þe water þ*a*t þys cerfoyle ys soden ynne þus shal he destroye that sykenes .

THe docke ys clepyd paradilla & lappaciu*m* yn latyn bothe . There ben foure manerys of dockes & þeye all ben al most of euen u*er*tu yn medycynes Al þuse dockes ben feruent & hoot & styf & storne yn u*er*tu . The fyrst u*er*tu docke Iuys I drunke co*m*for || *f.52r* tyth þe stomak & puttet oute bollyng wynde þ*a*t ys closed yn þe stomak . The ij u*er*tu dockes eten as wortes byndyth þe wombe . The iij u*er*tu þe water þ*a*t docke ys soden ynne wol destroye þe huge & bytynge ycche & þe scabbe eke þ*a*t brekyth þe skyn by ofte bathynges &

1467 colde] for the feuer of colde *ext. marg. H3* **1470** to pysse] for the uryn *ext. marg. H3* **1484** docke] xxxuij *ext. marg.* **1492** scabbe] for the scabe *ext. marg. H3*

1475 Cerfoyle] Cherfoyle MS.

wasshynges . The iiij u*er*tu þe rootes of hem soden yn wyne & leyde to þe place wol abate þe kernels & þe knobbes þ*at* rysen oft tyme yn feuers . The u u*er*tu þe decocc*i*on of dockes rolled aboute yn þe mouthe wol destroye þe toþe ache & hele also þe uua . yf she be swolle . The uj u*er*tu þe rootes of dockes hanged aboute þe necke wol suffre no kernel . ne feuer knobbe for to ryse ne waxe yn þe body The uij u*er*tu þys decocc*i*on dronke . ys good for hem þ*at* han þe blody {menyson} . or dessese yn þe thyes . The uiij u*er*tu þ*ys* decocc*i*on leuke laued yn to þe ere wol destroye þe ache of þe ere . The ix u*er*tu || docke rootes soden yn strong uynegre & *f.52v* þan stamped & after warde leyde unto þe splene wol represse þe swellyng of yt though yt be ryght gret & þys wol drye up þe humours þ*at* noyen þe splene . The x u*er*tu þe wyne or wat*er* þ*at* þ*ys* rootes be soiden ynne & drunke wol staunche woma*ns* floures . & put outte þe stoon . And þys also puttyth away þe Iaundyse .

KOckull ys clepyd yn greke lollyu*m* & yn latyn Nigella . The fyrst u*er*tu kockul grunde w*ith* Raphanus þ*at* ys w*ith* nepes & a lytel salte & þere of made a plastre to þe cancres wol clense hem & cure fretyng & etyng wondes And eke þ*at* maner of lepre þ*at* ys clepyt ȝerna . Thys lepre ys lyke þe scabbe þ*at* ys cleped Serpigo . It helyth also oþer lepres . The ij u*er*tu kockull brymsto*un* coluer dyrte & lylye seed all þuse grunden to gydres w*ith* wyne a plast*er* þere of wol hele þe forseyd syknesse & so wol a oynement made of || þe same . The iij *f.53r* u*er*tu þys same wol yn þe self wyse . sprede a broode kernelles & breke postomes & bocches & also yt wol make nesshe other hardnesse . The iiij u*er*tu aplaster of kockul seed yn mulsa & grunden smal w*ith* encense & safero*un* wol hele

---

1510 Kockull] xxxiij *ext. marg.*

1501 menyson] nenyson MS.

scyetica passio . The u u*er*tu A subfumygac*io*n of kockul wol do a woma*n* sone for to be delyuerd & a lysse hyr throwes .

HEmlok ys yn kynde colde & dedly The fyrst u*er*tu hemlok sleeth hem þ*a*t drynken yt yn amaner of a colde uenym And who so euer be uenemed wi*th* he*m* lok . hys skyn ys sp˻o˼tty wherfor by þys sygne . me may preue þ*a*t maner of uenym thorgh þe wyche a body dyeth . Thys drenke sumtyme was como*un* & open peyne to dampned me*n* atte Athene The greke Socrates was don unto ˻þe˼ deth wi*th* þys uenemous drynke of hemlok . But how þys poyson shuld be made . yt fallyth not us for to telle for þy þat no þynge shold be tolde *f.53v* here oute || neþer y taught . þe wyche myght noye but only thylke þ*a*t shal helpe & p*ro*fyte to ma*n* . If eny man be poysened þerwi*th* Drynke he stronge wyne chaufed & he shal a scape þe perell . But though þys herbe be perelouse for to drynke yyt she ys wonderly good to plastres & dyuerse medycynes . The ij u*er*tu a noynte þe soor eyen wi*th* þe Iuys of hemlok all aboute & so shalt þow do away þe feruours of heete . Or scrape hemlok leues grene & leye hem yn þe frount or face . & þey wol do þe same . The iij u*er*tu þys same cure wol hele þe holy fyre & thylke soor þ*a*t ys clepyd herpeta . The iiij u*er*tu Amasilaus sayth þat yf a mayde a noynte her tetes wi*th* hemlok Iuys fyrst whan þey begynne to waxe grete & bollne þey shuld after warde stonde styl small . The u u*er*tu þe hemlok grene stamped & bounde to þe tetes dryeth up þe mylke . The uj u*er*tu a plastre of hemlok leyde ofte to þe share quenchyth lecherye & al þe fluxe of þe || *f.54r* seed . The uij u*er*tu a plaster of hemlok medled wi*th* þe froth of {seluer} & swynes grece ys ryght holsom for þe hoot podagre . And þe self herbe by hyr self ys ryght good to þys

---

1523 scyetica] cietica *ext. marg. H3* **1525** Hemlok] <u>xxxix</u> *ext. marg.* **1552** podagre] for podagre *ext. marg. H3*

1551 seluer] seluel MS.

dyssese . The uiij u*er*tu wherto shal I reherse yche by yt self . The hemlok grounden & small broke & leyde to ys ryght good unto euery noyous heete .

PUlyoll or <u>Brother worte</u> ys hoot & drye yn þe thrydde degre as leches sayn . The fyrst u*er*tu yf þe woma*n* þ*at* ys w*ith* chylde drynke of þ*ys* herbe she shal awarpe hyr chylde . But natheles þys grounde smal & drunke yn mulsa wol putte outte a werplyng*e* of þe wombe . The ij u*er*tu pulyoll drunke w*ith* leuke wyne wol brynge oute womans floures And þe same wyse delyuere woma*n* of hyr after byrdon . The after byrdou*n* yn wom*m*an yn latyn ys cleped Secunda or Secundyna but for þys name ys unknowen to many folkes as y trowe þerfore I wol declare here & || expowne what yt ys . As *f.54v* a cheke þ*at* ys not yyt comefourthe hath þe yee shelle goynge aboute hym . Ryght so a chylde yn hys moders wombe ys couered aboute w*ith* a thynne skyn þ*at* ys made of þe moders seed . þe wyche skyn þe chyld brekyth co*m*mounly yn hys byrthe as þe chyke brekyth þe shelle whan yt comyth fourthe . The skyn ys called by leches Secundina . or secu*n*da . for þy þ*at* anoon after þe chelde ys oute of hys moders wombe . þys skyn cometh after by ryght of kynde . And yf þ*at* skyn tarye behynde yn þe moders wombe after þe chyld lender þan yt shulde . eyþer deth folewyth þan anoon . or elles som oþer gret sykenesse . The iij u*er*tu pulyoll grounden small w*ith* salt & hony & mad an oyeneme*n*t . wol helpe þe lymes þ*at* ben draw to gedre & shorted . yf þey be ofte a noynted þer w*ith* . The iiij u*er*tu þe pouder of pulyoll eten w*ith* hony or y dronke wol dys || solue or make þynne þe *f.55r* uyscouse humor*es* & caste hem oute by spettynges . The u u*er*tu pulyoll etyn fastyng or stamped & ydronke afterwarde wol hele all doloure of þe hert & of þe breste . The uj u*er*tu pullyoll eten or dronken w*ith* pusca or uenegre þ*at* be watery

---

1556 Pulyoll] <u>xl</u> *ext. marg.* **1561** floures] menstrua *ext. marg. H3*

wol cure & staunche þe keruyng & þe gnawyng of þe stomak . The uij u*er*tu pulyoll drunke w*ith* wyne wol destroye þe blak colre And yn þe same wyse . yt w*ith* stonde wol þe uenemous bytynges of addres . The uiij u*er*tu If aman þ*at* be syke . defayle by uyolence of þe feure or eny oþer sodeyn caas þe wyche aray ys wont amonge leches to be cleped malefaccio . Pullyol y grounde small & cast yn stronge uynegre & þan y putte to þe syke bodyes nose wol releue a syke body thorugh hys sauoure allone . The ix u*er*tu þe pouder of drye pulyoll or þe asshen of pulyoll wol co*n*ferme *f.55v* & fastne þe gomes of þe tethe . || The x u*er*tu grene pulyoll stamped & leyde to þe place wol staunche þe podagre & yt ys wonte to amende other bolnynges yf she be medled w*ith* floure & leyde to leuke . The xj u*er*tu pulyoll medled w*ith* acerote . wol putte oute þe pockes of þe body . The xij u*er*tu pulyoll leyde to þe splene w*ith* salte wol releue þe deednesse or þe dyssese of yt & do yt muche good . The xiij u*er*tu yf þe wombe . or nauel ake w*ith* ynfourthe bynde unto yt pullyoll & þ*at* woll hele yt . The xiiij u*er*tu pulyoll bounde to þe heed all aboute wol putte away þe heed ache . The xu u*er*tu þe decocc*io*n of pulyoll used ofte leuke wol destroye þe ycche yn þe body And yn þe same wyse It wol abate þe swellyng of þe matryce . The xuj u*er*tu pulyoll drunke w*ith* leuke wyne wol stau*n*che þe kowhe & yt wol make abody wel to pysse But better yf yt be soden yn þe same wyne & þan y drunke . The same yt wol do yf yt be grounde smal & medled w*ith* oyle & *f.56r* þer of mad a plast*er* . The xuij u*er*tu || pulyoll w*ith* wyne wol helpe to destroye þe stone . The xuiij u*er*tu pulyoll rotes grounden & medled w*ith* stronge uynegre wol staunche by a plastre all bolnynges of þe syde . The xix u*er*tu pulyoll drunke w*ith* wyne wol destroye addres uenym . And þe same wyse taken . yt wol scure to lechere as leches sayn . The xx u*er*tu In þe same wyse yt doth good to þe dyssese of þe lunges

---

1594 pulyoll[2]] wol *exp.*

& of þe mawe . And yeueth þe norce mylke y now . The xxj u*er*tu þe grene herbe w*ith* hony curyth houndys bytyng yf she be drunke w*ith* wyne & leeyde to yn plast*er* . The xxij u*er*tu þe serpentes eten pulyoll & so ameden þey her syght whefor yt ys preued here by þ*a*t yt wol do good to mannys eyen & also by exp*er*yence yt ys preuyd The xxiij u*er*tu take þe Iuys of pulyoll rootes . & medle yt w*ith* fresse galle & caste þer to pyp*er* & grynde hem small to gydre Thys oynement ys good for ache || yn þe lendes of þe reynes & also þe thyes . *f.56v*

PErsely ys cleped Serpillum yn latyn for þy þ*a*t as who sayth yt crepyth forthe ney by þe erthe . persely ys hoot & drye . The fyrst u*er*tu Grynde p*er*sely yn uenygre & oyle of roses & w*ith* þys oynemen*t* anoynte þe frounte of þe heed þ*a*t akyth Thys wol destroye þe heed ache . The ij u*er*tu þe smoke of p*er*sely dryuyth away serpentes & al oþer bestes þ*a*t cast uenym oute atte her mouthe And þerfor yt ys þe maner of kepemen to mele p*er*sely yn þe metes for to kepe away uenemous bestes specyly whan þey ben aslepe . The iij u*er*tu p*er*sely drunke helyth deedly bytynges . yf yt be all so leyde to yn plastre . The iiij u*er*tu p*er*sely p*ro*uokyth uryn & a swagyth þe fretynge of þe bely . The u u*er*tu p*er*sely dronke w*ith* uynegre wol helpe þe splene . The uj u*er*tu p*er*sely drunke w*ith* uenygre & hony wol helpe hem wonderly þ*a*t speten || blod . The uij u*er*tu p*er*sely drunke w*ith* wyne wol *f.57r* staunche þe ache of þe mawe & delyuer a wo*m*man sone of hyr floures .

THere ben to maners of Centory þe moor & þe lasse But for þe more ys unknowe to þe most party of me*n* & wel fewe knowen yt of hyr þerfore I lete passe ouer And of þe lesse I

1626 ache] for ack*es* of lendes of colde *ext. marg. H3* **1627** Persely] xlj *ext. marg.* **1638** bely] for the belye & uryn *ext. marg. H3* **1639** splene] for the splene *ext. marg. H3* **1641** speten] blod *bot. marg.* **1644** Centory] xlij *ext. marg.*

wol say þe u*er*tues & I trow alle folke knowen her . The lasse Centory ys drye yn kynde & she ys cleped ofte februfuga þ*at* ys to say afeuer {chas*er*} . The fyrst u*er*tu she wol clense wel newe wondes & a playst*er* of yt wol cycatryce þ*at* ys to say close w*ith* a seeue þe wolde wondes yn short tyme . The ij u*er*tu þe decocc*io*n of þys centory under putte þ*at* ys to say put yn atte erse w*ith* a clystrer wol p*ro*fyte hem muche þ*at* han sciatica passio . The iij u*er*tu centory þe lasse drunke w*ith* wyne helpyth wonderly all wondes . The iiij u*er*tu þys centory staunchet þe blood of a wonde & a batyth anoon þe ache . by batynge or bekyng yn hyr decocc*io*n . The u u*er*tu *f.57v* þys decocc*io*n || wol helpe yn þe same wyse þe sore synowes . The uj u*er*tu þe Iuys of þys centory drunke wol delyuer oute wo*m*me*n*s floures & purge oute a werplyng yf þere be eny . The uij u*er*tu þys centory drunke w*ith* wyne as yt sayde wol purge all euel medycyns doun*e* by þe wombe The uiij u*er*tu as yt ys seyde þ*at* þys Centory drunke w*ith* wyne wol destroye uenym & þ*at* hath be preued . The ix u*er*tu take þe Iuys of þys centory yn heruest tyme & drye yt atte so*n*ne & kepyth yt wel for yt wol be so good to all þe for seyd causes & ryght holsom & p*ro*fytable .

Camedrios yn greke ys sayd Germandrya yn latyn . & yt ys ⌞an⌟ hoot herbe & drye bothe yn þe iij degre . The fyrst u*er*tu þys herbe drunke w*ith* wat*er* wol delyuer a woma*n* of hyr deed chelde The ij u*er*tu she ys good to drynke w*ith* uenygre for brusynges . The iij u*er*tu þys herbe drunke w*ith* wyne dryth þe splene & purgyt womans floures And yn þe *f.58r* begy*n*nyng she wol heele þe dropesye þ*at* ys || cold . The iiij u*er*tu In þe same wyse maner she wol warysshe uenemous

1660 floures] menstrua *ext. marg. H3* **1664** uenym] for the breste *ext. marg. H3* **1668** Camedrios] xliiij *ext. marg.* **1673** splene] for the splene *ext. marg. H3*

1649 chaser] chast*er* MS.

bestys & deedly also . The u u*er*tu to all þuse causes for seyd þys helpyth yf she be powned & leyde to . The uj u*er*tu þys herbe grounde small w*ith* hony wol clense a wonde thought yt be oolde yf she be leyde to þe place . The uij u*er*tu An oynement made of þe Iuys of þys herbe & of hony wol make þe eyen clere & put away þe dasewenesse by ofte anoyntynge . The uiij u*er*tu medle þys herbe grounde small w*ith* oyle & þer w*ith* anoynte þe body þ*at* ys colde for þ*at* wol putte oute þe colde & ynduse heet yn to þe body ayen .

DRagouns . Addristuncte ys spotted lyke a snake . The fyrst u*er*tu þ*ys* may dryue away þe uenym of snakes . The man anoynted w*ith* þe Iuys of dragons rotes . þere shal noon adder greue hem . The ij u*er*tu dragons drunke w*ith* wyne wol heele addrys bytynges . || The iij u*er*tu þe Iuys of dragons *f.58v*
medled w*ith* oyle . helde yn atte yeres wol hele þe ache of he*m* The iiij u*er*tu dyppe yn þe Iuys welle . & leye yt to þe nose & þ*at* woll staunche þe syknes þ*at* called ys polypus . The u u*er*tu In þe same wyse yt ys a greet helpe unto cancres . The uj u*er*tu þe Iuys of dragons rootes dryueth away þe duskenes of þe eyen . yf þow wolt anoynte þyn eyen w*ith* þe Iuys allone or elles melle yt w*ith* hony . The uij u*er*tu It ys sayd þ*at* xiij cornes of dragons seed drunke w*ith* pusca wol put away þe duskenes of þe yen . The rootes y rosted & eten doth good to þe eyen . The uiij u*er*tu yf þe wo*m*ma*n* þ*at* ys w*ith* chyld smelle þe sauor of dragons floures whan yt wellyth . yt wol delyuer her of a werplyng . And yt wol do . yf þe rotes of dragons be under put to þe matryce . The ix u*er*tu þe pouder of dragons rootes medled w*ith* hony wol destroye þe kowhe & þe pose . yf yt be eten ofte . The x u*er*tu þys same ys greet helpe to hem þ*at* speten blood & also yt co*n*sumyth þe wyckednes of þe brest for euermore . The xj ||

1683 colde] for the feuer of colde *ext. marg. H3* **1685** Dragouns] xliiij *ext. marg.*

f.59r u*er*tu to þe same whan þey be rosted or decocte þey ben good. The xij u*er*tu dragon rotes drunke w*ith* wyne . scuryt to lecherye & p*ro*uokyth uryn & clensyth foule wondes & curyth þe fest*re* . id est siringam & helyth wondes . The xiij u*er*tu dragons w*ith* uenygre allone wol destroye spottes . The xiiij u*er*tu þe water þ*a*t dragon rotes be soden yn . wol hele þe kebe or moule yn þe hele . by ofte wassyng þere yn . The kebe cometh of colde . In latyn yt ys p*er*uyo . for þ*a*t yt noyeth & greueth unto þe hele . It ys also clepyd comenly mula .

ASclepius co*m*mendyth gretly {Camomille}. It ys clepyd Camomula & camomilla yn latyn þys herbe ys soot yn {sauor} & shrot yn {substa*u*nce} . Thys ys muche lyke an herbe . þ*a*t ys called amarusca . for þ*a*t she stynketh & ys bytt*er* . Autores sayn þ*a*t þere ben iij maneres of camomylle & by coloures of hyr floures only þey may be knowe Alle þey haue a yelowe floures yn þe meddel but yche of þuse iij haue *f.59v* leues of dyuerse coloure a boute þe yolow yn þe mydel || þe wyche ben whyte . blake & purpul . He þ*a*t hath a boute hys yelow floure p*ur*pel leues ys called p*ro*pyrly autem*us* þys ys þe most & strongyst of alle þuse iij kyndes . The ij ys cleped lenchemon & she þ*a*t hat wyth floures or leues aboute þe yelownesse . The iij ys cleped {Crisantemona} & he hath blak leues or floures abowte hys yelownesse . Alle iij ben hoot & drye yn þe iij degre . The fyrst u*er*tu þuse ydrunke ofte w*ith* wyne p*ro*uoken uryn & breken þe stoon yn þe bladdre & purgen wo*m*mens floures An so þey do yf þe matryce be beket yn þe water þat þys herbe ys soden yn . The ij u*er*tu In

---

1717 Camomille] <u>xlu</u> *ext. marg.* **1721** camomylle] for the belye *ext. marg. H3*

1717 Camomille] Canomille MS. **1719** sauor] sauar MS. substaunce] sulsta*u*nce MS. **1729** iij] u*er*tu *exp.* | Crisantemona] Crisautemona MS.

þe same wyse yt staunchyt þe fretyng & þe bolnynge of þe stomak And by þys drynke þow mayst do away þe spottes . or frakles of þe skyn . The iij u*er*tu þys also wol yt do yf yt be grounde smal w*ith* hony allone & bounde to . The iiij u*er*tu þe decocc*i*on of þys herbe dronke doth p*ro*fyth to þe Iaundese & helpyth wonderly to þe dysseses of þe mawe . The u u*er*tu Camomylle wol delyuere a wo*m*man of hyr ded chylde . The uj u*er*tu sethe Camomylle yn oyle & þer w*ith* anoynte hem þat hat þe fe || uers þ*ys* oynement wol destroye þe colde of þe *f.60r* feuers & of tyme þe self feuere . The uij u*er*tu þy*s* oynement dryueth away þe euel þ*a*t bolnyth þe flanke . The uiij u*er*tu Autem*us* drunke a dragme weyght w*ith* wyne destroyeth uenemouse bytynges & dedly . The ix u*er*tu plini*us* co*n*fyrmyth þ*a*t who so drynkyt þys camomylle tweyne dragme wyght yche day duryng fourty days w*ith* tweyne Ciates of ryght good & clene whyte wyne yt wol purge all þe splene . yf he also wasse þe place w*ith* þe same . The x u*er*tu þys Authem*us* cheude & leyde to . wol hele þ*a*t maner of lepre þ*a*t ys called Egilopa & also yt clensyth foule wo*n*des . The xj u*er*tu þys camomylle ys wo*n*t to hele þe heed þ*a*t ys greued w*ith* heet of þe feuer . Th*e* xij u*er*tu of tymes rysyth yn þe heed postemes or bocches of þe humours gadred to gyder þe wyche bocches þe greke clepyth exantimata . þan take grene camomylle . & sethe yt yn oyle . If þow may haue no grene . tak drye & wete yt ryght wel yn || uynegre & þer *f.60v* w*ith* anoynte þe heed alaboute for þer ys noon oynement þ*a*t helpyth þe heed more .

WOdebynde ys clepyd yn latyn Caprifoliu*m* & ligustion also . & so yt ys clepyd for þy þ*a*t yn þe cuntre of lygurye growyth most plente of þys herbe . It ys hoot & drye bothe yn þe iij degre The most u*er*tu of þys herbe . ys yn þe root &

1751 splene] for the splene *ext. marg. H3* **1754** heed] for the hede *ext. marg. H3* **1762** Wodebynde] xluj *ext. marg.*

seed & þey ben of euene u*er*tu & myght yn medycynes . The fyrst u*er*tu þys herbe drunke yn wyne wol abate þe bolnynge of þe stomak & also yt helpyth þe dygystyoun . The ij u*er*tu In þe same wyse yt helpyth sores of þe entrayles & of þe ynner partes þus þey p*ro*uoke uryne & purgyth wo*m*mans floures The iij u*er*tu al þuse herbes helpyn ayenst uenemouse bytynges yf þey ben solued wel yn wyne & þan grounde smal & dronken a partye of þys herbe þus stamped be leyde un to þe place . The iiij u*er*tu þys herbe etyn & drynke bothe wol *f.61r* do hem muche good þ*a*t han || þe colica passio & not only she but þe decocc*io*n of her rotes y drunke . The u u*er*tu þys decocc*io*n ys good also . to alle þe dysseses þ*a*t ben seyde before . yf yt be drunke . The uj u*er*tu þe seed of þys herbe helpyth hugely for to defye . S⌞t⌟rabus affermyth þ*a*t þys herbe ys noyose un to þe syght . bothe yn drynke & eke yn sauoure . And þ*er* for he comau*n*dyth for to use þe seed allone of þys herbe yn medycynes . But I wote not whether he sayth þus of hym self or þ*a*t he hadde yt of oþere autores bokes But þys I wot wel þ*a*t oold me*n* han hugely co*m*mendyd & preysed þys herbe . Neyther I haue mynde þ*a*t euer I radde eny boke þ*a*t accordyth unto Strabus seyng*e* yn thys matre .

HEre endyth þe fyrst Boke of Mac*er* & now folewyth here þe secu*n*de boke wyche fully conteyneth oþer twenty dyuerse herbes wit*h* her uertuys & proprytee*s* Of þe whyche . Sorell wit*h* hys nyne uertues þe formust y*s* þe fyrst . ||

f.61v Iubarbe ij
Purslane iij
Bysshopys worte iiij
Langedebeef u
Pulyoll haunt uj
Horehounde uij
Cost oþer moleyne uiij
Cyperus ix

Pyone	x	
Hony soucle	xj	
Groundeswely	xij	
Celydonye	xiij	
Gwayde	xiiij	
Ellebur whyte	xu	
Ellebur blak	xuj	
Uerueyne	xuij ||	
Morell	xuiij	*f.62r*
Hennebane	xix	
Hocke	xx	

SOrell or Surell orþer Soure docke ys clepyd yn latyn Acedula & yn greke Ayȝon And yt ys cleped as men trowe*n* for hys sauor ys tarte as ys uenygre . Thys herbe ys founde comounly i*n* grauely medes . & by syde þe watres . Many me*n* eten bysely in uer tyme . And þey sayn þ*a*t þey haue founde by experyment þat yt hath do hym muche good And destroyth yn hem many greuaunces . Thys herbe ys ryght colde & drye bothe yn þe thrydde ˪de˩gre . The fyrst u*er*tu aplastre of þys wol destreye þe holy fyre & þe malady þ*a*t ys {cleped} {herpeta} mordax . þys ys a bytynge scabbe & gnawyng . also yt wol helpe þe bolnyng of þe ˪e˩yen . The ij u*er*tu þys wol represse þe bocches þat crepyth furthe & yt curyth brennynges . And as men sayn yt doth muche || good to þe hoot podadre . yf þe place be couered w*ith* hyr grene leues . or yf þuse leues be stamped & medled w*ith* floure & leyde þer to . The iij u*er*tu It ys seyd þ*a*t þe Iuys of sorel medled w*ith* oyle of roses wol do muche good to þe olde heed ache . The wyche ache ys seyd yn greke Sephalargya . The iiij u*er*tu sorel eten or drunke w*ith* wyne wol stau*n*che þe flux of þe wombe what manere euer yt be . And also yt staunchyt

f.62v (margin, beside "brennynges . And as men sayn yt doth muche || good to þe")

1811 Sorell] i *ext. marg.*

1819 cleped] cheped MS. **1820** herpeta] hepeta MS.

wommans floures yf þey haue hem ouer muche If þe sorer be stamped grene & leyde to þe matryce . yt wol do þe same . The u u*er*tu sorel ydrunke *with* wyne . wol sle þe wormes yn þe bely þ*a*t ben round . And also yt *with* stondyth al uenymis . The uj u*er*tu sorel Iuys anoynted makyth a body glad chered . The uij u*er*tu Men sayn þat ho so beryth sorel a boute hem . no scorpyo*un* wol hurte hym . The uiij u*er*tu Sorel Iuys helden ynne atte ere helpyth hugely þe heryng . & destroyth þe ache of þe ere Thys yt doth by hem self or elles *f.63r* medled *with* þe oyle of roses . The ix || u*er*tu of þys herbe sorell eten ofte wol do he*m* muche good þ*a*t speten blode .

IUbarbe ys amaner of sorell but for þy þat she ys euer grene & fresshe she ys called Iubarbe & Synegrene . Thys ys þe lasse sorell plinius sayt þ*a*t ys lyke on to þat oþer sorell & þ*a*t þys as so good & as p*ro*fytable to all þe causes before sayd as ys þe forsayd herbe . Thys u*er*tu yt hath atte morwe . Su*m*me eye leddes ben wont for to be closed fast to gydre *with* amaner glewe of flume . so þ*a*t unnethe þey may be unclosed . The Iuys of þys herbe anoynted aboue upoon þe eyelyddes dyssoluyth wonderly þ*ys* fleume .

PUrselane ys cleped comounly ffolefote . & yn greke adg*ra*nus . Thys ys cold yn þe secunde degre . & moyst yn þe thyrde . The fyrst u*er*tu þys ys good for þat maner of feuer þ*a*t yn greke ys cleped Causon & to þe stomak also yf yt be stamped leyd þerto . The ij u*er*tu to þe same ys þe Iuys of þys *f.63v* herbe good yf yt be drunke & þe self herbe || yf yt be eten . The iij u*er*tu ete þys herbe as wortes & yt wol putte away ynmoderat hete . The iiij u*er*tu þys herbe etyn or drunken wol staunche þe ful fluxe of þe wombe . The u u*er*tu þys herbe wol putte away þe egghynge of þe tethe þ*a*t chewyth her . The uj u*er*tu to þe eyen þ*a*t ben swol she doth gret

---

1842 Iubarbe] ij *ext. marg.* **1845** good] for the yche *ext. marg. H3*
1851 Purselane] iij *ext. marg.*

good yf she be stamped & leyde þer to . The uij u*er*tu þys herbe eten wol not suffre þe heet of þe sonne to done hym harme þ*at* etyth hyr & she makyt þe wombe laxe . yf she be eten wit*h* salte & wyne . The uiij u*er*tu þys herbe eten wol staunche þe ache of þe bladdre . And she ys ryght holsom to hem þ*at* spetten blood . yf she be ofte eten . Plinius sayth þe souredocke þat ys sorel hath all most þe same u*er*tu þ*at* hath þys herbe & boþe yn effecte .

BYsshopisworte ys cleped Struccyon thys ys hoote & drye . The fyrst u*er*tu þe roote of þys herbe stamped & drunke wit*h* wyne . wol abate all þe syknesse of þe mawe & þe bolnyng of þe splene & þe || Iaundyse . The ij u*er*tu In þe same wyse she *f.64r* puttyt away þe hardenesse þ*at* ys cleped yn greke Sclirosys . & brekyth þe ston of þe bladdre & {puttyth} hym oute & purgyth wo*m*mans floures . The iij u*er*tu In þe same wyse she makyt a body to pysse fast and destroyet þe kowe . The iiij u*er*tu In þe same wyse also yt helpyth hem þ*at* spetten blood yf yt be drunken ofte . The u u*er*tu she wol delyuer a woma*n* of hyr ded chylde yf yt be underputte to þe matryce . And þ*at* same wyse It wol also brynge oute wo*m*mans floures whan þey caryn . as me*n* sayn . The uj u*er*tu þe Iuys of þys herbe meddled wit*h* uenygre & floure wol clense lepres . yf yt be wel anoynted on þe place . The uij u*er*tu A plast*er* of þe Iuys of þys herbe medled wel wit*h* barly floure wol hele euery whelke . The uiij u*er*tu *þys* herbe confecte wit*h* uenygre & floure & þe Iuys of scabiose & a noynted uppon þe scabbe wol hele yt . The ix u*er*tu þe Iuys of þys herbe medled wit*h* hony . & gronde wel || to gydre purgyth þe humours of þe *f.64v* heed yf yt be drawen yn atte nose . The x u*er*tu þe pouder of þys herbe casteyn atte nose wit*h* þe Iuys of whyte elebur wol make þe for to snese faste . The xj u*er*tu þe same pouder

---

1870 Bysshopisworte] iiij *ext. marg.*

1875 puttyth] puttyht MS.

medled wit*h* wom*m*ans mylke drawen yn at nose helpet hem hugely þ*a*t han the Iaundyse .

LAngedebeef þ*a*t ys oxe tonge ys good for to putte oute þe redde colre bre*n*t wit*h* huge hete . yf she be of tyme drunke wit*h* wyne . The ij u*er*tu In þe same wyse . yt wol hele hyn þ*a*t ys cardiacus for plente of blac colre . The iij u*er*tu þys herbe drunke ofte wol do away all þe wyckyt humo*ur*s of þe lunges . The iiij u*er*tu þe Iuys of þys herbe drunke wit*h* leuke water wol helpe hem wonderly þ*a*t han Sciatica passio . The u u*er*tu wyse me*n* sayn þ*a*t þe wyne þ*a*t þys herbe hath leyen yn . wol kepe þe stryngthe of a mans mynde yf he drynke yt . The uj u*er*tu þe decocc*i*on of þys herbe wol gladen hem þ*a*t
f.65r eten or drynke of yt . The || uij u*er*tu þys herbe drunke wit*h* hyr root & seed þ*a*t she beryth wol hele he*m* þ*a*t han t*er*cia*n* & eke q*ua*rteyn .

PUlioll haunt ys cleped oryganu*m* yn latyn yt ys drye & hoot bothe yn þe iij degre . The fyrst u*er*tu þe decocc*i*on of þys herbe drunke yn wyne curyth all deedly bytynges . The ij u*er*tu þys decocc*i*on drunke wit*h* mulsa . doth hym good þ*a*t hath drunke uenym þ*a*t ys cleped Acincuma . And yn þe same wyse as men sayn . yt ys good ayenst many . oþer uenomus . The iij u*er*tu þys herbe ys good for bruserys yf she be ofte eten or drunken . The iiij u*er*tu þys herbe drunke repryssyth & dryeth up bolnynges of þys dropese . The u u*er*tu þys herbe wit*h* mulsa wol do away þe blak colere . The uj u*er*tu a drynke of þys herbe . or a decocc*i*on of yt woll brynge oute wo*m*mens floures . The uij u*er*tu þe poudre of þys herbe eten wit*h* hony wol destroye þe kowhe . The uiij u*er*tu of bathynge yn þe decocc*i*on of þys herbe wol do away ychynge & nayles þ*a*t waxen yn þe heed & þe spottes of þe

1895 Langedebeef] u *ext. marg.* **1898** cardiacus] for the harte faynte *ext. marg. H3* **1905** The] uij u*er*tu *bot. marg.* **1908** Pulioll] uj *ext. marg.*

skyn . And þe Iaundse also . yf þe decocc*io*n be drunke yn || *f.65v* þe self bathynge . The ix u*er*tu þe Iuys of þ*ys* grene y drunke . wol helpe bothe þe bolnynges of þe uua & of þe chekes . The x u*er*tu þ*ys* same herbe holden wel yn þe mouthe & rolled often aboute þerynne wol hele þe blastres of þe mouthe . The xj u*er*tu þe Iuys of þys herbe helde yn atte nose w*ith* þe oyle of gladen . wol make þe blood renne oute þ*a*t noyeth þe heed . The xij u*er*tu þys Iuys helden yn atte eue wol staunche al þe ache of hyr w*ith* þe mylke of a woma*n* helde þ*er* w*ith* . The xiij u*er*tu þys Iuys medled w*ith* oynouns & rose mary . & set atte sonne yn a bras pot fourty days whan Sirius brennyth yt wol dryue away all noyus bestes . yf yt be set under þe hed of a body as men sayn . The xiiij u*er*tu þys Iuys drunke w*ith* good wyt wyne wol helpe hem wel þ*a*t han a combred her stomak so þ*a*t þey may not wel defye . The xu u*er*tu þys Iuys also drunke w*ith* hoot water wol a bate þe gnawyng of þe stomak & þys hath be preued . The xuj u*er*tu drye & open wolle wete & drenche yt atte full yn þe Iuys of þys herbe medled w*ith* oyle & uenygre || *f.66r* & leyde to þe place wol helpe hugely boþe brusours scaldynges & scabbes . The xuij u*er*tu þys herbe grunde p*ro*uokyth uryn & dryueth oute þe wormes of þe bely . The xuiij u*er*tu þe tethe þ*a*t chewen þys herbe shull not ake . The xix u*er*tu þe Iuys of þys herbe drunke helpyth all þ*a*t ys yn þe body w*ith*yn . The xx u*er*tu drynke yn þe Iuys of a fyge grunden small . & þys wol opene þe poures & make þe swot to renne oute þere as yt ys seyd The xxj u*er*tu aplastre madde ⌞of⌟ þe Iuys w*ith* w⌞h⌟yte mele & leyd onto þe thyes wol ofte tyme represse & do away þe ache of he*m* .

1930 heed] for the hed *ext. marg. H3* **1937** stomak] for the stomack *ext. marg. H3* **1942** brusours] for brusynge *ext. marg. H3* **1944** tethe] for the tethe *ext. marg. H3* **1950** thyes] for the thye*s* *ext. marg. H3*

HOrehounde ys clepyd yn latyn Marubium yn greke prassion It ys hoot & drye bothe . yn þe secu*n*de degre . The fyrst u*er*tu þe decocc*i*on of þys herbe al togydyr . or of hyr seed drunke . helpyth hem hugely & wonderly þ*a*t han þe ptisyk . The ij u*er*tu þys drynke wol abate many & dyuerse syknesse of þe brest . & bettre she worchyth yf gladen be putte þer to . *f.66v* || The iij u*er*tu þys herbe drunke w*ith* olde wyne wol sone destroye all uenym . It helpyth also þe chynke ofte & also þe comou*n* cowhe . The iiij u*er*tu It wol also shorte a woma*n*s trauelynge & bregghynge her throwes yn þe same wyse . And eke hastely brynge oute þe after byrdou*n* . The u u*er*tu þys herbe medled w*ith* hony . wol clense wondes & hele bocches þ*a*t freten þe flesse . The uj u*er*tu It ys seyde þ*a*t þys drynke wol staunche þe ache of þe sydes . The uij u*er*tu to al þuse ys good þe Iuys of þys herbe yf yt be dryed and kepte . The uiij u*er*tu þys Iuys drynke yn water wol dryue away þe feuere & þe pose . The ix u*er*tu þys Iuys medled w*ith* wyne . or w*ith* hony wol do so good unto þe eyen þ*a*t ben dasewed . The x u*er*tu þys Iuys cast yn atte nose . helpyth hem þat han þe Iaundyse . The xj u*er*tu Men sayn þat þys Iuys w*ith* oyle of roses caste yn atte ere . The xij u*er*tu Men sayn It ys not good to ette . nor drunke horehounde for hem þ*a*t han dyssese yn þe *f.67r* bladder . or yn || þe reynes . The xiij u*er*tu yf þow wolt sle þe malyce of horehonde ete after yt feenel seed & þat wol kepe the .

COste or moleyne ys clepyd yn Greke asaru*m* & yn latyn wlgago þys ys boþe hoot and drye yn þe thrydde degre . The fyrst u*er*tu þys herbe drunke p*ro*uokyth uryn & purgyth wo*m*mens floures & helpyth þe doloures of þe maw . The ij

---

1952 Horehounde] uij *ext. marg.* **1955** ptisyk] for þe tysyck *ext. marg. H3* **1960** comoun cowhe] for the chyne cuw *ext. marg. H3* **1972** ere] for the ere *ext. marg. H3* **1977** Coste] uiij *ext. marg.*

u*er*tu þys herbe drunken ofte wol hele þe dropesye & scietica passio . The iij u*er*tu þe decocc*i*on of þys herbe helpyth þe syknesse . & þe sores of þe kunte . The iiij u*er*tu It ys seyde þ*at* þys decocc*i*on dru*n*ke wol destroye þe Iaundyse . The u u*er*tu þys decocc*i*on purgyth þe entrayles w*ith* a uomyte . as doth elebur but þys purgac*i*on ys not so uyolent . as of þe elebur . Thys purgac*i*on ys not to be dradde yf she be yone yn þys wyse . Or þat þow yeue yt þow shalt consydre þe age & þe
strengthe of þe rese || uyo*ur* & loke what tyme yt be of þe *f.67v*
yere . And whether þe regyon þ*at* he ys ynne . be wel hoot or wel colde . or temp*er*at y now . ffor chyldryn & feble men & to olde men þow shalt yeue but alytel . To myddel age þow shalt yeue moor . And to fat men & stronge moor þan to lene & feble me*n* yn what age so eu*er* þey be . In cold regyoun þow shalt yeue moor þan yn an hoot . To hem þ*at* ben hardded yn eny labore yeue þow hem moor þan hem þ*at* ben yn rest & quyete & Idelnesse If þow wol be holde wysely suche poyntes & co*n*sydre suche oþer mo . þow shalt be syker for to yeue not only þys herbe . but also all oþer herbes þ*at* purgen w*ith* uomyte . ether soluen þe stomak or þe wombe .

Now haue I seyde generaly how þow shalt yeue all maner herbes . But now wol I say yn what wyse þys herbe shal be p*ro*pyrly yeue Thow shalt cake thrytty fresse leues of þys herbe & cast to hem as muche wyne as þey may be heled
ynne & lete hem lye & soke wel all a || nyght yn þ*at* wyne At *f.68r*
morwe take oute of þe wyne þuse leues & grynde hem small þan resolue hem yn þat same wyne þ*at* þey were soken yn And lete hym drynke as muche as he wold of good whyt wyne & strong And clense thurgh a clothe þe Iuys of þys herbe & yeue hym for to drynke . Thys nombre of leues ys y now for fatte & stronge men To oþer þat be not myghty &

1981 scietica…1982 passio] for the gowte yn the hyppe *ext. marg. H3* stronge yeue lesse after her myghte & age & suche oþ*er* co*n*dyc*i*ons before sayde .

LEches sayn þ*a*t þe herbe wyche ys cleped Ciperus yn latyn ys hoot & drye yn þe secunde degre The fyrst u*er*tu þe drynke of þys herbe purgyth & laxyt þe wayes of þe uryn . The ij u*er*tu þe decocc*i*on of þys herbe wol putte oute þe ded chylde as Apelledorus seyth yf a woma*n* wasshe & bathe hyr þere ynne . The iij u*er*tu þe same sayth . þat þe smoke of þys herbe wol co*n*sume þe splene . yf yt be ofte drawe yn atte mouthe . The iiij u*er*tu þys clerke sayth . þ*a*t yf an hoole man make *f.68v* hy*m* || þer of a subfumygac*i*on yt wol sadde & lyghte hym also . The u u*er*tu þe Iuys of þys herbe medled w*ith* oyle & a noynted . helpyth þe uyces & þe sores of þe armepyttes . The uj u*er*tu þe Iuys drunke ofte . dryeth up ouer muche humours . & sup*er*flue . The uij u*er*tu þe pouder of þys allone or medled w*ith* hony wol purge hugely bocches & roten wondes The uiij u*er*tu þys pouder ys also good to bleynes of þe mouthe . yf yt be drunken And so yt comfortyth þe stomak þ*a*t ys feble & helpyth þe dropesye yf yt be ofte y drunke . And by þe uryne yt purgyth watery humours . The ix u*er*tu Grynde smal þys herbe . & putte þer to stronge uenygre & þ*a*t wol destroye þe crepynge bocches .

PYonye ys hoot & drye yn þe secunde degre . The fyrst u*er*tu þys herbe drunke w*ith* well grounde almoundes & mulsa wol helpe þe splene . þe mawe & þe reynes . The ij u*er*tu In þe same wyse It purgyth wo*m*mens floures & staunchyt þe fluxe . The iij u*er*tu þe decocc*i*on of þys herbe drunken ofte yn wyne wol staunche þe gret ache of þe . bladder . And also *f.69r* || yt helpyt þe heed ache þ*a*t ys cleped {scotosys} & þe ache of þe stomak . The iiij u*er*tu þys same helpyth muche þe ache

---

2014 Leches] ix *ext. marg.* **2034** Pyonye] x *ext. marg.*

2040 scotosys] stocosys MS.

of þe sydes & þe Iaundyse also . The u u*er*tu pyony drunke ofte wol do away brusurs & other dyssesys . þ*at* dremes don to men by nyght tyme . The uj u*er*tu pyony {born} . & ofte tymes eten wol hele hym þ*at* ys lunatyke . The uij u*er*tu þe rote of pyone honged aboute a cheldes nek þ*at* hath þe fallyng euel wol take yt away & cure hym . ffor Galien sayth he preued yt by a chylde of uiij yere of age . ffor whyle þ*ys* rote was aboute þe chyldes necke þ*at* had þe fallyng euel he fyll not þan . he toke yt away . & a noon he fyll yn to þe euel And þan he henge yt ayen aboute hys necke & þus sone he was hoole ayen . Diascorides sayt þe same of þe hangynge aboute þe necke And so he sayth . yt wol do þe same yf yt be ofte y drunke . The uiij u*er*tu xu red cornes of pyone seed drunke yn wyne wol || staunche þe fluxe of þe matryce . The *f.69v* ix u*er*tu þe blake cornes of pyone seed . be wont to do away þe dyuerse syknesse of þe matryse yf þe wom*m*an pacyent drynke þer of xu cornes yn wyne atte nyght whan she goth to bedde . There ben ij maneres of þys herbe þe moor ys chepyd þe male . The lasse ys clepyd þe female . The root of þe moor ys twey palme longe & gret as a fynger . The root of þe lasse . ys dyuyded yn to many rotes as yt ys sayde Thys drunk ⌞w*ith*⌟ wyne after þe byrdoun woll clense wel þe matryce . In al oþer þynges boþe þe moor & þe lasse han all oo uertu .

HOnysoucle . ys clepyd yn greke Mellisophilos . In latyn comou*n*ly she ys cleped Baraces . oþer doracus . Amonge alle herbes þys ys most leef unto Bees . for þey maken moost of þys floure . The ij u*er*tu . If þat þe hyue be anoynted w*ith* þe Iuys of þuse leues . þe bees shul not goo away . And þe better yt ys . yf swete mylke be putte þer to for housebo*n*de men don þys . The iij u*er*tu þys herbe stam || ped & leyde to þe *f.70r* styngyng of þe bees . Anoon wol hele yt wel & fayre And yn

2065 Honysoucle] xj *ext. marg.*

2044 born] boru*m* MS.

þe same wyse þe styngyng of a waspe & of a spyder & of a nattercoppe . The iiij u*er*tu þys herbe stampyd wi*th* salt wol a bate þe olde bocches of þe brest & to helpe þe foule uyces . The u u*er*tu a woma*n* ys cured wi*th* þe Iuys of þys herbe soden wi*th* salte & wi*th* suche a drynke ys warysshed all noyous bolnynge . The uj u*er*tu þe decocc*io*n of þys grene herbe y dronke ofte . wol helpe þe syknesse þ*at* ys clepyd anteryke . And staunche þe blody menys*ou*n & do hem good þ*at* han dyssese yn her flankes & eke unto kowhers ide*m* . asmaticos & orthonoici . The uij u*er*tu þe same decocc*io*n purgyth þe bocches & puttyth oute þe sores of þe toon . The uiij u*er*tu þys herbe stamped wi*th* salte & leyd unto an houndes bytynge wol hele yt . The ix u*er*tu þe same decocc*io*n wol purge wo*m*mans floures thorugh o f t e bathynge & boylynge & yt wol stau*n*che þe tothe ache yf yt *f.70v* be holde longe yn || þe mouthe . The x u*er*tu plinius sayth þ*at* þe Iuys of þys herbe wi*th* hony & a noynted wol clense þe eyen of her derkenes .

<u>GRoundeswely</u> we clepen yt yn latyn Senacion And þe greke yrenosshe It ys clepyd Senacion . for her floure ys lyke hyreres Thys herbe growyth co*m*mounly on walles & yn gardyenes . Thys herbe ys colde . hys root shal not be putte yn use of medycynes Thys herbe mayst þow take & gadre by þe morowe . or at myd day . The fyrst u*er*tu þys herbe stamped wi*th* swynes grese & leyde to þe place wol asswage þe bolnynge or swellyng of strokes . The ij u*er*tu Grynde to gyder þe leues of þe floure of þe herbe . þan helde þer to a lytel of swete wyne & make þer of a plaster & laye yt hoot to þe bolnynge of þe erse & of þe ballokkes & þ*at* wol make hym hool . The iij u*er*tu putte to al þuse frankencense . & make of all a plaster & wol hele lyghtly þe soor synowes & all

2087 tothe ache] for þe toth ack *ext. marg. H3* **2091** Groundeswely] <u>xij</u> *ext. marg.* **2098** swellyng] for swelynge *ext. marg. H3*

wondes . The iiij u*er*tu þys herbe grounde wi*th* swynes grese & leyde to þe || place wol hele awonde though yf yt be olde . *f.71r* And yt wol staunche þe hoot potagre & maner hoot doloures & greua*u*nces of þe legge . The u u*er*tu to all þuse causes wol decocc*io*n of þe capytell of þys herbe {helpe} & {hele} . The uj u*er*tu so*m*me me*n* sayn for sothe . þ*a*t þys herbe þow schalt not drynke . for þ*a*t she wol strangly & choke hym þ*a*t drynkyth hyr But plinius sayth ayenst hem . for he sayth . þ*a*t so*m*me men hath youe hyr to drynke wi*th* wyne unto hym þ*a*t haue hadde þe Iaundys . & yt dyde hem muche good . The uij u*er*tu plinius sayth þ*a*t þys herbe drunke wi*th* wyne wol do huge good to þe seknesse of þe bladder & he sayth . þ*a*t many men haue p*ro*ued þys soth . The uiij u*er*tu þe saam sayth also þ*a*t many me*n* haue yeuen hyr yn þe for seyde wyse . for uyces & syknes of þe hert & of þe mawe . The ix u*er*tu plinius sayth also . þ*a*t þys herbe drunke wi*th* uino passe wol abate þe fretynge of þe wombe & many other || syknesse *f.71v* þ*a*t fallen yn þe bowles . The x u*er*tu also þys same wol do þys grene herbe yf she be putte yn uenygre & so eten . The xj u*er*tu þys herbe also medled wi*th* salte & leyde to þe place . ys good to destroye þe bocches & þe postemes of þe brest . The xij u*er*tu plinius also sayth . who so deluyth al aboute þys herbe root & takyt away þe erthe al aboute hys root wi*th* outen eny yren & wi*th* þ*a*t touche hys tothe . þ*a*t akyth thre tymes & after euery touche spete oute And þan sette ayen þys self herbe yn þe same place where she grewe before tyme And yf so be yt þ*a*t þys herbe lyue & growe as she dyde before þ*a*t tothe shal no more ake .

2120 fretynge] for fretyng*e ext. marg. H3*

2108 helpe] helped *final d deleted* | hele] heled *final d deleted*
2114 plinius] sayth *exp.*

<u>CElidonye</u> hath twey spyces þe fyrste ys cleped of leches þe
moor . þat other ys cleped þe lasse . The fyrst u*er*tu bothe
ben good for þe eyen . ffor as plinius sathe þ*at* þe swalowe
w*ith* þ*ys* herbe wol make hys byrdes to see ayen . though þey
be blynded . or though her yen were putte oute of her ||
f.72r heddes Men sayn þ*at* þys herbe spryngyth whan þ*at* swalowes
comen . And whan þey gon away . þan uanysshyth þys herbe
& dryeth up And she ys cleped <u>Celidonia</u> for celidoyne yn
greke . sygnyfyeth a swalowe The ij u*er*tu þys herbe grounde*n*
smal & soden yn butter ys a specyal oynement to þe ache of
þe heed . yf þe body be wel ybaþed yn þe water þ*at* þys herbe
ys soden ynne . The iij u*er*tu þe Iuys of þys herbe whan she
flouryth & sethe yt yn bras uessel & take of all þe scome &
sethe yt tyl yt be as thyk as hony þ*at* ys fyne . leches sayn þ*at*
þere ys no better medycyn for þe yen þ*at* ben dasawyd &
duske . yf þey ben often anoynted þer w*ith* . The iiij u*er*tu
Celidonye rootes y grounde w*ith* anyse & drunke w*ith* wyth
wyne . ys good for þe Iaundyse . The u u*er*tu as men sayn .
þys herbe gronde smal & leyde un to þe place . wol destrye þe
tothe ache . The uj u*er*tu a plaster of {celidonye} leues
grounde w*ith* wyne wol destroye & wype away þe spotte⸤s⸥ &
fracles .

<u>GWayde</u> ys cleped yn greke ysaccis & yn latyn she ys cleped
f.72v comounly Gwaisdo . Thys herbe makyth dyers for || to
wynne gretly . The fyrst u*er*tu þys herbe grounde small &
drunke yn water helyth address bytynge yf þere be leyde to þe
place aplaster made of þe leues of þ*ys* herbe stamped allone .
The ij u*er*tu a plaster maad of þe leues of þys herbe grounden
small closyth wondes though þey be*n* grete & stanchyth þe

2132 Celidonye] <u>xiij</u> *ext. marg.* **2135** to…ayen] for þ*e* yone syȝte *ext. marg. H3* **2136** putte oute] Be it knowne *bot. marg. H3* **2146** yen] yene dasewyd *ext. marg. H3* **2154** Gwayde] <u>xiiij</u> *ext. marg.*

2151 celidonye] celiodyne MS.

blood þ*at* rennyth oute of hem & batyth all maner bolny*n*ges . The iij u*er*tu þys herbe grounde smal w*ith* hony wol purge foule wondes & do away þe spottes & frakles & helpyth þe holy fyre . The iiij u*er*tu þys herbe sta*m*ped w*ith* þe gleyre of egges & leyde to þe place wol hele sone þe breche of bones & þe ache . & dryueth away þe scabbe the wyche leches clepen Inpetigo .

Ellebur hath two maner of spices . One ys whyt & purgyth abou Another ys blak & purgyth by nethe . It ys bothe hoot & drye yn þe thrydde degre But þe whyt ys moor uyolent þa*n*ne þe blak . þerefor fyrst I wol telle þe u*er*tues of whyt Ellebur . The fyrst u*er*tu whyte ellebur under putte yn what maner || euer yt be yt wol delyu*er* a wo*m*man of hyr chylde *f.73r* þ*at* ys ded yn hyr wombe . The ij u*er*tu þe pouder of þys drawen ynne at nose wol make a body to snese . & so he doth away þe syknesse from þe heed . Leches sayn þ*at* yf þys pouder be medled yn þe confecc*i*on or oynementes þ*at* purgen þe yen . yt doth hem muche good . The iij u*er*tu þ*ys* pouder medled w*ith* potage wol sle mys . The iiij u*er*tu þys same pouder youen w*ith* hony . wol destroye fleume . The u u*er*tu þys pouder eten eyþer drunken . wol purge w*ith* a uomyte . many & dyu*er*se wyckyt humours And as leches sayn yt dryuyt away olde syknesse dyssese þ*at* ys clepyd uertygo . The uj u*er*tu þys ytake ys good to wodeme*n* & to malen colyke & to hem þ*at* han þe fallynge euell & to lunatyke It doth muche good to þe dropesye yn þe begy*n*nyng . The uij u*er*tu It clensyth þe lepre yt dryuyth away þe dyssese {tetan*us*} & þe podagre . The uiij u*er*tu It co*n*fermyth & staunchyt hem þ*at* quaken yn þe palesey . It curyth þe frety*n*g || of þe wombe . The ix u*er*tu It doth good *f.73v* to dyu*er*se sykenesse of þe stomak & un to scietica passio &

2168 Ellebur] xu *ext. marg.* **2173** maner] euer *bot. marg.*

2188 tetanus] techan*us* MS.

to an olde kowhe . And to feuers yt p*ro*fytyth aboue all þynges . The x u*er*tu þys ys medycynall to hem þ*at* haue hadde þe quarteyn many yeres plinius monestyth hym þ*at* shal take þys herbe or hyr pouder . þ*at* he ordyne hym seuen dayes afore warly . & most metes & no drynke . & þ*at* he soupe not atte euen þ*at* shal take þys medycyne . or hyr pouder on þe morwe . Plinius co*m*maundyth also . for to aspye an hoot & a clere & a bryght day þe wyche be not wyndy Plinius eke sayth . who þ*at* takyt þys herbe . hyr pouder eyther hyr Iuys & obseruyth not þys techynge . he shal not ascape w*ith* outen an longe dyssese . Also plinius comaundyth þ*at* þys herbe be all way taken soden fyrst yn potage . & yn þe maner of corne þ*at* ys called lenſtis . And as plinius sayth who þ*at* takyt þus . yt shal do hym noon harme . Plinius furthermore sayth þat þys herbe shal be youe *f.74r* to no yonge chyl || dryn . ne to olde . nor feble folkes neyþer to nesshe & tendre men . but to femynyne men Other men co*m*maunden to taken þys yn þe Iuys of a ptisan . or yn mulsa ouþer y bake yn bred & so yt ys p*ro*fytable as þey sayn . It ys sayde þ*at* plybo wrote aboke & taught þere yn . how we shuld take þe Ellebur . & Ipocras yn hys afforismes makyth me*n*cyoun of þys herbe allone . And many oþer me*n* han wryte of þe u*er*tues of þys herbe & taught how þys herbe shuld be taken & {ete} I fynde not a clerke þ*at* co*m*maundyth to take þys herbe by eny certeyn wyght . And natheles I haue radde many bokes þer for . I trowe þ*at* þey semed þ*at* þey seyden y now where he sayde þ*at* yt shuld be take after þe myght & age of þe pacyent & after þe tymes . But me semeth not sykerly ydone to co*m*maunde for to yeue abody suche amedycyne þ*at* myght bry*n*g hyn yn to sodeyn perell .but yf a certeyn weyght or mesure were *con*ssegned . || *f.74v* As plinius hath wretyn þe mysore was wont to youe þe Ellebur by dragmes weyght And he confyrmed also þat þe

2215 ete] yete *initial y deleted*

leches þat folowed after than foure dragmes of Ellybur . but yit natheles yt semyth not þ*a*t he ordeyned yn þ*a*t . by what weyght yt shuld be takyn . But natheles sythen he comau*n*dyd for to yeue adragme . or foure scrypules of þe blak ellebur att most . me semeth þ*a*t wold sygnyfye þ*a*t we shuld yeue þ*a*t halfe wyght of þe wythe Ellebur þe wyche ys moor uyolent þan þe blak ellebur .

Of the blak Ellebur yt ys not so muche to drede . as of þe whyte . The fyrst u*er*tu olde men co*m*maunded to sethe þys yn þe corne þ*a*t ys cleped lens ouþer yn thylke þ*a*t ys cleped muscelly . & þus þey sayn yt ys medycynall to hem þ*a*t ben wode . yf þey eten yt or drynke yt . The ij u*er*tu In þe same wyse yt doth good to þe podagre & to þe dropesye whan þe feuerys meued . The iij u*er*tu It hylpeth wonderly þe palesye yn þ*ys* wyse & puttyth away dyu*er*se syknesse of þe toon & of other dyu*er*se Ioyntes yf yt be dronken . The iiij u*er*tu It dryuyth oute thorugh || þe wombe dyu*er*se colre & flume . *f.75r* The u u*er*tu þe decocc*io*n of þys Ellybur . wol make eyen bryght & clere . yf yt be drunke . The uj u*er*tu a plast*er* of þys Ellybur . wol sette to gydre & mature hardnesse & purge hem . The uij u*er*tu A siroyne of þys Ellybur sette yn atte nek . wol hele þe festre þ*a*t ys cleped siringa & aft*er* tre dayes . þys syroyne shal be do away . The uiij u*er*tu Grynde þys herbe smal & medled þer w*ith* barly mely . & a plast*er* of þys wol drye up þe humours of þe dropesye . The ix u*er*tu þys underputte wol clense a woma*n* of hyr floures & brynge oute þe chylde þ*a*t ys ded yn þe moders wombe The x u*er*tu þys wol yeue hyryng to hem þ*a*t ben dombe by syknes yf yt be putte y*n*ne atte ere & after too dayes or tre taken away . The xj u*er*tu A plast*er* þys Ellybur leyde un to þe place wol destrye

---

2232 blak Ellebur] xuj *ext. marg.* **2237** podagre] for þe podagre *ext. marg. H3*

2244 Ellybur] wol make *exp.*

þe spottes & clense leppes & putte away al scabbes . The xij u*er*tu uenygre þ*at* þys Ellebur ys soden yn . holden yn þe *f.75v* moþe || longe tyme . wol abate þe tothe ache as men sayn . The xiij u*er*tu plinius co*mm*aundyd . for to {yeue} a dragme of blak Ellebur & so þ*at* wol meue þe wombe lyghtly . And plinius for bedyth for to take or yeue eny moor þan atte most foure scrypules obolus & scrybulus ben boþe of oo weyght .

UErueyne clepyth þe greke Ierobothanum & perysteryon As men sayn þere ben tweyne spyces of uerueyne & þo too haue all most oon effecte & u*er*tu yn worchynge . The fyrst u*er*tu me*n* sayn þat who so beryth yt yn hys honde . noo hound shal berke uppon hym where so euer he by come . The ij u*er*tu uerueyne dru*n*ke wi*th* wyne . wol helpe hen þ*at* han þe Iaundyse . The iij u*er*tu uerueyne stampyd wi*th* wyne & leyde to þe place wol hele deedly bytynges . Thys medycyne shal be renewed atte euere foure dayes ende . The iiij u*er*tu þe Iuys of uerueyne made leuke & rolled wel & longe yn þe mothe *f.76r* wol purge þe blastres & wondes || of þe mothe . The u u*er*tu þe same wol do þe fresshe & newe decocc*io*n of þys herbe & {thurght} þys decocc*io*n . ys putte away euery corrupcyo*u*n & rotnesse of þe mouthe . yf she ⌞be⌟ rolled faste aboute yn þe mouthe so þ*at* þe chekes sowne after . The uj u*er*tu þys self herbe stamped whyle she ys grene & layde unto þe place wol close afresshe wonde . The uij u*er*tu take þe rootes of uerueyne & as many of hyr leues resolue hem yn water & do þe pacyent for to drynke þuse before hys accesse þ*at* ys to say . to fore or þ*at* he fele eny cold . þys drynke ys good for a tercyan . The uiij u*er*tu uerueyne ydrunke wi*th* wyne wol destroye all uenymes . The ix u*er*tu In þe same wyse take & drynke foure rootes & foure leues of uerueyne & þ*at* wol destroye þe feuer quarteyne . The x u*er*tu þe decocci*o*un of

---

2262 Uerueyne] xuij *ext. marg.*

2258 yeue] eyue MS. **2274** thurght] thurglt MS.

uerueyne made yn wyne & caste a monge metes & drynkes . wol make hem all mery & glad . þ*at* eten of þ*at* mete & drynken of þ*at* drynke . ryght || as wol langedebeef . of þe *f.76v* wyche I haue wreten to fore . The xj u*er*tu take uerueyne yn thyn honde & aske hym þ*at* ys syke how dost þow . or how faryst thow . And yf he say ayen to þe wel . he shal leue . And yf he aunswere & say euel . or I wote not . þere ys noon hope of hys lyfe yn þys worle . The xij u*er*tu men haue co*m*maunded to putte a crowne of uerueyne aboute þe heed þ*at* akyth what so euere were þe cause & þey seyden þ*at* þys wol a noon abate þe ache . The xiij u*er*tu plinius affyrmyth þ*at* þys herbe ys holsom to þe bowels & ⌞to⌟ þe syknesse of þe sydes & ⌞to⌟ þe mawe & of þe brest & namely to þe causes of þe lunges & to þe ptysyk ys uerueyne medycynal as sayth plinius . The xiiij u*er*tu uerueyne grunde*n* smal w*ith* olde swynes grece & leyde to outher anynted . wol represse hastyly þe bocches & welkes þ*at* comen yn þe heed thurgh þe feuer . The xu u*er*tu take mylfoyle Byteyne & uerueny yleke muche grynde hym to gydre & drynke hem yn || water . men *f.77r* suppose þ*at* þere ys no better ne p*ro*phytabler medycyne for þe stone þan þ*ys* . The xuj u*er*tu plinius sayth þ*at* wycches co*m*menden & prysen hugely þys herbe . for þey . sayn þ*at* þys herbe ys good ayenst all syknesse And allso þey sayn þere shal noo fleys byte þ*at* p*er*son þ*at* ys wasshon yn þe wat*er* þ*at* uerueyn ys soden ynne or a noynte hy*m* w*ith* þe Iuys of uerueyn . þ*at* he þ*at* were a noynted w*ith* þe Iuys of ueruyne . he shuld graunte hym all þyng þ*at* he wolde aske And þ*at* he shulde mouhaue of all gret me*n* loue þ*at* he wolde & þ*at* he shuld not haue þe feuerys . And yf þe feuerys where uppon eny body anon as he were anoynted w*ith* þe Iuys of uerueny

---

2296 ache] for the acke of hede *ext. marg. H3* **2309** fleys] for byty*n*g of flei*s* *ext. marg. H3*

2302 &] we *exp.*

þe feuerys shuld leue hym for euer . And oþer suche many þeye sayn . thuugh p*er* auenture þe myghty nature may graunt yt . þus us semeth þ*at* þey ben ydell sayenges .

MOrell ys cleped yn greke Strignu*m* & yn latyn morella þys *f.77v* ys ryght colde . The fyrst u*er*tu It ys sayde || þ*at* þe Iuys of þys herbe helde yn þe ere a lytel & a lytel . wol staunche wonderly þe ache of þe ere . The ij u*er*tu a plast*er* of þys herbe wol do medycyne & hele thylke maner of lepre þ*at* ys cleped Eglopa . þus men sayn & trowe þ*at* þe saam plast*er* wol hele þe heed ache . The iij u*er*tu Grynde smal þys herbe & þ*er*wit*h* bred & salte & make of þu se a plast*er* & leye yt to . yt wol represse þe maladye þ*at* ys cleped p*er*yodyda . p*er*yodyda ys a knobbe þ*at* rysyth yn þe feuers . The iiij u*er*tu þe Iuys of þys herbe wol an*n*on destroye þe ycche . The u u*er*tu þe Iuys underput wol staunche womans floures þ*at* ys to say þe ynmoderat fluxe of hyr floures . The uj u*er*tu Grynde smal þe leues of þys herbe wit*h* floure & make þer of a {plast*er*} & yt wol hele þe holy fyre & þe euel þ*at* ys cleped herpeta mordax . And muche bett*er* wol þys medycyne be yf þow take to þys aforesayd þe frothe of seluer ceunse & oyle of roses .

HEnnebane ys cleped Iusq⌞i⌟amus & yn latyn caniculata þys *f.78r* herbe ys seyde to be ryght cold of þys herbe þere || ben thre maners One hath a whyte floure . The ij bryngyth forthe a samrede floure . but þe thrydde hath ablak floure she þ*at* beryth the whyte seed ys bett*er* & nobler þan þe toþer thoo . But yf þys may not be founde men taken of hym þ*at* beryth þe same redde floure . The leches þ*at* now ben wol not

---

2319 Morell] <u>xuiij</u> *ext. marg.* **2329** ycche] for þe yche *ext. marg. H3* **2334** herpeta mordax] for þe fyer on legg*s* *ext. marg. H3* **2337** Hennebane] <u>xix</u> *ext. marg.*

2333 plaster] past*er* MS.

worche *with* hyr þ*at* hath þe blak floure . The fyrst u*er*tu þe woman whos brestes aken . drynke she Iuys of hyr þ*at* beryt þe whyte floure & after warde anoynte she hyr brestes al aboute *with* þe same Iuys & she shal be alle hool . The ij u*er*tu Grynde smal þe leues of þys herbe & floure to gyder Aplast*er* of þys wol abate al maner bolnynges & þe hoot podagre . The iij u*er*tu þe Iuys helde ynne atte ere wol sle þe wormes þ*at* ben yn he*m* & abate many oþer doloures & dysseses of þe eres . The iiij u*er*tu It ys sayde þ*at* þe uenygre yn wyche þe rotes of þys herbe hath be soden ynne wol abate þe tothe ache though yt be gret . yf þys uenygre be luke . & hold longe yn þe mothe . The u u*er*tu || þe Iuys wrongen *f.78v* oute of þe seed of þys herbe whan yt ys grene grounden smal wol abate þe uyscouse & hoot rewme . yf þe pacyent anoynte ofte hys eyen þerw*ith* . The uj u*er*tu a scruple of þys seed & as muche of myconye seed drunken to gyder yn mulsa wol staunche þe fluxe of þe matryce . The uij u*er*tu men sayn þ*at* þys same drynke may helpe hem þ*at* casten oute blode at mouthe yf yt be oftyme y drunke . The uiij u*er*tu þe seed of henne bane grounde small *with* wyne & þer of madde aplast*er* wol hele þe tetes & þe ballockes of al bolnynges . The ix u*er*tu þys herbe & hyr seed allso doth muche good yn plastres & medycynes . But yf she be eten as wortes she wol brenge hyr eters ynto þ*at* maner of wodenes þ*at* ys cleped manya . And also wol hyr Iuys do yf yt be helde yn to a wonde what soeuere yt be .

OLde men sayn þ*at* þe hocke ys seyd malua for þy þ*at* she makyt þe wombe solubles . Sextus niger & also diascorydes sayt þ*at* þys ys euel for þe stomak but ether of hem sayth þ*at*

2345 brestes] for þe acke of brests of women *ext. marg. H3* **2349** hoot…2350 podagre] for þe hote podagre *ext. marg. H3* **2354** tothe ache] for þe toth acke *ext. marg. H3* **2370** Olde men] xx *ext. marg.*

f.79r yf she be eten as wortes she doth muche good to || al þe partyes þ*at* ben wit*h* yn ama*n*nys body The ij u*er*tu þus þey sayn yt wol do good to þe bladre & destroye all uenemouse drynkes . The iij u*er*tu these tweyn leches sayn þ*at* a plast*er* of hocke leues & of whyt uylowe . or wythy leues leche many of þe toon & of þe toþ*er* wol hele a bledyng wonde raþer & bett*er* þan oþer precyouse plastres . The iiij u*er*tu þey sayn also þat þe malowe grounde wit*h* olde grece helpyth myghtyly brusynges . The u u*er*tu þe root of þe malowe stok putte unto þe tothe þ*at* akyth . abatyth þe ache as yt ys seyde . The uj u*er*tu yf a wo*m*man bere an hocke root lapped yn blak wolle & bounden wit*h* flexe unto hyr thye . shal haue no dyssese yn hyr tetes . The uij u*er*tu It is wryte . þ*at* þys herbe wol dryue oute of a wo*m*ma*n* hyr deed chylde yf gose grece be medled þerwit*h* . & þan þey be sette under þe kunte as yt were a pessarye . The uiiij u*er*tu Grynde hocke leues wit*h* alytel salte & þ*at* wol destroye thylke lepre þ*at* ys cleped *f.79v* Egilop . The ix u*er*tu wit*h* hocke Iuys þow || mayst hele þe stynggynges of bees . And yf þow medle þe Iuys wit*h* oyle no bees shul noyen þe . yf þow a noynte þere wit*h* þy body . The x u*er*tu sethe malowes yn pysse & leye þ*at* to þyn heed . so shalt þow destroye þe foule nayles þ*at* waxen yn þe heed . & eke þe noyous scroof . or scalle þat ys called furfur . And þe same plast*er* wol quenche þe holy fyre & hele bry*n*nyges . The xj u*er*tu þe decocc*io*n of malowes . wol make nesshe þe hardnes of þe matryce & helpe þe causes & seknesse of þe guttes & of þe matryce & of þe erse wonderly wel . yf she be underputt to hem . The xij u*er*tu þys herbe prykyth & excytyth unto lecherye .

HEre endyth þe secu*n*de boke of macer . And now begy*n*nyth þe thrydde boke þe wyche tretyth of dyu*er*se spyces . And

2379 oþer] wol hele *exp.*

specyaly of {enleuene} moost used comounly yn nombre of þe wyche . Pepyr wi*th* hys u*er*tues ix ys þe fyrst .

Peletre . ij. ||
Com*m*yn . iij . f.80r
Galyngale . iiij .
Sedewale . u.
Cloue gylofre . uj.
Canell . uij .
Coste . uiij .
Spykenarde . ix .
ffrankencense . x .
Aloe . xj .

NOw haue I treted before of a fewe com*m*on herbes . Now wol I telle þe uertues of spyces þ*at* ben knowe almost unto al men . And wyche spyces leche crafte hath made knowe . And fyrst of pyp*er* þe wyche þe kychen hath made more knowen þan hath medycyne . It ys sayde þ*at* pep*er* ys hoot & drye bothe yn þe thrydde degre . Of pep*er* þere ben three maneres . Whyte . longe . & blak . But for þy þat tweyne ben knowe by us onlyche to || leches I wol telle of þe blak pep*er* a fewe u*er*tues þ*at* I knowe wel . The fyrst u*er*tu blak pep*er* soden or raw wi*th* hony medled . wol helpe þe myght of þe dygesty*ou*n of þe stomak . yt destroyeth þe greuance of þe mawe . The ij u*er*tu pep*er* wol hele deedly bytynges & many quareles & causes of þe brest . The iij u*er*tu It wol do away þe cold of þe feuer þ*at* ys cleped p*ar*odyda febrys . yf þe pacyent take yt before hys tremelyng . The iiij u*er*tu Grynde small lorer leues or hyr bayes & þys pep*er* to gydre & drynke all þuse luke warme þys wol staunche þe gnawynge yn þe bely . The u u*er*tu medle *þys* pep*er* wi*th* pycche & make of hem a plast*er* And þ*at* wol represse þe kernelles þ*at* ben called scrophee . The uj u*er*tu þys pep*er* ys good to be

(f.80v at line "knowe by us onlyche to || leches")

2404 enleuene] enlenene MS.

medled w*ith* alle þe medycyns þ*at* cleren þe eyen of her harde duskenes The uij u*er*tu Make of þys pep*er* & of nytrum aplastre & þ*at* wol do a way þe spites & frakles . The uiij u*er*tu þere ys no better ne p*ro*fytabler medycyne for þe || *f.81r* cancres as men sayn þ*at* han preued bothe þys & other . Take þan pouder of þys pep*er* & as muche of ma*n*nys dyrte brent un to pouder & melle wel boþe to gydre & þan leye yt uppon þe cancres . The ix u*er*tu no man may descreue ne tel þe u*er*tues of pep*er* þ*at* ys blak for yt wol ˪be˩ putte yn all medycynes almost . & for þy I trowe þ*at* þere be seyde þus fewe presynges of þys pep*er* allone . for yt ys so com*m*on to many precyouse medycynes ynnumerable .

PElletre ys hoot & drye yn þe fourþe degre . The fyrst u*er*tu yf a colde humour greue þe tethe & make hem ˪for˩ to ake . take & chewe wel pelletre on þ*at* toþe þat akyth & holde yt longe yn þy mouthe & þ*at* wol helpe yt . The ij u*er*tu In þys wyse yt repressyth þe bolnynge of þe tunge þ*at* comyth of fleume . & reryth up þe uua yf she be fallen doun w*ith* ouer muche humores . to many other uyces of þe mouthe . yt doth good yn þys wyse The iij u*er*tu It doth muche good & p*ro*fyt *f.81v* || to hem þ*at* han þe fallynge euel yf yt be eten or drunke yn hony . And also yt puttyth away þe palesey . The iiij u*er*tu It ys seyde þ*at* peletre honged a boute chyndryn neckes þ*at* han þe fallynge euell wol hele hem . And yt wol helpe hem also by hys odour allone . The u u*er*tu a noynte þy body w*ith* oyle þ*at* þys peletre ys soden ynne before þe accesse of þe feuere & so shalt þow mynuce & destroye þe sturdynesse of þe feuere . The uj u*er*tu þys oynement wol dryue a way þe ache ˪of þe˩ reynes . The uij u*er*tu þys oynement wol wonderly helpe to þe palesye yf þe pacyent be ofte þer w*ith* yfroted w*ith* hondes somdele harde & þys onynement wol make al hys body souple & esy . The uiij u*er*tu þys wol make þe swote to renne

2439 þe] cancres *bot. marg.* **2448** Pelletre] ii *ext. marg.*

oute largyly atte pores & opene hem . The ix u*er*tu þys wol
also hele þe stonynge of þe lymes . The x u*er*tu þys wol kepe
also þe body from colde . The xj u*er*tu þys wol dyssolue þe
dyssese & contracc*io*n þat ys cleped tethan*us* . The xij u*er*tu
as muche good doth þe peletre yt self grounde small w*ith* oyle
yf || yf þow anoynte & frote wel þe place þerw*ith* þat þow *f.82r*
wolt amende of þe dyssese & do medycyne to . Gyngyuer ys
of þe self u*er*tu yn medycynes þat ys peper . And þerefore y
speke no more of yt .

Comyn as leches sayn ys bothe hote & drye yn þe iij degre .
The fyrst u*er*tu as leches sayn þ*a*t comyn ytake yn eny wyse
wol destroye þe wynde þat greueth þe bowels & þe stomak .
The ij u*er*tu þey sayn also þ*a*t yt excytyth hugely þe hete of
þe stomak & of þe mawe þe wyche heete makyth
dygestyo*u*n . The iij u*er*tu þey sayn also þ*a*t yt destroyeth þe
lust of lecherye . The iiij u*er*tu It wol also bynde þe wombe
þ*a*t ys laxe yf yt be soden yn uenygre . The u u*er*tu comyn
drunke ofte ⌞*with*⌟ pusca wol helpe he*m* wonderly þ*a*t ben
cleped ortonoici . Pusca ys whos twey partes be water & þe
thrydde uenygre ⌞or⌟ stronge wyne . The uj u*er*tu þys I
drunke w*ith* wyne ys good for uenemous bytynges . yf þys
comyn be grounde small & medled w*ith* been mele . || The *f.82v*
uij u*er*tu Comyn grounde smal w*ith* hony wol abate sodenly
þe bolnynges of þe ballockes yf yt be leyde to hem . The uiij
u*er*tu comyn drunke w*ith* pusca wol staunche wo*m*mens
floures . The ix u*er*tu comyn eten alytel & a lytel wol make
hem euel couloured þat eten yt .

Galyngale resoluyth þe flume of þe stomak yf yt be eten And
yf he be fleumatyke þat etyth yt . yt confyrmyth & strengthe
hym . The ij u*er*tu galyngale eten or drunken dryuyth oute þe
wynde þ*a*t ys closed yn þe bowles w*ith* yn furthe . The iij
u*er*tu It helpyth þe dygestyon & doth medycynes to coleryca

2477 Comyn] iij *ext. marg.* **2495** Galyngale] iiij *ext. marg.*

passio . The iiij u*er*tu It amendyth þe sauoure & odoure of þe mouthe yf yt be eten ofte

Cedewale as leches sayen wol do huge remedye ayenst uenenis þat men han eten or drunke . The ij u*er*tu drynke cedewale & yt wol hele þe bytynges of crepynge bestes . The iij u*er*tu It confortyth þe stomak yf yt be eten ofte & *f.83r* destroyeth þe dysseses of þe brayne || & puttyth away þe noyus wynde by bolny*n*ge & worchyth men muche hele . The iiij u*er*tu yf he þ*at* hath longe dyssese yn hys stomak & doloure wol chue yn hys mouthe fastynge cedewale & swolwe doun lytel & lytel yn to hys body hys spotel & þe moysture þ*at* fallyth yn hys mouthe thorugh þys yt wol hele hym of hys doloure . The u u*er*tu þys drunke wol destroye wormes yn þe wombe . And yt doth oute of þe mouthe þe stynche of garlycke & þe greet sauoure of wyne . þ*at* leueth yn a body whanne he {dry*n*kyt} muche wyne .

Cloue gilofre as men sayn ys hoot & drye yn þe secunde degre . The fyrst u*er*tu cloues drunke wol conforte & strynthe þe stomak & þe mawe And yt ys good almost to alle þe entrayles of man The ij u*er*tu It helpeth underly þe degestyon & makyt þe wombe coste . The iij u*er*tu a dragme weyght of þe pouder of cloues drunke wol scure to lechyrye . The iiij u*er*tu þe cloues grounden smal & drunke wit*h* fresshe cowe mylke oftentymes wol conforthe þe memorie & *f.83v* þe brayne yn þe || whyche ys þe myght of þe mynde .

CAnel hat thre spyces but þe best of hem ys she þ*at* ys most sotell & þe wyche bytyth best þe tunge & hath þer wit*h* a maner of swetnes . The fyrst u*er*tu It dryeth up þe humoures of þe stomak & confo⌞r⌟teth yt & strengyth yt . The ij u*er*tu

---

2502 Cedewale] u *ext. marg.*
2516 Cloue gilofre] uj *ext. marg.*
2525 Canel] uij *ext. marg.*

2515 drynkyt] dy*n*kyt MS.

þys wol make þe stomak for to defye sone metes & drynkes þat ben yn yt . The iij u*er*tu canel eten eyther drunke helyth þe lyuer purgyth wo*m*mens floures & makyth for to pysse faste . The iiij u*er*tu canel wol stau*n*che þe moyst cowhe & þe pose . The u u*er*tu þys wol represse þe spyce of þe dropesye þe wyche ys clepyd Tympana & þe ache of þe reynes also . And hele þe bytynges of crepyng bestes . The uj u*er*tu yf canell be Ioyned to þe medycynes þ*a*t helen þe eyen yt dryeth up þe wyckyd humoures & watery . The uij u*er*tu Canel grounden wel small & meled w*ith* stronge uynygre & y leyde to wol delyuer þe face of blake spottes & frakles & also destroye þe syknesse & þe scabbe þat ys y cleped Impetigo || The uiij u*er*tu Grynde wel & smal canell & tweyne dragmes *f.84r* of þys pouder drunke w*ith* colde water wol staunche þe fluxe of þe Emoraudes yf yt be drunke fastynge .

COste hath twey maners one ys heuy & red & þ*a*t comyth oute of Inde . That other ys lyght & not bytt*er* & somdele whyte yn coloure þys comyth outo of Inde . The fyrst ys moor p*ro*fytable þan ys þys . The fyrst u*er*tu þuse bothe purgen urynes & putten away tho þ*a*t wyth stonden hem þey curen þe splen & þe lyuer & dryuen away þe ache of þe sydes yf þe pacyent drynke hem yn swete wyne . The ij u*er*tu þuse wol purgen wo*m*mens floures yf þe woman make þere of a subfumygac*i*on And yn þe same wyse þey wol staunche þe ache of þe kunte yf þe woman putte under hyr a pessarye of these . The iij u*er*tu Grynde smal þuse w*ith* wyne & þys ornement or oynement . wol purge & clense þe face of frakeles & putte oute þe wormes of þe bely . The iiij u*er*tu þuse wole scure to lechyry yf þey be drunke yn mulsa þ*a*t ys leuke . || The u u*er*tu þe oyle þ*a*t coste ys soden ynne wol *f.84v* destroye & put away þe colde of þe feuer yf þe pacyent be anoynted þer w*ith* before þat þe cold come uppon hym . The

---

2544 Coste] uiij *ext. marg.*

uj u*er*tu þys oynement ys a souereyn medycyne for scietica passio & to þe {membres} þat ben astoned . The uij u*er*tu þe pouder of þys herbe wol hele an olde wonde wel & sone .

SPykenarde ys hoot & drye as wyse men sayn . The fyrst u*er*tu þe decocc*i*on of þys spicys y drunke co*m*fortyth þe mawe & a batyth þe doloures of þe stomak & purgyth þe reynes . The ij u*er*tu It helpyth þe bladder It dryueth oute bothe wo*m*ma*n*s floures & þe uryn . The iij u*er*tu It doth good to hem þat han þe Iaundyse yt wit*h* stondyth þe euel humo*urs* þ*a*t fallen fro þe brest by þe uua . The iiij u*er*tu It doth away þe pryckynges & bytynges of þe entrales . The u u*er*tu spykenarde drunke wol dryue outhe þe wynde þ*a*t ys closed wit*h*yn þe stomak And yf she be underput . she wol staunche þe fluxe of þe matryce . The uj u*er*tu spykenarde *f.85r* drunke wit*h* colde water || wol abate bolnynges of þe herte & staunche brakynges . The uij u*er*tu spik*n*arde drunke wit*h* thylke lycore þ*a*t ys cleped sapa . wol excyte to lechyre . yf yt be ofte ydrunke . The uiij u*er*tu þe decocc*i*on of þys spycys woll resolue þe hardenesse of þe matryce . yf þe mouthe of þe matryce be oftymes beked þere ynne . The ix u*er*tu Anoynte ofte þyn eyen wit*h* þ*a*t decocc*i*on leuke & yt wol destroye þe bytt*er* akynge of hem & þe heres of lyddes ben hugely comforted þer wit*h* . There ys amaner of narde þ*a*t ys cleped nardus celtica . Thys growyth oonly yn þe Rygyon of peple þ*a*t ys cleped þe peple of celte . Thys narde may do alle tho thynges þ*a*t may spykenarde . though men seme þ*a*t yt hat lasse uertu yn myght þan hath spykenarde .

FRankencence ys bothe hoote & dry yn þe ij degre . The fyrst u*er*tu encense claryfyeth þe syght . yf yt be resolued yn þe whyte of an eye or y gro*u*nde smal wit*h* fresse wo*m*mans

---

2564 Spykenarde] ix *ext. marg.* **2588** Frankencence] x *ext. marg.*

2562 membres] menbres MS.

mylke . The ij || u*er*tu men sayen þ*at* encense y grunden *f.85v* small w*ith* uenygre & melled w*ith* piche or fresshe melke wol hele soueraynly newe wondes & fresshe . The iij u*er*tu encense medled w*ith* {swynes} grece ys good for brennynges . The iiij u*er*tu medlde encense w*ith* hony & yt wol do away þe dyssese of þe nayles þe wyche dyssese ys cleped pannaricu*m* . The u u*er*tu me*n* sayn þ*at* encense grunde smal . & resolued wel yn leuke wyne wol do muche good to þe ere þ*at* akyth . The uj u*er*tu encense grounden smal w*ith* creta chimolea & medled w*ith* oyle of roses wol hele þe bolnynges of þe tetys . The uij u*er*tu leches trowen þ*at* þere be no þynge bett*er* for hem þ*at* speten blode þan ys encense drunke w*ith* wyne or w*ith* uenygre . The uiij u*er*tu Aplast*er* of encense grou*n*de w*ith* wo*m*mans mylke wol hele þe bocches þ*at* waxyn yn þe ere or yn eny oþ*er* place . The ix u*er*tu take encense & aloe & þe clere of þe whyte of an eye grynde þ*at* to gydre tyl yt be thyk & leye þys plaster to a ueyne þ*at* ys kutte . & do yt not away tyl þow trowe þ*at* þe kerfe be closed || to gydyr fast And yf yt be need . leey þys *f.85r*[b] medycyne uppon yt ayen tyl þat þere be a sadde seme upon þe place þ*at* was y kutte . Men sayn þ*at* no þyng may stau*n*che bett*er* blode a wonde þan may þys forseyde medycyne . The x u*er*tu encense comfortyth þe myght of þe mynde by hys odoure . The xj u*er*tu who so chewyth encense & pulyoll haund to gydre . yt wol do away alle wycked humours of þe heed by spettynge . The xij u*er*tu þys purgac*io*n of þe heed wol alyghte þe tunge þ*at* ys heuy . The xiij u*er*tu aplast*er* made of encense of gose grece eyþer dokes grece wol hele þe membres þat fyre hath y brent ouþ*er* hurte .

THere ben tow maneres of Aloe þat oon ys somdele whyte inne as lyuer whan yt ys y broke . And þ*ys* ys cleped aloe

---

2620 There ben] xj *ext. marg.*

2594 swynes] swnes MS.

epaticu*m* . And þys hath gret u*er*tu & strynthe yn medycynes That oþer ys of pycke coloure whan yt ys y broke þys ys of lasse u*er*tues yn medycynes . The fyrst u*er*tu aloe mun || *f.85v*^{b} dyfyeth þe stomak of flume & þe heed also And þys yt doth yn purgynge & dryuynge oute ryghtly by þe wombe noyous humours . The ij u*er*tu It purgyth hem þ*a*t han þe Iaundyse & yt helpyth þe ynner partyes of þe mawe . The iij u*er*tu þys wol helpe euery fresshe wonde fro*m* all rotynge yf þ*a*t þe pouder of yt be caste yn to þe wonde . And yn drynke yt wol helpe up safly . The iiij u*er*tu þys pouder wol specyaly hele þe bocches of þe wombe & of þe ballokes also as men sayn . The u u*er*tu aloe resolued yn water & leyde uppon þe leppes helpyth þe postomes of hem & of þe nose yf yt be leyde þere uppon And from þe eyen yt dryuyth away þe wannesse of hem . yf yt be a noynted aboute þe eyen . The uj u*er*tu aloe medled wit*h* uenygre & oyle of roses wol destroye þe heed ache yf þe frount be anoynted þerwit*h* . The uij u*er*tu þys oynement wol staunche þe ache of þe eyen . The uiij u*er*tu *f.86r* aloe || grunde small wit*h* wyne & hony wol helpe þe go*m*mes & þe tunge & þe uyces of þe mouthe yf þey be froted wel & ofte þer wit*h* . The ix u*er*tu aloe taken by hym self allone wol not solue þe wombe . but uribasius holdyth yt good to þe stomak . sethen al medycynes þ*a*t soluen þe wombe . doon harme to þe stomak {out taken} Aloe . The x u*er*tu he byddyth for to take twye dragmes of aloe wit*h* mulsa & yt wol purge bothe þe colre & þe flume . The xj u*er*tu urybasyus sayth þ*a*t yt were good & holsom for to take yche day after sowper thre pilles or tweyne . formed wit*h* þe Iuys of grene caule . of þe grettnesse of a been . Thys wol putte oute & purge þe wyckyd humo*ur*s wit*h* þe dyrte . not corrumpynge þe stomak ne doynge eny uyolence . The xij u*er*tu he þ*a*t ys ofte purgyd wit*h* þuse pilles . shal ounnethe eny tyme fele þe heed ache . The xiij u*er*tu & truste to me

---

2645 out taken] oun taken MS.

þere ys no þyng moor p*ro*fytable un to þe eyen þan ys þys
medycyne . The xiiij u*er*tu yf þow wolt solue || þe wombe þ*at* *f.86v*
ys costyf . un to two partyes of aloe . take oon parte of dyagredyu*m* & grynde hem wel to gydre & þys medycyne ys a noble & worþy laxatyf .

HEre endyth þe laste boke of Macer . Now folewen here after afewe dyu*er*se herbes þe wyche ben not yfunde yn þe bokes of Macer . And of tho ben foure and twenty yn nombre brefly or shortly wreton .

Of þe whyche sanicle ys þe . i
Baldemoyne . ij
Tansey . iij
Lauryel . iiij
Lyquoryce . u
Notemygge . uj
Myrtus . uij
Saffero*un* . uiij
Careway . ix
Saxifrage . x
Benette . xj
Diteyne . xij
Federfoy . xiij ||
Bawme . xiiij *f.87r*
Mille morbia . xu
Nepe . xuj
Radiche . xuij
Sclayre . xuiij
ffemygreke . xix
Gyth . xx
Alara . xxj
Ualeryan . xxij
Lupinus . xxiij
Ambrosia . xxiiij

SAnicle ys so called . for she helyth wondes . The fyrst u*er*tu þys herbe wol seche bothe boon & wonde & yn þe wonde wol she shewe hyr all suche as þe pacyent drynkyth hyr . But I moneste te þ*a*t þow be ryght wel ware how þow drynkest þys herbe . ffor she comyth not oute of þe wonde . she as cendyth yn to þe heed & yn to þe brayne & brekyt þe skyn of þe brayne þ*a*t ys y clepyd pia mater & so she sleeth þe pacye*nt* . ||

f.87v BAldemoyne helpyth þe hert releuyth þe brest & norysshyt þe stomak . Baldemoyne y founde yn þe myry doth yn medycynys all þ*a*t oþer boughte medycynes doon . Baldemoyne y uethte frely . wyche þ*a*t oþer medycynes yeuen for huge & gret pryse .

TAnsey though yt be bytter . yit yt ys a good medycyne to þe brest & alyght . The ij u*er*tu It purgyth not only þe bryst . but all þe pares wi*th* yn ama*n*nys body .

LAuriall ys lyke un to lorer bothe yn hys rynde & yn hys leues & eke yn hys greenesse . Thys herbe ys euermore grene she ne welkyth for noon heete of þe sonne . ne fadyth for noo colde . Persins cleped þe seed of þys herbe Cononidion & so don many poetes & leches also . Of þys seed ys made a noble pocyoun . þe wyche purgyth by þe nether partyes of a man all þe ynner partyes of a manys body whath so euer greue þe stomak . or þe bowels or þe lightes . Thys herbe wol helpe & hele yf eny grete {greu*u*se} cause make þat a pocyou*n* p*ro*fyte nott to sykenesse . nowonder . for why leche

f. 88r crafte || takyth nothyng þ*a*t ys alway soth . & ou*er*all be fall

---

2688 Sanicle] j *ext. marg.* **2696** Baldemoyne] Baldemoyne Baldmoy *top marg.* | ij *ext. marg.* **2701** Tansey] iij *ext. marg.* **2704** Lauriall] iiij *ext. marg.* **2714** crafte] takyth *bot. marg.*

2712 greuuse] grou*u*se MS.

men lyke . but natheles þys pocyoun shal neuere do eny harme .

Lyquoryce ys swettyst of all herbes Thys ys of so temp*er*at kynde þat she ys unnethe moyst . ne unnethe colde . unnethe she may be yn þe fyrst degre of these two . Thys ys good to all causes . & to noon harme full wherfor she may say to mankynde I am youre helthe . The fyrst u*er*tu þe decocc*io*n of *þys* lyquoryce medled wi*th* penydyes . & eten of þe pacyent . wol purge & moste þe syke lunges . þe wyked kowhe . þe hard & streyght brest . þe sore throtes . & þe sore ueynes of þe uoyce . There ys no þyng þat purgyth so wel þe brest . as doth þys medycyne . The ij u*er*tu lyquoryce soden yn water tyl she be nesshe . þan pressyd wel & ofte ydryed . ys cleped helum whan yt ys þus ydryed . þys wol helpe þe lunges & a bate þe || styfnesse . & þe dysseses of yt . There ys *f.88v* no spyce so p*ro*fytable un to þe stomak whan yt ys brent as ys þys . The iiij u*er*tu no medycyn hylpyth swyfther þe ynstrumentys of þe lunges . ne of þe brest . þan doth lyq*u*orice . Thuse ynstrumentes helpyth lyq*u*oryce wonderfully . not yn turmentynge . as doth coste ne yn fretynge as doth aloe . but yn softe lyky*n*ges .

THe Notemygge ys bothe hoot & drye yn þe secunde degre . The fyrst u*er*tu þys curyth þe styngkynge mouthe & staunchyth þe fluxe & byndyth þe wombe . It strengthyth þe lyuer . & þe stomak yt helpyth . The ij u*er*tu It puttyth oute þe wynde þ*at* greuyth þe entrayles . & yt encrescyth good dygesty*ou*n . The iij u*er*tu Galyen sayth þ*at* þe notemygge makyth fayre þe skynne . It curyth þe splene . & eke þe bolnynge of þe lyuer . The iiij u*er*tu þys wol ouercome þe

---

2717 Lyquoryce] u *ext. marg.* **2736** The Notemygge] uj *ext. marg.*

f.89r goute {maysterly} . as yt ys seyd || It wol also clense wondes fayre & wel .

MIrtus ys abunda*u*nt yn þe fer northe she growyth yn colde myres . & yet she ys hoot yn kynde . The fyrst take þe decocc*io*n of myrte w*ith* tisane & w*ith* þe Iuys of play*n*teyn . sethe hem to gydre yn to þe thrydde parte þys wol hele þe blody menyson And syke men þ*a*t ben cleped Ciliaci . If þow wolt take p*er*auenture boldely a moor strenger medycyne wolt abate þe fretynges of þe body yf yt be nede .

SAfferon ys good to putte away sykenesse & to metes also & unto many oþer dyuerse þynges . The fyrst u*er*tu saferon floures medled w*ith* wo*m*mans mylke . & kepte longe . wol hele sore eyen . yf þey be anoynted þer w*ith* . And yt wol also destroye uenym . The ij u*er*tu medle safro*u*n & frankencense & kockull & sethe hem to gydre yn mulsa & þan leye he*m* all unto the thyghe þ*a*t ys greued w*ith* scietica passio & þ*ys* wol dryue away þat dyssese . ||

f.89v CArewey & Cerfoyle ben lyke yn couloure . yn fygure or shap & u*er*tu . Ca reweye ys ryght hoot & sharpe . Careweye leues ben of cerulde colowre . & so ben þe sedes of Cerfoyle . Cerules ys yelowe as waxe or grene . or blak to gydre . as p*ro*pyrly whan yelowe ys seie w*ith* blak as ys þe seed . Carewey leues ben ragged & so ben also Cerfoyle leues . The fyrst u*er*tu þys delyueryth & bryngyth furthe hastely wo*m*mens floures & yt hath aryght wel lykynge sauoure and tast .

SAxifrage ys so ynamed . for she brekyt þe stone So*m*me me*n* clepen yt petrocylyum . The fyrst u*er*tu Grynde to gydre Saxifrage & cherystones & yeue þ*a*t hym to drynke þ*a*t hath

---

2746 Mirtus] uij *ext. marg.* **2753** Safferon] uiij *ext. marg.*
2761 Carewey] ix *ext. marg.* **2769** Saxifrage] x *ext. marg.*

2744 maysterly] maystely MS. **2765** blak] to gydre *exp.*

þe stone yn hot water . ffor þe tendre stone þere ys noo bett*er* medycyne as me*n* sayn . But for þe harde stone of longe tyme y gadred . þow moost take a strenger medycyne The ij u*er*tu leches sayn þ*a*t yt ys holsom to hem þat han þe feuers . ||

Benette ys cleped harys heer . The fyrste u*er*tu þys wol clense *f.90r* a wonde & after warde clense yt w*ith* good flesshe & coloure yt wel . The ij u*er*tu It ys good for þe goute .

Dytayne ys abunda*un*t yn þe southe . uirgil sayth whan Eneas was y shot w*ith* an arowe he cowde not haue yt oute w*ith* drawynge And þan he putte þe wonde ful of dyteyne & þ*a*t drowe þe arowe hed oute .

FEderfoye ys so cleped . for she dryueth away þe feuers . & þer of dowted neuer leche . And yn þys wyse ys hyr name sette yn olde bokes .

BAwme ys ryght fayre & wel sauorynge swote yn smellynge . Thys was cleped som tyme Ceralis . som tyme simbria . The fyrst u*er*tu for þe feuere yeue þe pacyent two scripules of þys drynke yn hoot water . The ij u*er*tu If þow haue an ache or dyssese yn þe bladder or þe strangurye þe wyche streynyth þe wayes & þe places of || þe uryn . þ*a*t yt makyth aman ofte to *f.90v* haue dyffyculte to pysse . þan drynke he w*ith* wyne þe Iuys of þys herbe & he shal be all hoolle .

MIllemorbia ys so called . for she ys good for a thowsand syknesse & she ys cleped also other whyse Nymfee & su*m*tyme fyala . The fyrst u*er*tu þys ys as good to wondes . as ys comfery & bett*er* . The ij u*er*tu In þe maner of rewe she claryfyth þe syght . The iij u*er*tu þys ys as good for þe wode goude as ys þ*a*t herbe þ*a*t ys cleped auricula leporyna . The

---

2776 Benette] xj *ext. marg.*
2779 Dytayne] xij *ext. marg.*
2783 Federfoye] xiij *ext. marg.*
2786 Bawme] xiiij *ext. marg.*
2794 Millemorbia] xu *ext. marg.*

iiij u*er*tu þe herbe þ*at* hath þe name salisea . dryueth not away ne destroyeth colde uenym ne bett*er* þan doth þ*ys* herbe . The u u*er*tu It hath y*n*numerable u*er*tues .

NEpe ys cleped yn latyn Raphan*us* Thys herbe ys good for þe cancre yn þys wyse . ffyrst bynde to þe cancre a frosshe . all þe tyme of a nyght þys wol so wonderly co*n*sume & drye up þe
f.91r cancre þ*at* þow shalt haue won || der by þe morwe so drye þe skyn shal be . Than take away þ*at* & leye to yt þe nepe root kowe pysse . þe floure of rye & þuse wol sle þe strengthe & al þe myght of þe cancre . þan hele þow up þe cancre . as þow woldest hele a noþer wo*n*de & yn þe same wyse .

RAdiche hat þe same or lyke u*er*tu to þe nepe . but yt ys alytel weyker . The fyrst u*er*tu þys ys good for to make abody wel for to pysse . The ij u*er*tu þys co*m*fortyth þe brest & strengthyth all þe ynner partyes w*ith* yn a mans body . The iij u*er*tu . who so etyth þe root of þys herbe yn thylke tyme þ*at* Mars regnyth yt wol lenþe hys lyfe .

Sclayre as leches sayen ys good for þe hoot goute . The ij u*er*tu sclayre claryfyeth her uoyce þ*at* ben hoos And she ys ryght good bothe to þe lunges & to þe mawe & to þe bowelles . And ful many other good uertues She . hayth . ||

f.91v FEmygreke wol make nesshe þe postemes bocches & resolue þe knobbes & gaderyng to gyder wol do þys by hys oon . but yt wol daunte yt þe bett*er* . w*ith* hockes & wylde malowe . The ij u*er*tu a plastre of femygreke lynsede & floure wol destroye thylke euel cleped Eucatesma . The iij u*er*tu a plast*er* of femygreke & of caule grounden smal wol make esy & nesshe þe euel & þe aches þat ben cleped arthetici dolores . wyche ben goutes & yt hylpyth to þe podagre .

2803 Nepe] xuj *ext. marg.* **2811** Radiche] xuij *ext. marg.*
2817 Sclayre] xuiij *ext. marg.* **2821** Femygreke] xix *ext. marg.*

Gyth hath foure corners or pykes eyþer hornes growynge upwarde coddes yt hath . & yn hem cornes whyche maken bred byt*er* . It ys good for many causes .

ASara ys bytwene an herbe & a tree The fyrst u*er*tu þys wol aswage do laures þat ben w*ith* ynne þe body & aches . The ij u*er*tu grynde smal þe rotes of þys herbe & drynke hem w*ith* wyne þys wol anoon drawe gret uomytes & putte away þe syknesse . But þys medycyne || shalt þow not do but where *f.92r*
þow seest þ*a*t oþer medycynes p*ro*fyten not for þys ys a gret & stronge medycyne .

UAleryan ys of gret u*er*tu . she hath a gret top & smal sedes . A porcyo*u*n of hyr y grou*n*den smal . ys good for many causes . Thys y drunke w*ith* wyne wol wanysshe þe from the feuers .

LUpinus ys an herbe þ*a*t growyth a boute yn þe feldes þ*a*t beryth large & sharpe pryckes . who so etyth þys yn potage he shal not be drunke lyghtly Take þys lupyn & wermode & þe hey hony . of eueryche ylke muche medle hem wel to gydyr & þys pocyoun wol sle wormes yn the bely .

AMbrosia wol dryue oute of þe body þ*a*t bledyth ynwarde . as muche blod as þe pacyent drynkyt Iuys of þys herbe .

2829 Gyth] xx *ext. marg.* **2832** Asara] xxj *ext. marg.*
2839 Ualeryan] xxij *ext. marg.* **2843** Lupinus] xxiij *ext. marg.*
2848 Ambrosia] xxiiij *ext. marg.* **2849** herbe] Laus deo Amen . *ext. marg.*

1 Here] The text is headed by the traditional Christogram symbol of western Christianity, derived from the first three letters of the Gr. name of Jesus (*ie.* IHC). This divine monogram becomes a typical heading in many mediaeval manuscripts (see also GUL MS Hunter 328).

51 for...52 þat] Derived from OE causal marker *for þȳ þæt/for þǣm (þe)*, *for þy þat* becomes the most frequent causal conjunction in H497 (12×).

53 hath] Participial form of *yeven* 'to give' (see also 1988). According to the *LALME* (1986: 412), this is the characteristic form of *yeven* in the East Midlands.

54 þe wyche] Of northern origin, *the which* gained ground throughout the 14th century in southernly texts, to the extent that it became the most frequent relativiser, even more than plain *which*, in 15th-century prose (Mustanoja 1960: 198-199). It mostly occurs with non-personal reference, and in non-restricted clauses (Raumolin-Brunberg 2000: 212).

65 An] Reduced form of conjunction *and*, a characteristic form in the middle south of England (McIntosh et al. 1986, IV: 313). See also 803 and 1734.

69 make...pysse] The verb *maken* is elsewhere followed by a *to*-infinitive in H497, in examples like *make þy nose to blede* (204), *make þe to swete* (224), *make þe skyn to glytere* (537-38), etc.

71 medleyt] The neuter pronoun *yt* is sporadically linked to the verb, *ie. beyt* (444) and *streyneyt* (737).

78 It...seyde] Even though somewhat frequent in the early ME period, impersonal passives became more and more common towards the end of the period (Mustanoja 1960: 438). It becomes a recurrent construction in H497, as shown in 309-310; 394-395; 756; 878-879; 1697-1698; 1827; 1965; 1984; 2353; 2421; 2458-2459; etc.

80 mogwort] Even when vowel <u> predominates (*mugwort(e)* 4×), to avoid the sequence of minims vowel <o> is also an orthographic variant, though preserving the same high back vowel as in OE *mucg-wyrt*.

87 mayny] Although considered an erroneous spelling of lemma *manī* in the *e-MED*, this variant is localised in *LALME* as a unique spelling of the county of

Essex (McIntosh et al. 1986, IV: 27). Its occurrence is, however, sporadic in H497 (1×) if compared with the standard form *many* (52×).

92 be] The use of the subjunctive mood gains ground throughout the 13th and 14th centuries in conditional clauses depending on a main clause in the indicative, particularly in texts of northern influence. In southern dialects, however, the indicative is still active until late in the 15th century (see Mustanoja 1960: 469). In light of the East Midlands provenance of H497, the text shows a prevalent use of the subjunctive mood in this type of clauses (see also 292).

99 entrall] Derived from OF *entraille* and eventually from ML *intrālia*, this word shows two different stems in H497. The diphthongised forms *entrails/entrayles/entraylles* (12×) are of French origin whilst monophthongal forms like *entrall/entrales* (3×) replicate the spelling of the Latinate cognate.

106 leymes] Derived from OE *lim* (masc.), this word is rendered in ME by means of vowels <i, y>, the latter preferred in the neighbourhood of minims. In H497, the standard spelling of this word is *lym(m)es* (5×). According to Jordan (1974: 234-235), the 15th century witnesses a neutralizing process by means of which *i* > *e*, especially before a nasal consonant. This explains the use of *leymes*.

111 eyen] The author fluctuates between the use of the strong and the weak plurals (*eyes* vs. *eyen*). Still, weak plurals predominate, as *–n* forms amount to 40 occurrences, if compared with a single occurrence of the strong plural morpheme *-(e)s*.

120 euere so] Used as a generalising relative, *what* is often reinforced by means of *euer so* 'in whatever so manner', where *wyse* splits *wat* and *euere* (Mustanoja 1960: 192-193).

131 shalt þu] V – S order is generally observed after adverbs, particularly those of time, place, and manner, *i.e. afterwarde, allone, also, as, better, elles, how, not, now, ofte(n), propyrly, so, þan, þere, þerwith, þus, unneþe* and *wherto*. Several instances can be found in the text, as shown in 55-56; 61; 73; 150; 226-227; 512-513; 577; 1789; 2661; etc.

137 Ssho] In H497 feminine pronoun *she* (165×) predominates over *ssho* (1×). According to the *e-MED* and the *LALME*, the latter is considered to be a

typical form of the North and North-Midland dialects (McIntosh et al. 1986, IV: 7).

138 hym dare] Verb *durren* occurs in a subjectless clause wherein the animate experiencer (*hym*) is in the oblique case. Although common in OE, this construction was rarely used in ME, being eventually superseded by those with a nominative subject (Molencki 2005: 149). In H497, a nominative experiencer is also found in the construction *þey dare not goo* (1062).

149 eny] The fronting of *eny* gives rise to the base order O – V – S, topicalised for emphasis. The author is methodical as to the use of this base order in this case of frontings. However, if a light-weight monosyllabic subject, the commonplace S – V order is the rule, as in 1840; 1847; etc.

150 goyn] Infinitival form of the verb *gōn*, wherein vowel <i> works as a diacritic to indicate vowel length, pronounced as /ɔ:/.

165 for…166 slepe] Even though originally an indicator of purpose, *for to* soon developed the function of an infinitive marker, to the extent that it is a mere alternative to a *to*-infinitive in the 13th century. From a statistical standpoint, this marker begins to lose ground throughout the 14th and 15th centuries, being eventually displaced by the *to*-infinitive construction. H497 contains a total of 53 occurrences of *for to*, a negligible figure if compared with the overwhelming preference for *to*-infinitives. Fischer (1992: 318-321) argues that *for to* constructions are, to some extent, favoured in particular contexts, *i.e.* if in subject position or if in reference to a future action.

166 un…167 wytyng] Absolute construction consisting of a pronoun in the oblique case (*hym*), functioning as the subject of the participle. An imitation of the Latin absolute ablative, this structure is rare in early ME. It spread again, however, from the second half of the 14th century, as a result of the powerful influence of French and Latin, gaining considerable ground by the second quarter of the 15th century, when the oblique case is superseded by the Nominative case (Mustanoja 1960: 114-115). In spite of this, H497 still shows the use of the oblique case in the latter part of that same century.

171 tonge] Even though *u*-forms predominate in H497, *i.e. tung(e)* (7×), *o*-forms are also found (2×) to avoid the sequence of minims.

174 sownyng] Vowel /u:/ rendered as <ou>/<ow>, the latter being just sporadic.

178 yn[2]] Preposition stranded given the impossibility for relativiser *that* to take pied-piping positions (Fischer 1992: 300). The second preposition, in turn, introduces the phrase *yn hys modrys wombe*. As a general rule, examples like this are mostly avoided in ME MS composition inasmuch as scribes recur to the use of a punctuation symbol, particularly the period, so as to avoid any likely misunderstanding. Preposition stranding is a frequent device in H497, as shown in 58; 411; 601; 819; 873; 940; 1353; 1424; 1483; 1492; 1508; 1735; 2008; etc.

181 wermode] From OE *wermōd/wærmōd/wyrmōd*, variant *wermod(e)* is the most representative (20×), followed by *wormod(e)* (10×) and *warmod(e)* (3×). The PDE form *wormwood*, according to the *OED*, is an altered form from the original *wermod*, interpreting a false association with *worm* + *wood*.

183 wreton] The strong participial morpheme *-on(e)* is, according to the *LALME*, a distinctive northern spelling even though also sporadically attested in the East and West Midlands, particularly in the latter (MacIntosh et al. 1986, I: 469). Despite the use of this form, the standard morpheme *–en* is the most frequent choice, as in *dronken* (193), *y sodden* (202), *eten* (389), etc.

189 for] The most frequent causal subordinator in H497 is *for/ffor* (60×), followed by *for þy (þat)* (12×), *for þat* (3×), *for by cause* (1×) and *for why* (1×).

193 of…herbe] Note the particular noun phrase order wherein the prepositional postmodifier *of þe self grene herbe* is topicalised for emphasis. The Stockholm MS shows *so is also þe self grene herbe ius* (Frisk 1949: 65). Plausibly stemming from a common source, the author of H497 preserved the original noun phrase order with the inclusion of the *of*-genitive, of a more widespread use in the 15th century.

197 parodyda] A Latinate borrowing from *parōtis*, *parōtidis*, rendered as *parodyda* (2430), *peryodyda* (2328), *parodycas* (1474). In contrast, there is just a single occurrence of the regular ME spelling *parotida* (329).

198 boon] The weak and the strong plural morphemes co-occur with noun *bōne* 'bone', although *-en* forms outnumber the plural form *bones*.

208 þe…nettell[2]] Compare the use of the *of*-genitive *þe Iuys of nettell* with the zero-morpheme *nettell leues* (Görlach 1991: 83).

211 þuse] Variant *þuse* 'these' (4×), either demonstrative, determiner or pronoun, is the characteristic variant of the South West, *i.e.* Devon, Dorset, Somerset and Gloucestershire, also spreading to areas of the South West Midlands, *i.e.* Hertford, Monmouth, Worcester and Warwickshire (McIntosh et al. 1986, IV: 6).

236 pylees] Verbal noun from ME *pilen* 'to remove the peel or rind from (sth.); to peel'. Note the use of digraph <ee> in unstressed position, which contrasts with the conventional spelling *pyles/pilles* used elsewhere in H497. In light of the absence of other similar instances, the digraph could be deemed as another writer's slip instead of *pyles*.

238 bytyn] Participial form of the verb *bīten* 'to bite, sting'. The *–yn* morpheme in strong verbs, together with *-in(e)* and *-yn(n)e*, is a characteristic feature of the East Midlands and the northern varieties of ME (McIntosh et al. 1986, I: 469).

244 To...same] As above, V – S order is also observed after a fronted adverbial adjunct, thus complying with the V2 rule of English, as shown in this example where the prepositional phrase *to the same* is fronted for emphatic purposes. This practice is frequently observed in H497, *i.e.* 380; 427; 559; 889; 1765; 1856; 2108-2109; etc.

260 Stampe] Plausibly from OE *stempan* 'to mash (an ingredient)', the ME form arises from *i*-umlaut before a nasal, hence *stempan* > *stampen* /stampən/ (Jordan 1974: 58).

270 sharpe...spere] Stereotyped comparison *as sharp as a spear* (see Calle-Martín 1996: 64-84).

276 fluxe] From OF *flux* (L *fluxus*). OF <u> /y/ persisted in the West Midlands, not merging with OE /y/ as the latter was perhaps more tense. In the other dialects, OF <u> /y/ was replaced by /u:/, represented as <u> or <i> /i/, hence two-foldly represented as *flux(e)* and *flyxe* (below) (Jordan 1974: 209). On a statistical basis, the former is more frequent (20×) if compared with *flyxe* (4×).

278 ache] The copula is inadvertently omitted. The Stockholm MS reads *þat is with ache* (Frisk 1949: 69).

284 cornels] From OE *cyrnel* 'any pathological lump or growth', this word is rendered as *kernel* (6×) and *cornel* (1×) in H497. The former results from the unrounding and lowering process of OE /y/ to ME /ɛ/ <e>, characteristic of the south East Midlands. The allograph *cornel*, in turn, is derived from the West Midlands form *curnel* inasmuch as OE /y/, before covered <r>, yields both <ur> and later <or> (Jordan 1974: 69; 72; see also *OED*). H497 shows the typical form of the South East Midlands, setting *cornel* apart as an influence of the West Midlands.

285 ys] Subjectless clause, plausibly as a result of a scribal error.

292 where as] Use of relative adverb *where* followed by pleonastic *as*. Following Kivimaa, Fischer explains the origin of *as* in these constructions in semantic terms: both *there* and *where* expressed temporal meaning, thus belonging to the same paradigm as *as*, which functioned as a temporal conjunction. Consequently, the relative adverbs began to be used where one would expect *as*, and *as* was used instead of these adverbs, henceforth deriving in the pleonastic use noted here (1992: 305).

293 Ignys sacer] From L *sacer ignis* 'sacred fire, St. Anthony's fire', the latter coined in the Middle Ages after the monks of the order of St. Anthony who were particularly successful at treating this ailment. The illness consists in swollen and gangrenous blisters producing a progressive rot. Both *holy fyre* and *sacer ignis* co-occur in H497.

300 Hange] From OE *hangian*, this word is rendered as *hange* (7×) and *honge* (4×). The back sound /ɔ/ <o> was retained exclusively in the West Midlands, whilst the other dialects preferred /a/ <a> (Moore 1929: 79).

306 yit] Even when sporadically used in the south, *yit* 'yet' is a typical spelling in the Midlands and the northern dialects in ME (McIntosh et al. 1986, I: 365).

316 quarteyn] As a trace of the French system, the adjective appears in postposition, a frequent structure in borrowings. Note also the use of *feuer tercyan* (315). Sometimes the adjective may even keep the French plural morpheme –*s* (Mossé 1968: 64).

317 eye shelle] From OE *ǣg-scyll* 'the outer shell of an egg', it is spelt as *eye* and *yee* (1567) in H497.

318 my] 3rd p. sing. of verb *mouen* 'may, to be able to' followed by infinitives *cŏnteinen* and *hŏlden*. This rare form is recorded in *LALME* as typically northern (McIntosh et al. 1986, IV: 215).

322 nesse] OE *hnesce* 'soft, tender', the spelling <ss>, from OE <sc>, is sporadically found in the Midlands. This practice, however, is sporadic in H497 insofar as the standard spelling <sh> is more frequent. See also *unwasse* (682), *wasse* (820), *fresse* (1315), etc.

331 secundyne] From L *secundīnæ*, a borrowing to denote the afterbirth, particularly 'the placenta extruded from the womb after the expulsion of the fœtus in parturition' (*OED*).

333 a...goyng] The Stockholm MS reads *and a-swage þe foot ache of going* (Frisk 1949: 73), the noun *going* standing for 'the act of walking'.

335 resons] From OF *raisin/resin/rosin* 'a grape, a cluster of grapes', the original accent is advanced to initial position throughout the ME period. As a result, Jordan (1974: 206-207) argues that the unaccented vowel became a sound between /i/ and /ɛ/, or even /ə/, as in *gentil* vs. *gentel*. Vowel <o>, however, is rare in these contexts.

338 Rewe] The author alternates the use of the feminine pronoun *she* and the neuter form *yt/it* for the anaphoric references to *rewe*, from OE *ryge* (masc.), and ultimately from OF *rue*. Note also the unrounding and lowering to /ɛ/ in *rewe*, typical of the Kentish and South East Midlands varieties.

349 mothe] Though spelling <ou> predominates in the rendering of OE /u:/ (*mouthe* 3×), vowel <o> (*mothe*) is used to avoid the likely sequence of minims in this word, preserving the same high back vowel as in OE *mūþ*.

350 Helde] Imperative form of *hŏlden* 'to hold, keep', from WS *healdan* and Angl. *haldan*, the latter without breaking and pronounced as /æ/. Vowel <e> in *helden* is the result of an intrinsic development of the Angl. dialect by means of which original /æ/ raised to /ɛ/, thenceforth subjected to homorganic lengthening. In H497, the form *helde(n)* (20×) predominates over *holde(n)* (10×), the latter coined on the basis of WS *heald* > *hald*.

361 eyne] As in OE, the weak plural morpheme (46×) outnumbers the strong form *eyes* (1×).

364 yn...365 garnet] *i.e.* 'with the peel of a pomegranate'.

372 destre] From OF *destruire* (L *dēstruere*), the regular development of the OF diphthong is <o>, pronounced as /ø:/ in ME. This sound later merged with the outcome of OE <ēo> which, once unrounded, became /e:/ <e>, as in *destre* (Jordan 1974: 211-212).

374 hym...375 drede] Verb *drēden* in a subjectless clause with an oblique animate experiencer (*hym*). Dummy *þar* appears clause-initially, thus filling the original subjectless position inherited from Anglo-Saxon (Fischer 1992: 235).

385 an hoot] *An* is regularly used before vowels and consonants <l> and <h>, regardless of its phonological implication. See, for instance, *an oxe* (174), *an longe dyssese* (2203), etc.

392 ne] Coordinate conjunction *neyther* ... *ne*. In ME, both *nor* and *neither* can also correlate with *neyther*. The former is overwhelmingly used in H497.

395 of...maneres] Prepositional noun adjuncts, particularly with *of*, were generally postpositive in late ME. The inverse order is not uncommon, *i.e. of uyoletes thre maneres* (Mossé 1968: 124).

403 ynne] Following the OE restrictions as to the use of relativisers *þe* vs. *se/sēo/þat*, prepositions are systematically stranded with relativiser *þat* (Fischer 1992: 391).

410 moder] The author refers to the anatomical sense of noun *mōder* (from OE *mōdor*, fem.) 'the uterus of a woman, womb'. The feminine oblique pronoun *hyr* is used for its anaphoric reference.

416 ixe] A Roman number with a superscript <e> used for an ordinal. This is a frequent practice among ME scribes "particularly with reference to years, days of month [...] and in the numbering of chapters in a book" (Mustanoja 1960: 306). As a matter of fact, there are many a case in H497 when the author numbers the different virtues of a given plant. See, among many others, ordinal *ij* (532), *iij* (513), *iiij* (461), *u* (463), etc.

428 þere...429 yn] Scribal error in the rendering of the adverb. Even though committed to make use of the form *þere of*, the author realises that locative adverb *þere yn* was more appropriate to denote the particular location of the sound, eventually forgetting to omit *of* therefrom.

436 do] Verbs *dōn* and *māken* share the same semantics, with the meaning of 'to cause (sb. to do or experience sth.), have (sth. done)', *māken* outnumbering *dōn* in these contexts.

440 boon] From OE *bāne* 'poison, venom', *i.e.* 'the poison wol make (you) sleep again'.

443 swolewe] According to Jordan (1974: 59), the stem vowel <o> is justified in terms of a reconstructed OE infinitve **swolgian*, hence deriving *swolwen*. PDE *swallow* with <a> is yet coined from *swalgh* 'gullet'.

445 þe spedyer] According to Mustanoja (1960: 282), this is a proportional comparative consisting in the use of *the*, from the OE instrumental case *þe/þȳ* followed by a comparative, a construction used for emphasis.

453 drynke] From OE *drincan* (*dranc/druncon/druncen*), the conventional participial form in ME is both *drunken* and *dronken*, the latter as a mere orthographic change to avoid the likely sequence of minims in a word. The form *drynke(n)*, however, is not recorded as a participial form in the *e-MED*, deemed as an erroneous rendering formed on the basis of the vowel of the infinitive.

465 gladyn] From OE *glædene/gledene* (fem.), the spelling <y> in atonic positions is a clue as to the provenance of the text. Jordan argues that since the 13th century post-tonic /ə/ adopted a middle sound between /i/ and /ɛ/ in the Midlands and the South (1974: 138).

482 stryngthe] From OE *strengþ/strengþu* (fem.), vowel <e> in closed syllables raised to /i/ <i, y> under the influence of apical sounds, especially before covered *n*, in the North and Midlands, but with a clear withdrawal in more southernly texts (Jordan 1974: 59–60). H497, therefore, gives evidence of the standard spelling *strengthe* (5×) together with the raised forms *stryn(g)the* (3×).

482 somme] The Stockholm MS reads *somme men* (Frisk 1949: 80).

493 thylke] Derived from OE *se ilca* 'the same', this variant is the result of the erosion of the vowel of the article before *ilke* (Mustanoja 1960: 176). This form was in use until the late 15th centure, eventually superseded by *same*.

511 þys...root] Uninflected genitive, *i.e. þys herbe root*.

534 boor] Participial form of *bēren*, from OE *beran* (*bær/bǣron/boren*).

541 þat...yaf] Appositive phrase to refer back to the main authority of this first virtue of leek. The *punctus* is here used at clause level as a linking device of the subject *ypocras* and the clausal verb *yaf*, the appositive phrase remaining in-between.

543 Emoptoycy] From ML *haemoptoicus* 'a person suffering from a disease characterized by bloody sputum'.

549 furthwith] The Stockholm MS reads *with-ynne-forth* here (Frisk 1949: 84). Note the use of *with ynne* (f. 20v, 1) clause-finally to convey exactly the same meaning as the adverb of the Stockholm MS.

565 dystroy] From OF *destruire* (L *dēstruere*), French <ē> is considered to have been tenser than the native counterpart, which explains the raising process to /i/ <i> in some sporadic ME words (Jordan 1974: 206). This accounts for the existence of a form such as *dystroy* in the text. However, its occurrence is negligible (1×), if compared with the standard spelling *destroien*, ammounting to 145 occurrences in H497.

565 addres] From OE *nædre* (fem.), the initial <n> was lost at the beginning of the 14th century by a mistaken division of *a nadder*, hence producing *an adder*.

571 destryth] Plausibly vowel <y> in an unstressed syllable is a clue as to a Midland provenance of the text, wherein post-tonic /ə/ adopted a middle sound between *i* and *e* (Jordan 1974: 138).

578 consounde] Hypercorrected form of verb *consouden* 'to heal (a wound or fracture) by promoting cicatrization or knitting'. Consonant <n> is mistakenly added, plausibly as a result of a false association with the adjective *sŏund(e* 'healthy, cured or healed after illness or injury' (*e-MED*).

586 methe] From OE (WS *medu*, Angl. *meodu*) 'mead'.

588 before or] Temporal conjunction *before* followed by pleonastic *or* expressing that the action of the main clause precedes that of the subordinate, a rare conjunction in ME if compared with *before* (*that*) and *er*/*or* (*that*). Although the verb *take* is uninflected, the subjunctive is the expected mood under these circumstances as a way to express non-factuality or a prospective event.

596 olyfaunt] From OF *olifant* (L *elephantus*), this borrowing undergoes an accent shift to initial position some time before the 13th century. As a consequence, <au> begins to appear from that time before a tautosyllabic nasal as a reflex of OF nasalized <a> (Jordan 1974: 205). This fact justifies the origin and development of the diphthong in this word not only in the East Midlands but also in the other dialect areas.

597 gretyst] The use of the superlative *grēt* without pre-positive *the*. This is a recurrent practice of the author, as in *hugest* (587) or *gretyst* (1192). In phonological terms, the superlative ending generally implies the doubling of the final consonant together with the shortening of the radical vowel, if long. However, the form *gretyst* does not give evidence of such a shortening process, plausibly because the long vowel of the positive degree was regularly reintroduced into the comparative and the superlative, particularly at the end of the period (Mossé 1968: 65).

601 with] Although prepositions *by* and *of* predominate for the expression of the agent in passive constructions, personal agency may be also expressed with other prepositioins, such as *from*, *mid*, *through* and *with* (Mustanoja 1960: 442).

609 unther] From Old Northumbrian *unþer*, hence giving ME *unþer/unther* 'under' (see also 747).

612 on…wyse] Prepositional phrase headed by both *on* and *in*. See also the structure *yn þe same wyse* (622).

623 lyke to] Herb *basīl(e* 'basil' is lacking here (Frisk 1949: 87).

625 Fenell] From OE *finol/finul* (masc.) and ultimately from ML *fēnuculum*, the ME word *fenel* has eventually adopted vowel <e> from its synonym *fenkel* 'fennel'.

630 she] From OE *nædre* (fem.), this noun preserves the OE gender.

642 hat] Consonant <t> for <þ>, characteristic among southern scribes, particularly in the East Midlands. This phonological change takes place with preceding <d> or <t> and mostly affects the 3. sg. pres. of verbs (Jordan 1974: 186).

646 greuaunces] From OF *grevance*, after the corresponding accent shift, <au> appears in the 13th century before a tautosyllabic nasal as a reflex of OF

nasalized <a> (Jordan 1974: 205). This fact justifies the origin and development of the digraph not only in the East Midlands but also in the other dialect areas. This process also accounts for the use of the spelling *staunche* (653), *commaunde* (806), *coryaundre* (1086), etc.

676 destryeth] A French borrowing from *destruire* (L *dēstruere*), the present form *destryeth* may be explained on account of its falling intonation, becoming <u> in English, pronounced as /y:/, and later spelt with <i> (Jordan 1974: 215-216).

685 us semeth] Verb *sēmen* in a subjectless clause with an oblique animate experiencer (*us*).

689 Rosa canina] The author is erroneously referring here to the plant *rosa canina* 'dogrose', a variable rose species native to Europe, northwest Africa and Asia. This kind of rose is the flower of Hampshire.

715 oleum rosaceum] Taken from L *oleum rosacium* 'an oily substance obtained from the maceration of fresh roses in olive oil'.

721 felthe] From OE *fȳlþ*, the stem vowel results from the unrounding and lowering of OE /y:/ to ME /ɛ:/ <e>, characteristic of the south East Midlands.

735 eek] The Stockholm MS does not show such a word in front of the participial form of *streinen* (Frisk 1949: 93). Therefore, <ee> has been interpreted here as a mis-spelling of adverb *ēk* 'too, also, in the same manner', where the final consonant is lacking.

736 streyneyt] The pronominal object *yt* is attached to the imperative of the verb. It should be therefore interpreted as *streyne yt*.

754 yn yn] Scribal dittography.

758 bloed] From OE *blōd*, the spelling <oe>, of French influence, is occasionally employed in the late ME period as a long sign for /o:/ (Jordan 1974: 86).

787 spette] From OE *spǣtan* 'to spit', digraph <tt> gives evidence of a close syllable shortening, which accounts for PDE *spit* /spit/ after a raising from /ɛ/ to /i/ initiated in ME (already in the 13th century in the south East) and continuing into the 15th century (Dobson 1957: 567).

839 puttyth] The verb *putten* is systematically rendered with <tt>, amounting to 75 occurrences, if compared with a single instance of *putyth*.

842 knowhers] Derived from noun *cough* 'one who coughes'. Plausibly hypercorrected, not recorded in the *e-MED*.

849 cowe] Coined from the OE verb *cohhettan*, the spelling of this noun in H497 is the result of a labialising process of the lengthened velar group <hh>, originally western and eventually spreading through the eastern varieties (Jordan 1974: 181), which explains the use of word-final <w> here.

851 þe þe] Scribal dittography.

856 meled] Allographs *meled* and *melde* appear. The first stems from the omission of OF <d> under the influence of the ensuing consonant. The latter shows metathesis *dl* > *ld* to ease the pronunciation of this verb. The former outnumbers the latter in H497.

859 tweynte] The allograph *twein-/tweyn-* is characteristic of the Midlands, particularly in its eastern variety (McIntosh et al. 1986, I: 443).

860 thrydede] In the same fashion, *thrid-* and *thryd-* types spread from the southern part of the East Midlands dialect to the very north of England, extending well into the West Midlands (McIntosh et al. 1986, I: 508).

862 fleume] Allographs *fleume* and *flume* alternate here. The first preserves the OF diphthong /ɛu/ whilst the second is deemed as an occasional 15th century spelling of the French digraph (Jordan 1974: 216).

869 streyght] Participial form of verb *streighten* 'to straighten, stretch', final *–t* appears after the assimilation of the two dental consonants.

870 furth] From OE *forþ*, the spelling *furth* in H497 stems from a neutralising process of *o* > *u* before /r/ (Jordan 1974: 62).

877 nesestrelles] From OE *nosþryle*, this word is the result of the dissimilation of <þ> to <t> after a fricative, becoming *nostrel* already in late OE. Vowel <e>, in turn, may be accounted for as an erratic lowering process of /ɔ/ to /ɛ/ in areas of the south of England, which Jordan explains as *i*-umlaut of *o* (1974: 62).

910 colluryes] From OF *colire/colure* (L *collȳrium*) 'any medicine applied to the eye, collyrium'. The stem vowel, on the one hand, is the regular development of OF <u> /y/, which becomes <u> /u/ in ME, with the exception of the West Midlands where it was still pronounced as /y/ (Jordan 1974: 209). On the other hand, the unstressed *y*-spelling is retained as a reflex of the L cognate, pronounced as /i/.

919 clof thunge] From OE *cluf-þung(e)* 'crowfoot, hellebore'. According to the *e-MED*, the standard rendering of this word is, among others, *clof-thung/clof-tonge*.

930 a brood] *i.e. sparclen abrōd(e* 'to spread (sth.) out, stretch out, extend'.

930 uennes] From OE *wenn* 'A lump or an excrescence on the human body'.

934 ys...to] Impersonal passive *þys rose* [...] *ys seyde to hele*.

951 þys[1]] Plural form of demonstrative *þys*, a variant recorded in *LALME* as a typical spelling of the middle South of England (McIntosh et al. 1986, IV: 6). However, it has been interpreted here as a scribal error in view of the outstanding occurrence of variants *these*, *þese* and *thes* in H497.

962 stomake ys] A detached genitive ending (*stomake ys*), a scribal practice recorded in *LALME* as a characteristic southern form, particularly in those counties under the influence of the South West (McIntosh et al. 1986, IV: 322).

965 ys ys] Scribal dittography.

972 to...973 sege] *gōn to sēggĕ* 'to ease oneself'.

973 Aneys] From OF *anis* (L *anīsum*), the <ey> spelling is a 15th century orthographic practice to represent /i:/. Jordan (1974: 239) argues that this digraph is likely the result of imitating other ME forms such as *eyȝe/ei* 'eye' or *heygh* 'high'. Compare it with *anyse* (959), showing the conventional rendering of ME /i:/.

1021 dyrknes] From OE *deorcnes* (fem.), variant *dyrkness* is a development of an alternative OE form *dyrknes*, mostly Angl.

1026 greuonce] From OF *grevance*, the word is three-foldly represented in H497. Setting aside the *a*-forms (*i.e. greuance*) which replicate the spelling of the OF cognate, *au*-forms (*i.e. greuaunce*, f. 50v, line 4) appear in the 13th century, after the corresponding accent shift, before a tautosyllabic nasal as a reflect of OF nasalized <a>. Third, *o*-forms are typically found in southern areas as a reflex of the French back realisation /ɔ/ (Jordan 1974: 205).

1030 pepyr] The *y*-spelling in unstressed positions is a typical feature of the Midlands, wherein post-tonic /ə/ adopted a middle sound between *i* and *e* (Jordan 1974: 138).

1041 profyth] From OF *profit* 'benefit, advantage', where word-final <th> indicates a late ME aspirated pronunciation (Jordan 1974: 183).

1047 flume] Variant *flume* here is an occasional 15th-century spelling of the French digraph <eu, ew>. The PDE orthography, however, stems from the disappearance of vowel <u> before a labial, eventually causing compensatory lengthening: /flɛmə/ > /flɛːmə/, a systematic change that affected all French <u> diphthongs around 1300 (Jordan 1974: 216; 244).

1061 þey dare] Unlike other previous instances in H497 with an oblique animate experiencer (138), verb *durren* occurs with a nominative subject (*þey*).

1077 methe] From OE *medu* (masc./neut.) 'mead'.

1093 þat…caule] Restrictive relative clause introduced by *þat*. Still, its antecedent is possessive *his*, thus implying 'whose, of which'. This construction may be tentatively compared with Chaucer's *The Man of Lawe his tale*, of current use in the late period, wherein the inflectional genitive is substituted by possessive *his* (Fischer 1992: 230). This case is structurally different, however, in the sense that *hys pysse* precedes the relative, being the factual subject of verb *ys*. The same reading is offered in the Stockholm MS (Frisk 1949: 110).

1121 femygreke] From OF *fenugrec/fengrec*, variant *femigreke* is consistently used in H497 (5×). Even though recorded in the *e-MED*, we consider *femygreke* to be an orthographic misinterpretation of the French cognate, wherein minims in <nu> are mistakenly re-spelt as <mi>. This view is corroborated by the subsequent development of this word in the sense that the alternative *femygreke* does not have any phono-orthographic repercussion in PDE *fenugreek*.

1132 hys] 3rd p. s. pres. of the copula. The *LALME* records this form as a typical feature of the Middle south of England, particularly the whole of the East Midlands and the southern varieties (McIntosh et al. 1986, I: 339).

1132 hoos] *i.e.* *hōs* 'harsh, ungrateful to the ear'. According to the *OED*, although written evidence for *r*-forms date back to c. 1400, the PDE spelling implies the existence of an unrecorded OE *hārs*, beside *hās*.

1142 Oynouns] From OF *oignon*, final <ou> is the typical spelling of OF /u:/ <u, o> in the vernacular if in contact with a nasal consonant (Jordan 1974: 208), hence the consistent rendering as *oynouns* in H497 (25×).

1171 hosen] From OE *hosa* (masc.) 'leggings or stockings', this noun still preserves the weak plural morpheme, i.e *hosen*. Likewise, *shone* 'shoes' displays an *n*-plural notwithstanding the OE strong plurals *scōs/sceōs* (Hall 1960: 296).

1190 presyd] From OF *preisier* 'to praise'. In H497 the original diphthong is retained in *preysed* (f. 61r, 14) whilst the participial form *presyd* gives evidence of monophthongisation from /ɛi/ to /æi/ and eventually to /ɛ:/, hence the <e> spelling (Jordan 1974: 213).

1195 self] *Self* as a premodifier with the meaning of 'itself'. The Stockholm MS shows that the determiner *þe* has been accidentally skipped by the author when copying from the original (Frisk 1949: 116).

1201 fnesynge] From OE *fnēosan* 'to sneeze', the change from <fn-> to <sn->, according to the *OED*, is attributed to a possible misreading or misspelling of the ME word *fnesen* as *snesen* after the initial combination <fn-> became unfamiliar. Barnhart (1988: 1026), however, considers that it is more likely that the initial sound was gradually lost in ME, producing *nesen* in the early 14th century, a form which was later influenced by words like *snort* and *snore*, thus adopting initial <s->. On a chronological basis, therefore, the spelling <fn-> is not the typical 15th-century rendering, being instead interpreted in H497 as an orthographic reflex of the source text. Compare this spelling with *snese* (1893; 2176).

1208 brest] Infinitive of verb *bresten* 'to break, burst, be broken', from OE *berstan*, after metathesis.

1209 seche] From OE *swylc*, variant *seche* is a discriminating spelling as to the author's provenance in the sense that *sech* and *selk* types are prototypical forms of the Midlands (McIntosh et al. 1986, I: 321). It co-occurs with *suche*-forms (1211).

1219 syth þat] Even though exclusively a temporal conjunction in early ME (from OE *siþþan þæt*), its causal meaning gained most of its ground throughout the 13th century.

1221 how þat] Nominal clause introduced by *how that*, the latter pleonastically used.

1226 þe sharper] Proportional comparatives *þe moor ... þe sharper* and *þe moor bred þow castyst ... þe moor feble & weker* denoting parallel increase. Note the use of the periphrastic comparison with a two-syllable adjective (*moor feble*).

1264 so...as] Comparison of equality *so ... as* in a negative clause.

1272 breche] From OE *brǣc* (neut.) 'a fracture'.

1300 drunk] Note the systematic omission of the prefixal past participle marking in H497. There are just 100 instances of prefixal forms out of 1223 past participles in the text, a form leading to its complete obliteration towards the end of the 15th century. In this same fashion, Wojtyś states that in the 15th century prefixal marking was frequent in the West Midlands and London whilst in the eastern part of the Midlands prefixless forms are a choice. Its use is, however, consistent in the southern dialects throughout this same century (Wojtyś 2007: 285).

1311 kersen] From OE *cressa* (masc.), after metathesis.

1317 yt] The order S – O – V is found in ME, particularly when the object is a pronoun or a demonstrative (Mossé 1968: 129).

1330 lecour] Borrowed from OF *licor/licur*, this word is rendered as *lycore* and *lecour* in H497, with the stress in final position. Vowel /i/ is unlengthened, particularly in the Southern varieties, hence explaining variant *lycore* /liku:r/. The unstressed position, on the other hand, gives rise to another orthographic variant in the vernacular, *i.e. lecour* /ləku:r/, as the French pre-tonic vowel behaves as its native counterpart (Jordan 1974: 201).

1336 wythe] In light of the recurrent use of the spelling *wyth(e)* (6×), the possibility of a scribal error must be tentatively ruled out. Jordan (1974: 183) is the only source which provides a fairly convincing explanation for this practice, arguing that OE <t> in final position often becomes <th> to indicate a late aspirated pronunciation.

1337 toþer] Coined from a mis-analysis of *that* and *ōther* 'the other, the second, latter'. Generally preceded by determiner *þe* in ME, as here *þe toþer good sauore*, a redundant habit in view of the existence of *þe* and *þat*.

1346 attones] Adverbial phrase *at ōnes* 'together, at one and the same time'.

1362 yn…wyse] A recurrent ME placement of the prepositional object (*yn þe same wyse*) between the inflected auxiliary verb and the infinitive, acting as an adverb of manner (Mossé 1968: 129).

1369 chyres] Lemma *chīth* (*e-MED*) is also represented in ME as *chide* or *chire*. Possibly the scribe interpreted a letter <s> in *chyses* instead of the original <r>, which is precisely the spelling found in the Stockholm MS (Frisk 1949: 124). Other extant versions, however, give evidence of this *s*-form (Hatton 29 and Cambridge Ee.I.15). This spelling is not recorded in the *e-MED*.

1373 erse] From OE *ears* 'anus, rectum', the ME form lengthened to become *ers(e)* /ɛ:rs/, whose pronunciation is connected with a southern weak articulation of <r> before <s> typically Angl. (Jordan 1974: 44).

1380 mounke] *i.e. thēr-among(e* 'in addition to these, along with them, with them'. The occurrence of <nk> for <ng> is recorded in *LALME* as a typical spelling of the middle south of England, particularly from the southern and the East Midland varieties, later spreading to some western counties like Warkick and Worcestershire (McIntosh et al. 1986, IV: 321).

1390 costlewe] Note the omission of conjunction *and* in-between the adjectives *heue* and *costlewe*.

1401 sayle] Shortened form of verb *assail(l)en* 'to attack, assault' (*e-MED*).

1408 alay] From OE *ālecgan* 'to allay, alleviate'.

1437 atte] Use of *atte* 'at the' where the fricative is blended to /t/ under the influence of the preceding dental (Jordan 1974: 186). This produces, in turn, the co-occurrence of two determiners (*þe* and *þat*) within the same noun phrase. Therefore, *atte* is mis-spelt instead of preposition *at*.

1440 rennynges] This same noun is rendered as *rennyng* in 551 and *rennynges* in 1442. From OE *rynnyng*, the unrouding and lowering to /ɛ/ of the stem vowel gives evidence of the southern provenance of the author, as the <e> territory of OE /y/ covers mostly Kent and part of the East Midlands –Norfolk, Essex and Suffolk in particular (Jordan 1974: 66).

1451 shal mowe] *i.e. shullen + mouen* 'shall be able to'.

1453 hyn] The oblique masculine pronominal *hyn* as a characteristic East Midland spelling (McIntosh et al. 1986, IV: 314). See also 1898; 2222.

1458 yt] Dummy *yt* used to fill the subject position before the verb in light of the existing separation between the actual subject *þys seed* and the clausal verb *helyt*.

1472 to…1473 gydre] The *i/y* forms in this word are recorded as a characteristic spelling of eastern England, particularly the south and the Midlands (McIntosh et al. 1986, I: 440).

1473 parodycas] A Latinate borrowing from *parōtis, parōtidis*, represented with the following allographs in H497, *parodyda* (2430), *peryodyda* (2328), *parodycas* (1474).

1514 ȝerna] From Arab. *zarníkh*, a medical term to denote 'a pustular skin disease characterised by scabby eruptions'. Etymologically connected with Sp. *sarna*.

1528 me…preue] Verb *prēven* in a subjectless clause introduced by impersonal *me* (from OE *man*). As in the case of *durren*, this construction, though frequent in OE, was rarely used in ME, being superseded by those with a nominative experiencer. There is no other example of impersonal *prēven* in H497. From an etymological viewpoint, this verb is borrowed from OF *prover/pruver/pruever*. On the one hand, *proven* (2117) is a reflex of OF close /o:/ before labials. On the other, *preven* is the result of the regular development of OF diphthong <ue>, which smoothed into /ø:/ > /e:/, thenceforth merging with the result of OE *ēo*, which accounts for the use of the *e*-form in *preue* (Jordan 1974: 207; 212).

1533 fallyth…us] Impersonal verb *fallen* appears with the animate experiencer (*us*) in the oblique case. In addition to this, a dummy *hit* heads the clause to fill the vacant position of the subject.

1551 seluer] Verbatim translation of L *spuma argenti* 'litharge of silver, a name given to it as being a by-product in the separation of silver from lead' (Frisk 1949: 264).

1557 ys...1558 chylde] *i.e. bēn with/mid child* 'to be pregnant'. PDE *to get with child, to go with child* (*OED*).

1566 yyt] Orthographic variant of adverb *yēt* 'yet'. In H497, this adverb is rendered as *yit* (5×) and *yyt* (2×). The former is considered to be a standard spelling of this word, found in almost every dialect area. The latter, however, is deemed as a rare form in *LALME*, to the extent that it has been localised just in two anchor texts, one from Derbyshire and the other from Worcestershire (McIntosh et al. 1986, IV: 73).

1572 chelde] *Chyld* and *chelde* coexist in the singular, amounting to 27x and 3x occurrences, respectively. OE /i/ undergoes homorganic lengthening before cluster *ld*, hence deriving in the standard form *chyld* /ʧi:ld/. Variant *chelde*, however, arises from a rare Southumbrian practice to neutralise /i/ to /ɛ/ in closed syllables and particularly in contact with labials, liquids and consonants /ʃ/ and /ʧ/ (Jordan 1974: 62). The resulting sound was later homoganically lengthened to /ɛ:/.

1637 a...1638 swagyth] From OF *assua(i)er* 'to alleviate, relieve pain'. Even though written solid elsewhere in H497 (5×), the initial vowel is split, as if a prefix. Word division is not subjected to such strict set of rules as in PDE, a fact leading to frequent associations and splittings without an etymological basis. See, for instance, *afeuer* > *a feuer* (1650), *a scape* > *ascape* (1538), *a batyth* > *abatyth* (1657), and the like.

1651 wolde] Adjective *ōld(e* 'old'. The odd spelling *wolde* is the result of a 15th century glide sound before covered /l/, thus producing the insertion of a transitional /u/ (Jordan 1974: 241). Notwithstanding this, the typical spelling for that same glide is <ow>, not <w>.

1661 yt sayde] The copula (*ys*) lacking before the participial form.

1675 uenemous...1676 deedly] Post-positive adjective as an imitation of the French model (Mossé 1968: 123). If the head of a noun phrase is modified by two attributive adjectives, the first is usually pre-positive (*uenemous*) and the second post-positive (*deedly*).

1678 thought] From OE (WS *þēah*, Angl. *þāh*), variant *thought* is considered as characteristically southern (McIntosh et al. 1986, IV: 57).

1689 bytynges] Compare the use of the inflectional genitive *addrys bytynges* with the *of*-genitive *uenym of snakes* (1687).

1692 called ys] Infrequent position of the past participle, which precedes the auxiliary verb *bēn*.

1719 sauor] From OF *savor*/*savour*, the original accent advances to initial position in ME, becoming *savour* /sa:vər/. In statistical terms, variants *sauo(r)r(e)* (8×) and *sauour* (8×) are preferred, if compared with a single instance of *sauar*, certainly mis-spelt.

1723 a...floures] The determiner *a* premodifies the plural head *floures*.

1724 yolow] From OE *geolu* 'yellow', diphthong <eo> retained a front round vowel /ø/, generally spelt <o, eo, oe, u> in the eastern part of England, agglutinating the Kentish dialect, the East Midlands and the north east (Jordan 1974: 96-97).

1747 uenemouse...dedly] See 1676-77. As if a cliché, the same adjectives appear (*uenemous* and *deedly*), the first pre-positive (*uenemous*) and the second post-positive (*deedly*).

1750 ryght...wyne] A sequence of three pre-positive adjectives. Note the use of intensifier *right*, a ME innovation which, though sporadic in the early period, gains ground throughout the 14th century, reaching its climax between 1420-1500 (Méndez 2007: 191-193).

1756 to...1757 gyder] Lemma *tōgeder* shows several variants in H497: *to gydre* (24×), *to gyder* (12×), *to gydyr* (3×), *to gydres* (2×), among others. As recorded in *LALME* (McIntosh et al. 1986, IV: 270), the first is clearly an East Midland variant, ascribed in particular to the counties of Cambridge, Norfolk, Suffolk, Essex and Lincoln.

1768 dygystyoun] From OF *digestion*, the original accent advances to the second syllable already in ME, thence short /ɛ/ <e> is the regular outcome in the vernacular as in *dygestyoun* (1421; 2427; etc.) and *degestyon* (392), for instance. However, infrequent *y*-forms like *dygystyoun* are the result of an intrinsic development of French /ɛ/ in English, which raised to /i/ because the vowel was tenser than the native counterpart (Jordan 1974: 206).

1783 of[2]...1784 bokes] Double genitive in *of oþere autores bokes*, wherein the inflectional genitive *autores* is in-between the *of*-genitive construction.

1820 herpeta mordax] From ML and ultimate from Gr. ἑϱπης, *herpeste(n mordax* refers to a skin disease characterised by gnawing and irritating herpes.

1822 furthe] From OE *forþ*, this variant is the result of a process, already initiated in OE, by means of which /ɔ/ is neutralised to /u/ before consonant /r/, thus *forþ* > *furth* (Jordan 1974: 62).

1836 ho] From the OE interrogative pronoun *hwā*, *ho* is the typical rendering of this generaliser in the middle south of England, both in the eastern and the western varieties (McIntosh et al. 1986, I: 539).

1845 þys] Note the use of *as* instead of the copula *ys* here. The Stockholm MS reads [...] *þat þis is as good and profitable to alle þe causes beforeseid as is þe foreseide herbe* (Frisk 1949: 148).

1860 egghynge] Coined from OE *ecg* (fem.) 'edge, point' (Hall 1960: 99), the word *eğğing* is used here to denote 'a stinging sensation of the teeth'. Even though <gg> is the conventional spelling for OE /ʤ/, the author is sometimes committed to rendering <ggh>. See also *bregghynge* (1962).

1875 puttyth] 3rd p. sing. pres. of verb *putten*. Even when *puttyth* (1509) and, to a lesser extent, *puttyt* (1875) are the most widespread forms in H497, the latter after the southern practice of assimilating <þ> to <t> before a dental consonant, variant *puttyht* is solely explained as a scribal error, rendered instead of the standard 3rd p. sing. morpheme <th>.

1891 casteyn] *i.e. caste yn* 'to put in (a place), bring into' after an irregular word boundary. The Stockholm MS thus reads *the poudre of þis herbe cast in at the nese* (Frisk 1949: 150).

1901 Sciatica passio] Borrowed from ML *sciatica passio*, it denotes 'a rheumatic or neuralgic affection of some part about the hip joint'. H497 alternates the use of *sciatica* (3×) and *scietica* (5×).

1907 quarteyn] Borrowed from OF *quartaine/quarteine*, these diphthongs generally smoothed to /ɛ:/, excepting word-final positions before a liquid or a nasal, where the diphthong remains. This explains spellings such as *quartaine* (4×) and *quarteyne* (1×) in H497, the latter as a reflex of its French cognate.

1916 repryssyth] From OF *represser* 'to counteract, overcome', where two phonological processes sequentially intervene in ME. First, the stressed vowel lengthens before consonant <s>, *i.e.* /rə'prɛs/ > /rə'prɛ:s/. Next, the resulting vowel raised to /i:/, the former being tenser than its native counterpart, *i.e.* /rə'prɛ:s/ > /rə'pri:s/ *repryssyth*. This variant, however, coexisted with the original short vowel /ɛ/, the latter being the input for PDE *repress*.

1930 atte eue] *i.e. ēve(n* 'evening, between sunset and darkness'.

1968 pose] From OE *gepos* 'a head cold; catarrh'.

1972 ere] Verb phrase inadvertently omitted by the scribe. As in the Stockholm MS, it should therefore read *caste yn atte ere helpyth yt* (Frisk 1948: 154).

1977 Coste] A scribal confussion with herb *soft(e* 'mullein, also *asarum europaeum* or a part of this plant used medicinally' (*e-MED*). *Cost* denoting 'costmary (chrysanthemum balsamita)' is properly dealt with in 2545.

1987 ys…be[1]] Periphrastic construction *to be (not) to* + infinitive denoting 'must not be'.

2000 ether] Correlative conjunction *eyther … or* (8×) is the typical spelling of the East Midlands whilst *ether … or* (1×) is rather a north East Midland spelling, Lincolnshire in particular (McIntosh et al. 1986, IV: 159).

2044 born] Participial form of *bēren* 'to bear, bloom, bring into existence'. The form *borum* may be taken as a scribal error on account of the use of letter <u> instead of letter <n> and the tilde, which has been interpreted as an abbreviated <m>.

2061 twey] Recorded in *LALME* as a typical allograph of the middle south of England, mostly a Midland form with sporadic ocurrence among southern scribes (McIntosh et al. 1986, I: 443).

2074 nattercoppe] From OE *atorcoppe* 'a spider', hypercorrected <n> added as a result of a false association with the word *nadder* 'a serpent'. Compare this with the mistaken division of *a nadder* as *an adder*, which responds to a different orthographic reasoning.

2080 anteryke] From OF *goute artetique* and ML *gutta artetica* 'arthritic, rheumatic'. The spelling *anteryke* here is evidently a corruption of the borrowed term, an error also replicated in the Stockholm MS. Likewise, the noun *syknesse* is also erroneous as the author is clearly referring to the persons suffering the above-mentioned illness (Frisk 1949: 223).

2094 gardyenes] From OF *gardin*, digraph <ye> must be taken as a reflex of short /i/ after the corresponding accent shift in ME. Note also the other posible allographs of this word in H497 as *garden* (1×) and *gardeyn* (1×).

2119 uino passe] From ML *uinum passum* 'raisin wine'.

2134 sathe] 3rd p. sing. pres. of verb *seien* 'to say'. From OE *sægþ*, palatal /j/ is lost in the present tense by analogy of the past tense, wherein that same consonant systematically disappears before /d/ and /n/, thereafter lengthening the preceding vowel /sɛ:de/ (Jordan 1974: 176).

2137 whan þat] Relativiser *whan* followed by pleonastic *that*. Fischer (1992: 302) argues that such constructions developed in English at the beginning of the 14th century, possibly "spreading from the free relative *wh-* form [*i.e. swā hw... swā*] to other *wh*-forms introducing subclauses", like *which þat*, *what þat*, *where þat*, and the like.

2161 batyth] 3rd p. sing. pres. of verb *bāten* 'to alleviate', a reduced form of verb *abāten*, ultimately derived from OF *abatre*. H497, however, shows an outstanding preference for *a*-forms as they amount to 44 occurrences altogether.

2169 abou] From OE *ābūfan* 'above'.

2183 yt...dyssese] A whole line may be missing as a result of an author's slip when copying from the source text because the Stockholm MS reads as follows: *it driueþ a-wey olde sikenesse, and be suche a vomyte is done a-wey þe disese þat is clapid vertigo* (Frisk 1949: 165-166).

2185 malen colyke] From OF *melancolique* and ML *malancolicus* 'one who has too much *black bile*', whose symptons were propensity to violent anger, mental gloom and sadness (*OED*).

2223 þe mysore] Hypercorrected form instead of *Þemison* plausibly assuming a false association with *þe sōr(e* 'pain'. *Þemison* was an authority who lived during the first century, known through a medical treatise "in which he developed a system of pathology and therapeutics that was accepted as the professional creed of the sect of the Methodici" (Frisk 1949: 330).

2226 yt semyth] Verb *sēmen* wherein the oblique experiencer is omitted, the subject position filled by a dummy *yt*. Compare it with *me semeth* (2221).

2238 hylpeth] Variant not recorded in *e-MED*. Allographs *hylp/hylpe/hilp* are noted in *LALME* as a feature of the South West (McIntosh et al. 1986, IV: 317).

2245 siroyne] From OF *siron* 'a sprout'.

2246 tre] Note the use of the plosive /t/ for etymological /Θ/ <th> as an East Midlands feature (McIntosh et al. 1986, IV: 320). See also the oblique pronominal *te* in 2692. This is yet an erratic practice in H497 as the *th*-spellings (*three* 1×), predominate if compared with the occurrences of *tre* (2×).

2248 barly mely] *i.e. mēle* 'a meal', hence *barlī-mēle* to denote 'barley meal'.

2261 scrypules] From *scrupūlus* 'a unit of weight of one twenty-fourth of an ounce'. H497 shows three different renderings, *i.e. scruples*, *scrypules* and *scrybules*. While the first is the regular development of French /u:/, therefore rendered as <u>, more controversial becomes the explanation for the *i*-forms. According to the *OED*, "the relation between the forms with *ū* and those with *ī* has not been satisfactorily explained, and some scholars dispute the identity of the word". Orthographically speaking, on the other hand, *scrybulus* must be deemed as an error instead of the etymological <p>.

2261 obolus] Borrowed from L, this terms denotes a small unit of weight equal to a halfpenny.

2263 tweyne] Allograph *tweyn-* (1x in H497) is a typical East Midland spelling.

2292 aunswere] From OE *andswarian*, consonant <d> disappears in ME before consonant /s/. The resulting variant, on the other hand, undergoes the same trend of development of French nasalised /a/, which becames <au> /au/ before /n/ + a dental consonant, thereby the form *aunswere* in H497 (Jordan 1974: 205).

2305 prophytabler] Synthetic comparison with a polysyllabic adjective. Even when the relevant literature agrees as to consider that "later in the 15th century comparison by *-er* and *-est* occurs less frequently in longer words" (Mustanoja 1960: 279), the use of the synthetic and the periphrastic models is still indiscriminate in H497.

2317 thuugh] From OE (WS *þeah* and Angl. *þah*) 'though', spelt as *þeigh* and *þaugh* in ME. These forms were eventually displaced by ON **þoh* (Jordan 1974: 95). Still, there is not a convincing explanation for variant *thuugh* in H497, which might be a hypercorrected form assuming a false relationship with preposition *thurgh*.

2317 myghty] Anomalous line-final division in ME (*myg-hty*). In H497 words are generally split into syllables, the writer being meticulous not to split letters standing for one sound. This deviation stems from the need to fill the entire length of the line and avoid unnecessary blank spaces in the margin (Calle-Martín 2009: 49-51).

2335 ceunse] From OF *encens* 'fragrance', variants *cense* and *ceunse* are found in H497. The former results from the regular development of the French cognate whilst the latter witnesses the appearance of /u/ before a covered nasal, hence *ceunse* (Jordan 1974: 205). PDE *scent*, however, develops in the 17th century perhaps by a mistaken analogy with verbs *ascent/descent* (Barnhart 1988: 966).

2338 ys...be] Impersonal passive *þys herbe ys seyde to be.*

2353 ynne] Preposition *yn(ne)* appearing twice, both in pipe-piping and preposition stranding positions.

2367 brenge] From OE *bringan* 'to bring, fetch', *e*-forms are explained as the Southumbrian neutralisation from /i/ to /ɛ/ in the vicinity of labials, liquids, /ʃ/ and /ʧ/ (Jordan 1974: 62).

2386 gose grece] Noun phrase containing an uninflected genitive *gose grece*. Compare this structure with the inflectional form *swynes grece* (326).

2404 enleuene] Word recorded in the *e-MED* as *elleven/endleven*. From a dialectal perspective, variant *enleuene* is recorded in *LALME* as a characteristic form of the East Midlands (McIntosh et al. 1984, IV: 160).

2433 pycche] From OE *pic*, this word is two-foldly represented in H497. On the one hand, variant *pic(c)he* (2×) after the adoption of the French writing

<ch> and <cch> with medial lengthening (Jordan 1974: 165). Variant *py(c)ke* (2×), on the other hand, is attributed to a Scandinavian influence.

2455 profyt] See also *profyth* (1042).

2456 fallynge euel] There were three types of *falling evil* in the Middle Ages: epilepsy, catalepsy and analepsy. The author is here referring to *epilepsy*, defined as "a sickness of the hinder part of the head, where the neck and the head are joined together", coming from cold corrupt humours (Dawson 1934: 135).

2458 chyndryn] Scribal error instead of *chyldryn*.

2481 þe wyche] Defining relative clause introduced by *þe wyche*. Note that the antecedent (*hete*) is repeated after the relativiser in order to avoid the misinterpretation of the preceding noun (*mawe*) as the factual antecedent of *þe wyche*.

2485 pusca] A Latinate borrowing to denote 'a mixture of vinegar and water'. Not recorded in the *e-MED*.

2489 been] Genitive plural morpheme *-(e)n* of *bē* 'bee'.

2499 coleryca...2500 passio] *i.e. colik passiŏun* 'a disease characterised by severe abdominal pain, the colik; a disease affecting the colon'.

2503 uenenis] Borrowed from OF *venim*, this word is elsewhere written in H497 as *uenym*.

2509 chue] Verb *cheuen* 'to chew, masticate' is written elsewhere in H497 as *cheuen/chewen*. Jordan (1974: 127) argues that the *eu*-diphthong stems from *ēo* + *w*, yielding /ø:u/ and eventually /eu/ <ew>. In the 15th century, coinciding with the raising from /e:/ to /i:/, the resulting diphthong /eu/ becomes /iu/. Variant *chue*, in turn, is sporadically used in H497.

2547 moor profytable] Periphrastic comparison with a polysyllabic adjective. The synthetic model is used with this same adjective in 2440 (*profytabler*). For comparison, see other instances of the periphrastic comparison in *moor feble*, *moor feruent*, *moor sharpe*, etc.

2572 outhe] From OE *ūt*, variant *outhe* witnesses a late aspirated pronunciation (Jordan 1974: 183).

2584 nardus celtica] *i.e.* 'Celtic spikenard'. In *De Materia Medica*, Dioscorides defines it as a small plant grown in the Alps having oblong and yellow leaves and a quince yellow flower (see Beck 2005: 10).

2596 þe wyche] Defining relative clause introduced by *þe wyche*. Note that the antecedent (*dyssese*) is repeated in order to avoid the mis-interpretation of the preceding noun (*nayles*) as the factual antecedent of *þe wyche*.

2620 whyte...2621 inne] *i.e.* *within(ne* 'in the interior', wherein the fricative becomes a plosive.

2621 aloe...2622 epaticum] A Latinate borrowing denoting 'hepatic aloes', *i.e.* any of the opaque and liver-coloured aloes, originally from East Indies, whose powder is of a dull yellow colour.

2622 strynthe] From OE *strengþu* 'strength', the stem vowel raises from /ɛ/ to /i/ in closed syllables from the beginning of the 13th century under the influence of neighbouring sounds, covered /n/ among them. The change is initiated in the Northern dialects whilst the middle South of England is at first reluctant to adopt it. In H497, *e*-forms (5×) outnumber *i*-forms (3×). The omission of the consonant <g>, on the other hand, is viewed as a transition from /g/ to /n/ which, initially velar, was pronounced as a palatal, hence *strynth* (Jordan 1974: 60; 178).

2667 Lauryel] From F *laurier* 'laurel', this herb is spelt as *lorer* (3×), *lauryel* (1×) and *lauryall* (1×) (2705). First, variant *lorer* stems from the regular development of the French cognate in the vernacular. Digraph <ie>, on the other hand, is justified as a typical 15th-century spelling of southern ME. *Lauryall*, in turn, is the result of the Anglo-norman development from <ei> to <ai>, initially pronounced as /æi/ and later smoothing to /ɛ:/ (Jordan 1974: 211; 213). According to the *OED*, final <l> arises from the common substitution of the original <r>.

2691 te] Oblique second person pronoun *þe*. The general substitution of <þ> for <t> is recorded in *LALME* as a characteristic feature of the South East (McIntosh et al. 1984, IV : 320).

2714 be fall] As in OE, impersonal verb *bifallen* 'to come to pass, happen' does not occur with the experiencer as subject (Traugott 1992: 211).

2715 lyke] Adverb *līk* 'equally, alike, in the same way'.

2717 swettyst] From OE *swēt*, the doubling of the consonant <tt> gives evidence of a shortening process in the comparative and superlative forms. As mentioned above, *þe* is lacking in the superlative. Compare this rendering with *gretyst* (598 and 1195), whose orthography implies the existence of vowel length.

2731 swyfther] Word-final <th>, from the OE voiceless plosive /t/, indicates a late ME aspirated pronunciation (Jordan 1974: 183). See other instances like *wythe* 'white', *outh* 'out', *profyth* 'profit', etc.

2736 Notemygge] From ML *nux muga* and OF *nois mugate* 'a nutmeg', the ME cognate is a partial translation of French *nois* 'nut' and *mugate* 'musk' (*OED*), the latter pronounced as /y/ as a reflex of OF <u> /y/, represented either as *notemuge* (Frisk 1949: 193) or *nottemygge*.

2750 menyson] *i.e.* 'dysentery'.

2776 heer] From OE *hāra* + *ēare* 'hare's ear', the name given to the common avens (*Geum urbanum*).

2799 auricula leporyna] Latin borrowing translated as 'hare's ears'. This term is used to denote a primula, any plant of the genus Primula, including primroses, cowslips and polyanthuses.

2820 hayth] From OE *hæfþ*, 3rd p. sing. pres. of *habban* 'to have'. This form is rendered in H497 as *hath* (2x2), *hat* (6×) and *hayth* (1×), the latter, according to *LALME*, characteristic from the East Midlands (McIntosh et al. 1986, IV: 190).

2825 Eucatesma] From Gr. ἐνκαϱθίς 'encanthis', *i.e.* a tumour in the inner corner of the eye (*OED*).

2827 arthetici...2828 dolores] Latinate borrowing to denote 'an affection of the joints, gout'.

2846 hey hony] i.e. *hei-hōve* 'the herb ground ivy, often used medicinally'.

Chapter 4. The Glossary

4.1. Conventions

This chapter contains a selected glossary of the terms found in H497. As this volume is ultimately designed for an academic readership, the present glossary disregards those words with which a Middle English scholar is familiar, mostly grammatical words like determiners, prepositions and conjunctions. The underlying impulse here is, therefore, the compilation of lexical words, both general and scientific, to offer an *ad hoc* tool for a successful reading of the text. Adverbs, in turn, are often fuzzily interpreted as to whether they are, strictly speaking, lexical or grammatical words. The glossary is restricted to listing adjuncts of manner insofar as, unlike other adverb types, they semantically modify the action expressed by the verb.

Exceptionally, however, we make room for particular grammatical items when their spelling is not fully transparent, thus not easily identifiable with its corresponding headword. The preposition *thorugh*, for instance, has been purposely recorded on account of its spelling, with the use of regular forms such as *thorugh/thorgh/thurgh* together with others which may be more problematic such as *þorfe* or *thurght*.

The entry structure sequentially displays the following information: a) the headword; b) the part of speech; and c) the meaning of the glossed items. In addition, the different allographs are also listed together with the number of occurrences.

Several conventions have been used in the layout of the entries. As cited above, the present research stems from a major project developed at Málaga University which pursues the diplomatic edition of late Middle English *Fachliteratur*. These editions eventually serve as the input for the compilation of an annotated corpus of Middle English scientific prose. Given the level of orthographic variation among Middle English scribes, the use of a uniform spelling was more than a must during the annotation process. For convenience, headwords show the most frequent variant in the text, which is taken as the nominative singular form in the case of nouns and adjectives. Verbs, in turn, are listed under the corresponding infinitive, accordingly based on the orthographic practice of the scribe.

If a word is not found in the *e-MED* (Kurath et al. 1956-2001), the headword is followed by a dagger (†). Part-of-speech tags, on the other hand, are italicised in the glossary by using the following notation: nouns (*n.*), adjectives (*a.*), verbs (*v.*), adverbs (*adv.*), conjunctions (*c.*) and prepositions (*p.*).

Meanings, in turn, are given according to the definition found in the *e-MED*. If a particular word is not recorded therein, we rely on Frisk's interpretation in his 1949 critical edition of the other versions of the text. On the other hand, when a particular tag phrase, collocation or prepositional verb deserves mentioning, these appear at the end of the corresponding entry preceded by two horizontal bars. For the sake of brevity, note that the implicit headword is shortened. Note, for instance, ‖ *goon to s.* 'to ease oneself' under the headword *sege* 'a seat; a chair, stool'.

As cited above, if a word shows an obscure allograph, not easily identifiable with its corresponding headword, we grant it the status of a headword to refer back to its factual entry. For simplicity, an arrow (→) has been used for these purposes. In this vein, the entry *þorfe* → thorugh, *p.* refers to the factual headword *thorugh*.

4.2. Glossary

A

abaten, *v.* To alleviate, allay
a bate (5×), *a batyth* (3×), *abate* (33×), *abatyth* (3×)

abrode, *adv.* Wide, open; broad
abrode (1×), *a brood* (1×), *abroode* (1×)

abundant, *a.* Many, much, abundant
abundant (2×)

accesse, *n.* An attack of illness characterized by fever, esp. of malarial fever or ague
accesse (5×), *axses* (1×)

accorden, *v.* To accord, come to an agreement
accordyth (1×), *acorde* (1×)

acedula †, *n.* Sorrel
acedula (1×)

ache, *n.* Ache
ache (79×), *aches* (3×)

ache, *n.* Any of a group of celery-like plants, as smallage, parsley
ache (1×)

acincuma †, *n.* A kind of venom
acincuma (1×)

acolden, *v.* To make (sth.) cold or cool
acoldyth (1×)

acombren, *v.* To harass or distress (sb.)
a combred (1×)

aculiphe †, *n.* Nettle
aculiphe (1×)

addre, *n.* Serpent, snake
adder (1×), *addre* (2×), *addres* (7×), *address* (1×), *addrys* (1×)

addris tuncte, *n.* Any one of various medicinal plants; the yellow gagea (Gagea lutea), wood lysimachia (Lysimachia nemorum), fenugreek (Trigonella foenumgraecum), or dragonwort (Dracunculus vulgaris)
addristuncte (1×)

adgranus, *n.* The European purslane
adgranus (1×)

adustyoun, *n.* Treatment with heat or burning
adustyon (1×), *adustyoun* (5×)

affermen, *v.* To establish, settle; to corroborate (a statement)
afferme (2×), *affermyth* (1×), *affyrmyth* (1×)

afforism †, *n.* Afforism
afforismes (1×)

aforesayd, *a.* Aforesaid, above-mentioned
afore sayd (1×), *afore seyd* (1×), *aforesayd* (1×)

afterbyrden †, *n.* After-birth; the bearing of a child in the womb, gestation
after byrden (3×), *after byrdon* (1×), *after byrdoun* (3×), *afterberden* (1×)

age, *n.* A person's age
age (7×)

aken, *v.* To ache, be painful
ake (4×), *aken* (2×), *akyn* (1×), *akyth* (8×)

akorous, *n.* Gladiolus root
akorous (1×)

akynge, *ng.* Pain, aching
akynge (2×), *akynges* (1×)

ale, *n.* Beer, ale
ale (1×)

alighten, *v.* To lighten, alleviate
alyght (1×), *alyghte* (1×)

allayen, *v.* To allay, alleviate
alay (1×), *allaye* (2×)

allenten, *v.* To alleviate, lessen
allente (1×)
allone, *adv.* all alone, solitary
allone (14×)
allopicia, *n.* Falling of the hair
allopes (1×), *allopicia* (1×), *allopiciam* (1×)
alltea, *n.* Wild malowe (Althaea officinalis)
alltea (1×)
almost, *adv.* Almost
al most (1×), *all most* (2×), *almost* (4×)
almounde, *n.* The fruit of the almond tree
almoundes (1×)
aloe, *n.* The juice or resin of the tree, aloes
aloe (12×)
aloe epatic, *n.* Hepatic aloes
aloe epaticum (1×)
Alsydes, *n.* Alcides
alsydes (1×)
al togydyr, *adv.* all in one group, all together
al togydyr (1×)
alway, *adv.* Always
all way (1×), *alway* (2×)
alym, *n.* Common or potash alum
alym (1×)
alyssen, *v.* To deliver, release
a lysse (1×)
amarusca, *n.* Stinking camomile
amarusca (1×)
Amasilaus, *n.* Amasilaus
Amasilaus (1×)
ambrosia, *n.* Ambrose, wild sage, wood germander
ambrosia (2×)
amenden, *v.* To cure (a disease, etc.); to recover from illness
ameden (1×), *amende* (4×), *amendyth* (1×)
amonge, *p.* Among
a monge (1×), *amonge* (4×)
amorwe, *adv.* In the morning
a morwe (1×)
aneyntisen, *v.* To destroy (sth.); to lessen, diminish (sth.); deplete
aneyntyse (1×)
aneys, *n.* The plant anise
aneys (6×), *anneys* (2×), *annyse* (1×), *anys* (1×), *anyse* (4×)
anon as, *c.* As soon as
anon as (1×)
anoon, *adv.* At once, instantly, immediately; shortly, soon
a noon (6×), *annon* (1×), *anoon* (5×)
anoynten, *v.* To apply a medicinal substance
a noynte (11×), *a noynted* (10×), *anoynte* (37×), *anoynted* (22×), *anynted* (1×), *noynted* (1×)
anoyntyng, *ng.* The action of applying medicinal unguents or lotions to a wound or sore
anoyntyng (1×), *anoyntynge* (1×)
anteryke → **arthetica**, *n. / a.*
anynted → **anoynten**, *v.*
anys(e) → **aneys**, *n.*
Apelledorus, *n.* Apelledorus
Apelledorus (1×)
apium, *n.* Wild celery or smallage
apium (3×)
apple, *n.* Apple
apples (1×)
arage, *n.* A plant of the genus Atriplex, esp. the garden orach
arage (6×)
aray, *n.* Order or position of things, arrangement, order
aray (1×)

Aristologia, *n.* One of several kinds of plants, including Aristolochia rotunda; also Chenopodium Bonus-Henricus
aristologia (1×), *osterlagya* (1×)
armepytte, *n.* Armpit
armepyttes (1×)
arnoglossa, *n.* Plantain
arnoglossa (3×)
arowe, *n.* Arrow
arowe (4×)
arthemesis, *n.* Mugwort (Artemisia vulgaris)
arthemesia (1×), *arthemesis* (1×), *arthemesys* (1×)
arthetica, *n.* / *a.* Arthritis, rheumatism; Arthritic, rheumatic || **goute a.** gout
anteryke (1×), *artetica* (1×), *arthetica* (2×); *arthetici* (1×)
aryght, *adv.* Correctly, truly
aryght (1×)
asara → **azara**, *n.*
ascapen, *v.* To escape
a scape (1×), *ascape* (1×)
ascenden, *v.* To rise
ascendyth (1×)
Asclepius, *n.* Asclepius
Asclepius (3×)
asken, *v.* To ask, enquire
aske (2×), *askyth* (1×)
aslepe, *adv.* asleep
a slepe (1×)
asmathicus †, *n.* Asmathic; asthmatic
asmathicus (1×), *asmaticos* (1×)
aspien, *v.* To look for, seek to discover
aspye (1×)
assenten, *v.* To agree, approve of (a suggestion, idea, etc.)
assente (1×)
asshe, *n.* Ash
asshen (3×), *asshes* (7×)
astoned, *a.* Dulled, benumbed, deadened
astoned (1×), *astonyed* (1×)
aswagen, *v.* To relieve pain; to mitigate, alleviate
a swagyth (1×), *asswage* (1×), *asswagyth* (1×), *aswage* (3×)
Athene, *n.* Athens
Athene (1×)
atter, *n.* Rotten matter, pus
attere (1×)
attones, *adv.* At the same time, simultaneously
attones (1×)
august, *n.* August
august (1×)
aunsweren, *v.* To answer
aunswere (1×)
auricula leporyna †, *n.* Primula, any plant of the genus Primula, bearing primrose flowers, including primroses, cowslips and polyanthuses
auricula leporyna (1×)
autemus, *n.* Purple camomile
autemus (2×), *authemus* (1×)
autor, *n.* Author, authority
autores (2×), *autours* (1×)
awarpen, *v.* To throw, cast down
awarpe (1×)
ayȝon †, *n.* Sorrel
ayȝon (1×)
azara, *n.* Asarabacca (Asarum Europaeum)
asara (1×), *asarum* (1×); *azara* (1×)

B

baken, *v.* To bake
y bake (1×)
baldemoine, *n.* A plant of the genus Gentiana (prob. either G. lutea or the native British G. amarella)

baldemoyne (4×)

ballok, *n.* Testicle

ballockes (3×), *ballok* (1×), *ballokes* (4×), *ballokkes* (1×)

baraces †, *n.* Honeysuckle

baraces (1×)

bare, *n.* A bare part of the body, bare skin

bare (1×)

bareyn, *a.* Unpregnant (animal)

bareyn (1×)

barly floure, *n.* The grain or meal of barley

barly floure (1×)

barly mele, *n.* Barley meal; meal made by grinding grain (usually wheat); the bolted meal, flour

barly mele (1×), *barly mely* (1×)

baten, *v.* To alleviate, allay

batyth (1×)

bath, *n.* Bath

bath (1×), *bathe* (3×)

bathen, *v.* To bath or wash

bathe (4×), *bathed* (1×), *bathen* (1×), *ybaþed* (1×)

bathynge, *ng.* Bathing, a bath

bathynge (4×), *bathynges* (1×)

batynge, *ng.* Beating

batynge (1×)

bawme, *n.* Aromatic oleoresin of the balm of Gilead and other shrubs of the genus Commiphora

bawme (2×)

bay, *n.* The berry-like fruit of various plants, trees or shrubs

bayes (1×)

becomen, *v.* To become (sth.); to come (to a place)

be come (1×), *by come* (1×)

bedde, *n.* Bed

bedde (1×)

bee, *n.* Bee

been (1×), *bees* (6×)

beef, *n.* Beef

beef (1×)

begynnen, *v.* To begin

begynne (1×), *begynneth* (1×), *begynnyth* (1×)

begynnyng, *ng.* Beginning

begynnyng (3×)

beholden, *v.* To look or gaze at (sth.); observe or watch (sth.)

be holde (1×)

beken, *v.* To warm (sth.)

beked (1×), *beket* (1×)

bekyng, *ng.* The process of baking

bekyng (1×)

bely, *n.* The belly of man or animal, abdomen

bely (13×)

ben, *va.* To be

are (2×), *be* (281×), *ben* (73×), *hys* (1×), *is* (3×), *was* (11×), *were* (13×), *where* (1×), *ys* (384×)

ben, *v.* To be ‖ **b. with child** to be pregnant ‖ **b. wont to** to be accustomed or inclined to

am (1×), *are* (2×), *be* (23×), *bee* (1×), *ben* (34×), *is* (1×), *was* (1×), *ys* (257×)

ben, *n.* The seed of the broad bean plant

been (1×), *benes* (2×)

benette, *n.* A medicinal plant, prob. the common hemlock (Conium maculatum)

benette (2×)

ben mele, *n.* Ground dried beans, bean meal

ben mele (1×), *been mele* (1×)

beren, *v.* To carry (sth.); to give birth to (a child)

bere (3×), *beren* (1×), *beryt* (3×), *beryth* (8×), *boor* (1×), *borum* (1×)

berken, *v.* To bark

berke (1×)

best, *n.* Beast; any living creature (non-vegetable)
best (2×), *beste* (2×), *bestes* (10×), *bestys* (1×)

beten, *v.* To beat
bete (1×)

beteyne, *n.* The European betony (Betonica officinalis); also medicines made from this plant
beteyn (6×), *beteyne* (25×), *byteyne* (1×)

blacken, *v.* To become black or dark in colour
blackyth (1×)

bladdre, *n.* Bladder
badder (1×), *bladder* (6×), *bladdre* (7×), *bladre* (1×)

blak, *a.* Black colour
blac (1×), *blak* (17×), *blake* (5×)

blak, *n.* The colour black, dark or black colour
blak (1×)

blak colre, *n.* Black Bile, one of the four primary 'humours'
blak colere (1×), *blak colre* (1×)

blak ellebur, *n.* Black hellebore; the dried root of certain species of Helleborus
blak ellebur (4×)

blastre, *n.* Blister
blastres (2×)

bleden, *v.* To lose blood, bleed
blede (1×), *bleden* (2×), *bledyth* (1×)

bledyng, *ng.* Bleeding, loss of blood; a hemorrhage
bledyng (1×)

bleyn, *n.* Inflammatory swelling or sore; blain, pustule, pimple, blister
bleynes (1×)

blod, *n.* Blood
blod (7×), *blode* (7×), *bloed* (1×), *blood* (1×), *bloode* (2×)

blody, *a.* With blood
blody (8×)

blynde, *a.* Blind
blynde (1×)

blynden, *v.* To grow or be blind
blynded (1×)

bocche, *n.* Pathological swelling, eruption or lesion, such as a boil, a tumor, a (running) sore, an ulcer
bocche (6×), *bocches* (33×)

body, *n.* The human body
body (60×), *bodyes* (3×)

boke, *n.* Book
boke (11×), *bokes* (4×)

boldely, *adv.* Boldly, courageously, fearlessly
boldely (1×)

bolkynge, *ng.* A belch, belching; retching, vomiting
bolkynge (1×)

boll, *n.* Ball, a spherical receptacle
bolles (4×)

bollen, *v.* To swell or cause to swell; to swell up, become puffed up or inflated
bolle (2×), *bollen* (3×), *ybolle* (1×)

bollyng, *ng.* Bloating, flatulence
bollyng (1×)

bolnen, *v.* To swell
bollne (1×), *bolne* (2×), *bolnyth* (1×)

bolnyng, *ng.* Swelling or distention (of some part of the body); a swollen part
bollnyng (1×), *bolnyng* (12×), *bolnynge* (11×), *bolnynges* (13×), *boluyng* (1×)

boon, *n.* Bone
bon (1×), *bones* (1×), *boon* (3×)

boon, *n.* Poison
boon (1×)

boter → **butter**, *n.*

boughte → **buyen**, *v.*

bouter → **butter**, *n.*

bowel, *n.* Human intestine
bowelles (1×), *bowels* (3×), *bowles* (2×)

bowen, *v.* To bend
bowed (1×)

boylen, *v.* To be agitated, surge, seethe, boil
boyle (1×)

boylyng, *ng.* Boiling
boylyng (1×), *boylynge* (1×)

brakyng, *ng.* Vomiting
brakyng (2×), *brakynge* (2×), *brakynges* (1×)

bras, *n.* Copper, brass
bras (2×)

brassica, *n.* A plant of the cabbage family
brassica (1×)

brayen, *v.* To break (sth.) into small fragments, as by stamping, crushing, grinding, chopping
brayde (1×)

brayn, *n.* Brain
brayne (4×)

brayn panne, *n.* The part of the skull that encloses the brain
brayn panne (1×)

breche, *n.* Breakage, fracture
breche (2×)

bred, *n.* Bread
bred (8×), *brede* (1×)

brefly, *adv.* In few words, briefly; concisely
brefly (1×)

bregghynge, *ng.* Shortcutting, termination
bregghynge (1×)

breken, *v.* To break (an object) into parts; to crush (the human body, etc.)
breke (2×), *breken* (1×), *brekyt* (2×), *brekyth* (5×), *broke* (3×), *broken* (2×), y *broke* (2×), *ybroke* (1×)

brekyng, *ng.* Fracturing or fracture (a bone or limb)
brekyng (2×), *brekynges* (1×)

brennen, *v.* To burn, burn down ‖ **b. up** to flame up
brenne (3×), *brennet* (1×), *brennyth* (2×), *brent* (8×), *y brent* (1×)

brennyng, *ng.* A burning sensation; inflammation
brennynges (3×), *brynnyges* (1×), *brynnyng* (1×), *brynnynges* (1×)

brest, *n.* Breast
brest (25×), *breste* (1×), *brestes* (2×)

bresten, *v.* To issue suddenly, spring forth ‖ **b. out** to blister (skin, flesh), produce an eruption
borst (1×), *brest* (1×)

brisen, *v.* To break (sth.) into small particles, as by crushing, stamping, or grinding
brosed (1×)

brotherworte, *n.* Pennyroyal (Mentha pulegium); wild thyme (Thymus serpyllum); wild marjoram (Origanum vulgare)
brotherworte (2×)

brow, *n.* Eye-brow
browes (2×)

brude, *n.* Sprout, shoot
brude (1×)

bruserys → **brusur**, *n.*

brusur, *n.* Wound, bruise
bruserys (1×), *brusours* (1×), *brusurs* (1×)

brusyng, *n.* Fracturing (of bones); bruising
brusynges (3×)

bryght, *a.* Clear, bright
bryght (5×)

brymstoun, *n.* Mineral sulphur
brymstoun (1×)
bryngen, *v.* To bring; to fetch
brenge (1×), *bryng* (1×), *brynge* (7×), *bryngith* (1×), *bryngyth* (2×)
brynnyng → **brennyng**, *ng.*
bryst, *n.* Evil deed, injury
bryst (1×)
buffet, *n.* Blow delivered with the fist or flat of the hand
buffet (1×)
bute, *n.* Beauty
bute (1×)
butter, *n.* Butter
boter (1×), *bouter* (1×), *butter* (1×)
buyen, *v.* To purchase, buy
boughte (1×)
bydden, *v.* To ask, beg
byddyth (1×)
bynden, *v.* To tie (sth.) up; gather or hold together
bounde (4×), *bounden* (2×), *bynde* (8×), *byndyth* (3×)
byrd, *n.* Bird
byrdes (1×)
byrdoun, *n.* Bearing of a child in the womb, gestation
byrdoun (1×)
byrthe, *n.* Birth
byrthe (2×)
bysely, *adv.* Constantly, incessantly
bysely (1×)
bysshopisworte, *n.* Betony
bysshopisworte (1×), *bysshopys worte* (1×)
byten, *v.* To bite or sting (sb.); injure by biting, jabbing or stinging
byde (1×), *byte* (2×), *bytyn* (1×), *bytyth* (1×)
bytter, *a.* Bitter
byter (1×), *bytter* (5×)
bytyng, *ng.* Biting; wound inflicted by biting
bytyng (6×), *bytynge* (10×), *bytynges* (20×), *bytyngges* (1×)

C

caas, *n.* Event, case
caas (1×)
caken, *v.* To do the cooking
cake (2×)
calamynte, *n.* A member of the genus Calamintha, the common calamint
calamentes (1×), *calamentum* (1×), *calamynt* (1×), *calamynte* (4×)
callen, *v.* To call (sth. by a certain name), name (sb. sth.)
calle (1×), *called* (24×), *callen* (1×), *callyd* (2×)
camedrios, *n.* A medicinal plant: the common, or wall, germander
camedrios (2×)
camomylle, *n.* The common camomile
camomilla (1×), *camomula* (1×), *camomylle* (7×), *canomille* (1×)
cancre, *n.* Cancer; an ulcerated non-malignant tumor, a spreading ulcer
cancre (5×), *cancres* (8×)
canell, *n.* Cinnamon (in powder, stick, or roll)
canel (4×), *canell* (3×)
caniculata †, *n.* Henbane
caniculata (1×)
capitellum †, *n.* A kind of poppy
capitellum (1×)
cappe, *n.* Cap worn under the helmet
cappe (1×)
caprifolium, *n.* The European honeysuckle
caprifolium (1×)
capytell, *n.* The head (of a herb, plant)

capytell (1×)
cardama → **cardamomum**, *n.*
cardamomum, *n.* A plant of the mustard family, a cress; esp., the common water cress
cardama (1×), *cardamomum* (1×)
cardiacus, *n.* A vein associated with the heart; prob. the median vein in the arm
cardiacus (1×)
carewey, *n.* The plant caraway (Carum carui)
careway (1×), *carewey* (2×), *careweye* (2×)
casten, *v.* To pour or sprinkle ‖ **c. in** to bring into ‖ **c. out** to force (a liquid) out of its place or channel
cast (1×), caste (9×), *casted* (1×), *casten* (1×), *casteyn* (1×), *castyst* (1×), *castyth* (2×)
castreon, *n.* Betony
castreon (1×)
Caton, *n.* Cato
Caton (6×)
caule, *n.* Cabbage, kale, colwort, rape, mustard, or some other plant of the genus Brassica
caule (19×), *caules* (8×)
cause, *n.* Cause
cause (4×), *causes* (25×), *cavses* (2×)
causon, *n.* A kind of chronic fever
causon (1×)
cedewale → **sedewale**, *n.*
celidonye, *n.* The greater celandine (Chelidonium majus); also, any of its parts used medicinally
celidonia (1×), *celidonye* (2×), *celidoyne* (1×), *celiodyne* (1×), *celydonye* (1×)
celte †, *n.* Celts
celte (1×)
cense, *n.* Incense, or its smoke or fragrance
cense (1×), *ceunse* (1×)
centory, *n.* The common centaury
centory (11×)
ceralis, *n.* The aromatic oleoresin of the balm of Gilead and other shrubs of the genus Commiphora
ceralis (1×)
cerfoyle, *n.* Honeysuckle
cerfoyle (15×), *cherfoyle* (1×)
cerote, *n.* An officinal ointment consisting of wax blended with medicinal ingredients
cerote (1×), *cerotes* (1×)
certeyn, *a.* Certain
certeyn (3×)
cerulde → **cerule**, *n. / a.*
cerule †, *n. / a.* Cerule; cerulean
cerulde (1×), *cerules* (1×)
ceruse, *n.* White lead, a compound used in pigments and medicaments
ceruse (1×)
cessen, *v.* To cease or desist
cesse (1×)
ceunse → **cense**, *n.*
chacen, *v.* To dispell, do away with; to expell ‖ **c. away** to repel (sth.), ward off ‖ **c. out** to expel
chace (1×), *chastyth* (1×), *chasyth* (1×)
chafed → **chaufen**, *v.*
chaster †, *n.* Glandular swelling resulting from fever
chaster (1×)
chastyth → **chacen**, *v.*
chasyth → **chacen**, *v.*
chaufen, *v.* To warm (sth.) by rubbing; to heat
chafed (2×), *chaued* (2×), *chaufed* (1×), *chawe* (1×)

chaungyng, *ng*. Modification, change, the act or process of altering
chaungyng (1×)
chawe → **chaufen**, *v*.
cheke, *n*. Jaw, jawbone
cheke (1×), *chekes* (3×), *chekys* (2×)
cherfoyle → **cerfoyle**, *n*.
cheryston, *n*. Cherry-stone, the stone or pit of a cherry
cherystones (1×)
chese, *n*. Cheese
chese (2×)
cheste, *n*. Chest
cheste (1×)
cheude → **chewen**, *v*.
chewen, *v*. To chew (sth.)
cheude (1×), *chewe* (4×), *chewen* (1×), *chewyth* (2×), *chue* (1×)
choken, *v*. To suffocate
choke (1×)
chue → **chewen**, *v*.
chyke, *n*. Chicken
chyke (1×)
chyld, *n*. Child, baby
chelde (2×), *cheldes* (1×), *chydryn* (1×), *chyld* (5×), *chylde* (22×), *chyldes* (2×), *chyldren* (1×), *chyldryn* (4×), *chyldryns* (1×), *chyndryn* (1×)
chyne, *n*. Cavity (in the body); gap (of a wound)
chynes (1×)
chynke, *n*. Asthma or whooping cough
chynke (7×)
chyse, *n*. Sprout, petal ‖ **safrom c.** sprouts of saffron
chyses (1×)
ciate, *n*. A measure of weight (equal to ten drams)
ciate (1×), *ciates* (4×), *ciatis* (1×), *ciatus* (2×)
ciatica → **scietica**, *n*.
cicatrice, *n*. Cicatrix, scar of a healed wound or sore
cicatrices (1×)
ciliac †, *n*. The person who suffers from the celiac disease
ciliaci (1×)
ciperus, *n*. The galingale or its root
ciperus (1×), *cyperus* (1×)
claryfyen, *v*. To make (the eyesight) clear; to free (respiratory passages) from phlegm
claryfye (3×), *claryfyeth* (2×), *claryfyth* (1×)
clene, *a*. Not foul or dirty, clean, unsoiled; free from (disease, infection, etc.)
clene (6×)
clenly, *adv*. Cleanly
clenly (1×)
clensen, *v*. To cleanse (sth.) of filth or dirt, wash, wipe; to remove (filth), wipe (blood) away
clense (24×), *clensed* (1×), *clensyt* (2×), *clensyth* (7×)
clepen, *v*. To apply (a name or designation to sb. or sth.)
cheped (1×), *chepyd* (1×), *clepe* (1×), *cleped* (67×), *clepen* (15×), *clepyd* (41×), *clepyt* (2×), *clepyth* (2×), *y cleped* (2×), *y clepyd* (1×)
clere, *n*. / *a*. The clear or clarified portion of a liquid; free from impurities, pure
clere (7×)
cleren, *v*. To make clear or clean, cleanse
cleren (1×)
clerke, *n*. Scholar, master (of some subject); man of letters, writer, author
clerke (3×), *clerkes* (1×)
clofunge, *n*. Crowfoot (Ranunculus); hellebore
clofunge (1×)
closen, *v*. To obstruct a passageway

clos (1×), *close* (4×), *closed* (5×), *closyth* (1×)

clothe, *n.* A piece of woven or felted fabric; a cloth
clothe (3×), *cloute* (1×)

cloute → **clothe**, *n.*

clove, *n.* A bulbil or clove, esp. of garlic
cloue (2×), *cloues* (3×)

clove gilofre, *n.* A bulbil or clove
cloue gilofre (1×), *cloue gylofre* (1×)

clunatis †, *n.* Smerewort
clunatis (1×)

clyster, *n.* Clyster, enema; any medicinal liquid administered through the rectum; the instrument for injecting such liquids, a sort of syringe
clyster (2×), *clystery* (2×), *clystrer* (1×)

coccion, *n.* Boiling
coccion (4×)

codd, *n.* A seed pod or capsule
coddes (1×)

col, *n.* Charcoal, or a piece of it
coles (2×)

colde, *n.* / *a.* A cold; cold
cold (12×), *colde* (38×)

colera → **colre**, *n.*

colera rubea, *n.* Yellow bile
colera rubea (1×)

colica passio, *n.* Colic passion, colic pains
coleryca passio (1×), *colica passio* (1×)

colluryes, *n.* Medicine applied to the eye, collyrium
colluryes (2×)

colon, *n.* Large intestine or colon (also including the rectum)
colon (1×)

coloure, *n.* Colour as an inherent property of matter
coloure (8×), *coloures* (2×), *colowre* (1×), *colure* (1×), *couloure* (1×)

colouren, *v.* To give colour to (sth.)
coloure (1×), *coloured* (2×), *colured* (1×)

colre, *n.* Bile, one of the four primary 'humors'
colera (1×), *colre* (7×)

colver, *n.* Dove, culver
coluer (1×)

colyke, *n.* Disease characterized by severe abdominal pain, the colic
colyke (1×)

comen, *v.* To approach, arrive or come ‖ **c. upon** to attack
come (5×), *comen* (4×), *comet* (2×), *cometh* (2×), *comyth* (5×), *cornyth* (1×)

comenly → **comounly**, *adv.*

comforten, *v.* To strengthen, revive (a part of the body, the functioning of an organ, etc.)
comefourthe (1×), *conforte* (1×), *comforted* (1×), *conforteth* (1×), *conforthe* (1×), *comfortyth* (10×), *confortyth* (1×)

commaunden, *v.* To command, prescribe
comaundyd (1×), *comaundyt* (1×), *comaundyth* (5×), *commaunde* (2×), *commaunded* (2×), *commaunden* (1×), *commaundyd* (1×), *commaundyth* (4×)

commenden, *v.* To commit or consign
commenden (1×), *commendyd* (1×), *commendyth* (1×)

comoun, *a.* Common, usual, ordinary
common (2×), *comoun* (5×), *comune* (1×)

comounly, *adv.* Frequently, commonly, usually
comenly (1×), *commenly* (1×), *commounly* (2×), *comounly* (7×)

comyn, *n.* The plant cumin

commyn (1×), *comyn* (9×)
comyng, *ng*. Arrival, coming
comyng (1×)
conceyven, *v*. To conceive, become pregnant
conceyue (3×), *conceyueth* (2×)
condempnen, *v*. To condemn, criticize
condempnen (1×)
condycion, *n*. Situation or state
condycions (1×)
confeccion, *n*. Preparation of a medicine
confeccion (6×)
confecten, *v*. To prepare (sth.) by blending or combining ingredients
confecte (3×)
confermen, *v*. To ratify, approve or confirm authoritatively
conferme (2×), *confermyth* (1×), *confyrmed* (1×), *confyrmen* (1×), *confyrmyth* (2×)
comfery, *n*. The herb comfrey
comfery (1×)
cononidion, *n*. Laurel
cononidion (1×)
consounden, *v*. To heal (a wound or fracture) by promoting cicatrization or knitting
consounde (1×)
conssegnen, *v*. To certify
conssegned (1×)
Constantinus, *n*. Constantinus Africanus
Constantinus (1×)
consumen, *v*. To reduce or destroy
consume (3×), *consumyth* (1×)
consyderen, *v*. To inspect, examine, or observe (sth.)
consydre (2×)
conteynen, *v*. To include (sth.)
contened (1×), *conteyne* (1×), *conteyneth* (1×)
contraccion, *n*. Contraction or spasm (of muscles)
contraccion (1×)
contrary, *n*. Adverse condition or difficulty
contrary (1×)
contynuall, *a*. Continual
contynuall (1×)
convenyent, *a*. Suitable or appropriate; convenient (under given circumstances or for a purpose)
conuenyent (1×)
corne, *n*. A crop of cereal-producing plants
corne (2×), *cornes* (8×)
cornels → **kernel**, *n*.
corner, *n*. Angle, corner
corners (1×)
cornyth → **comen**, *v*.
corrumpen, *v*. To corrupt, contaminate
corrumpynge (1×)
corrupcion, *n*. Disintegration, deterioration; a morbid condition, disease, or infection; pus, rot
corrupcion (2×), *corrupcyoun* (1×)
coryaundre, *n*. The plant coriander
coriaundre (1×), *coryandre* (2×), *coryaundre* (11×), *coryawndre* (1×)
coste, *n*. The herb costmary
cost (1×), *coste* (5×)
costlewe, *a*. Costly, expensive
costlewe (1×)
costumably, *adv*. Customarily, usually
costumably (1×)
costyf, *a*. Constipated, costive
coste (1×), *costyf* (9×)
counseylen, *v*. To counsel (sb.), advise, teach
counseyle (1×)
coveren, *v*. To cover (the body or its parts) with an article of clothing or armour
couered (2×), *ycouerd* (1×)
coveytously, *adv*. Covetously, greedily
coueytously (1×)

cowde → **cunnen**, *n.*
cowe, *n.* Cow
cowe (1×), *kowe* (1×)
cowe → **kouhe**, *n.*
cowhe → **kouhe**, *n.*
cowhen, *v.* To cough
cowhe (1×)
crampe, *n.* Violent contraction of muscles, a spasm; disease characterized by contortion or spasms
crampe (1×)
crepen, *v.* To creep
crepen (1×), *crepyth* (2×)
crepynge, *ng.* Crawling sensation in the body
crepyng (1×), *crepynge* (2×)
creta chimolea †, *n.* Cimolean chalk
creta chimolea (1×)
crisautemona †, *n.* Corn marigold, chrysanthemum
crisautemona (1×)
Crisippus, *n.* Chrysippus
Crisippus (1×)
crome, *n.* Crumb of bread; a small bit of broken bread or other food
cromes (4×)
croune → **crowne**, *n.*
crowne, *n.* Wreath of laurel, garland of flowers
croune (1×), *crowne* (1×)
cunnen, *v.* To have ability, capability, or skill, be able (to do sth.), be capable (of doing sth.), know how (to do sth.)
cowde (1×)
cunte → **kunte**, *n.*
cuntre, *n.* Country, land
cuntre (2×)
cuppe, *n.* Drinking vessel; bowl
cuppe (1×), *cuppes* (2×)
cure, *n.* Medical or surgical care, treatment
cure (2×), *cures* (1×)
curen, *v.* To cure, heal
cure (6×), *cured* (1×), *curen* (1×), *curyt* (1×), *curyth* (7×)
custumable, *a.* Customary, traditional
custumable (1×)
cycatrycen, *v.* To heal by forming a cicatrix
cycatryce (1×)

D

dampnen, *v.* To declare (sb.) guilty; condemn to death
dampned (1×)
dare → **durren**, *va.*
darte, *n.* Skin eruption; herpes
darte (1×)
dasewen, *v.* To grow dim ‖ **ben d.** (p.p.) to be dimmed
dasawyd (1×), *dasewed* (2×), *dasewen* (1×)
dasewenesse, *n.* Lethargy, sloth
dasewenesse (2×)
daunten, *v.* To subdue (an opponent); to defeat (an adversary)
daunte (1×)
day, *n.* Day
day (9×), *daye* (1×), *dayes* (9×), *days* (3×)
declaren, *v.* To tell about (sth.), tell (sb. sth.)
declare (1×)
decoccion, *n.* The process of thickening a liquid by boiling
decoccion (63×), *decoccioun* (1×), *decoccyon* (1×), *decocion* (1×), *decocyoun* (1×), *decoocion* (1×)
decocten, *v.* To boil
decocte (1×)

ded, *a.* Dead
ded (8×), *deed* (6×)
deedly, *a.* / *adv.* Subject to death, mortal; mortally, painfully
dedly (4×), *deedly* (6×)
deednesse †, *n.* Deadness
deednesse (1×)
defailen, *v.* To grow feeble, weaken physically
defayle (1×)
defaute, *n.* Lack, insufficiency
defaute (1×)
deffe, *a.* Deaf
deffe (1×)
defyen, *v.* To digest (food, drink)
defye (6×)
degestyon → **dygestyoun**, *n.*
degre, *n.* Degree (of heat, cold, moisture, or dryness)
degre (47×)
deliveren, *v.* To save (sb.), rescue, give relief to ‖ **d. out** to let out, free
delyuer (12×), *delyuerd* (1×), *delyuere* (5×), *delyuery* (1×), *delyueryd* (1×), *delyueryth* (1×)
delven, *v.* To dig (sth.), cultivate
deluyth (1×)
dep, *a.* Deep
depe (1×)
derkenes, *n.* Darkness, dusk
derkenes (1×), *dyrknes* (1×)
destroyen, *v.* To overcome or destroy (sth. evil or dangerous), to drive out or cure (an illness)
destre (1×), *destreth* (1×), *destreue* (1×), *destreye* (1×), *destreyth* (1×), *destroue* (1×), *destroy* (2×), *destroye* (1×), *destroyed* (1×), *destroyen* (1×), *destroyet* (3×), *destroyeth* (5×), *destroyt* (6×), *destroyth* (12×), *destrye* (3×), *destryeth* (1×), *destryth* (1×), *dystroy* (1×)
deth, *n.* Death
deth (4×), *dethe* (1×)
devel, *n.* Malignant spirit, demon, devil
deuels (1×)
Diana, *n.* Diana
Diana (1×)
diarria, *n.* Diarrhea
diarria (1×)
Diascorides, *n.* Dioscorides
Diascorides (3×), *diascorydes* (1×)
disnoicus †, *n.* Dyspanaic, affected with dyspnaea
disnoicus (1×)
docke, *n.* A plant of the genus Rumex
docke (5×), *dockes* (5×), *dokes* (1×)
dolaures → **doloure**, *n.*
doloure, *n.* Pain, suffering
dolaures (1×), *dolores* (1×), *doloure* (3×), *doloures* (5×)
domb, *a.* Lacking the ability to speak; mute; deaf and dumb
dombe (2×)
don, *v.* To do (sth.), carry on ‖ **d. away** to remove (sb. or sth.), put away
do (81×), *don* (4×), *done* (1×), *doo* (1×), *doon* (2×), *dost* (1×), *doth* (58×), *dothe* (1×), *doþe* (1×), *doynge* (1×), *dyde* (2×), *ydone* (1×)
Doracus, *n.* Doracus
doracus (1×)
doun, *adv.* Down
doun (5×), *doune* (1×)
dounfallyng, *n.* Downfalling
dounfallyng (1×)
doute, *n.* Doubt
doute (1×)
dowten, *v.* To feel uncertain, be in doubt
dowted (1×)
dradde → **dreden**, *v.*

dragme, *n.* A unit of apothecary's weight equivalent to one eighth of an ounce, a dram
dragme (6×), *dragmes* (4×), *drammes* (1×), ʒ (2×)

dragoun, *n.* Dragon tree
dragon (2×), *dragons* (10×), *dragouns* (1×)

drawen, *v.* To draw or withdraw || **d. in** to draw (nourishment, moisture), absorb || **d. out** to remove (sth.)
draue (1×), *draw* (3×), *drawe* (8×), *drawen* (5×), *drawyth* (2×), *drowe* (1×)

dreden, *v.* To be afraid
dradde (1×), *drede* (3×)

drem, *n.* Dream, vision
dremes (2×)

drenchen, *v.* To sink, drown
drenche (1×)

dronkenesse, *n.* The state of being drunk, intoxication
dronkenesse (1×), *drunkenesse* (1×)

dropesye, *n.* Dropsy
dropese (3×), *dropesye* (11×), *dropse* (1×), *dropsye* (1×)

dropsye → **dropesye**, *n.*

drunkenesse → **dronkenesse**, *n.*

drye, *a.* Dry
dry (1×), *drye* (58×)

dryen, *v.* To dry || **d. up** to lose moisture, become dry, dry out
drye (20×), *dryed* (3×), *dryeng* (1×), *dryet* (1×), *dryeth* (12×), *dryth* (1×), *ydryed* (2×)

dryenge, *ng.* Act or process of drying
dryenge (1×)

drynke, *n.* Beverage, drink
drenke (1×), *drunke* (2×), *drynk* (1×), *drynke* (23×), *drynkes* (4×)

drynken, *v.* To drink || **d. in** to swallow a drink
dronke (39×), *dronken* (8×), *dronkyn* (2×), *drunk* (3×), *drunke* (1×), *drunken* (12×), *drynk* (2×), *drynke* (107×), *drynken* (2×), *drynkest* (1×), *drynkyt* (3×), *drynkyth* (2×), *dynkyt* (1×), *I drunke* (2×), *y dronke* (19×), *y dronken* (1×), *y drunke* (8×), *ydronke* (3×), *ydrunke* (5×)

drynkyng, *n.* The action of drinking
drynkyng (1×)

dryven, *v.* To chase, pursue || **d. away** to get rid of, do away with || **d. out** to banish, expel
dryue (10×), *dryuen* (1×), *dryueth* (11×), *dryuyt* (2×), *dryuyth* (5×)

dryvynge, *ng.* The action of driving or chasing
dryuynge (1×)

durren, *va.* To have the courage (to do sth.), dare
dare (3×)

duske, *a.* Dark, not bright; dark-colored, dull
duske (2×)

duskenes, *n.* Darkness; dimness of eyes
duskenes (3×)

dust, *n.* Dust
dust (2×)

dyagredyum †, *n.* Diagrydium, an old name for a preparation of scammony, used in pharmacy
dyagredyum (1×)

dyen, *v.* To die
dye (1×), *dyeth* (1×)

dyer, *n.* Dyer, one who dyes cloth
dyers (1×)

dyffyculte, *n.* The quality of being difficult, hardness
dyffyculte (1×)

dygestyoun, *n.* Digestion of food and drink

degestyon (1×), *degestyoun* (1×), *dygestyon* (1×), *dygestyoun* (5×), *dygystyoun* (1×)
dyghten, *v.* To prepare
dyghte (2×)
dygystyoun → **dygestyoun**, *n.*
dyppen, *v.* To dip (sth.), immerse
dyppe (2×), *dypped* (1×)
dyrknes → **derkenes**, *n.*
dyrte, *n.* Excrement; dung; feces
dyrte (3×)
dyscoloryng, *ng.* Discoloration, changing of natural colour
dyscoloryng (1×)
dyslacion, *n.* Dislocation of a bone
dyslacion (1×)
dyssese, *n.* Physical hardship or suffering
dessese (3×), *dyssese* (27×), *dysseses* (20×), *dyssesys* (1×)
dyssolven, *v.* To decompose or destroy (sth.); to disintegrate; to break up or dissolve
dessolueth (1×), *dyssolue* (6×), *dyssoluyt* (1×), *dyssoluyth* (2×)
dystillacion, *n.* Application by drops, dripping; distillation; vaporization
dystillacion (1×), *dystyllacion* (1×)
dytayne, *n.* One of two medicinal plants: dittany of Crete (Origanum dictamnus) and/or white dittany
diteyne (1×), *dytayne* (1×), *dyteyne* (1×)
dyteyne → **dytayne**, *n.*
dyverse, *a.* Various
dyuerse (31×)
dyversly, *adv.* In a different manner, differently
dyuersely (1×), *dyuersly* (2×)
dyvyden, *v.* To divide, separate (sth.) into parts
dyuyded (1×)

E

effecte, *n.* Fulfillment
effecte (2×)
egges → **eye**, *n.*
egghynge, *ng.* Numbness (of the teeth)
egghynge (1×)
egilop, *n.* Ulcer or fistula in the inner angle of the eye; ?a kind of leprosy
egilop (1×), *egilopa* (1×), *eglopa* (1×)
elena, *n.* Elecampane, horseheal
elena (1×), *elenum* (1×)
elephancya, *n.* Leprosy
elephancya (1×)
ellebur, *n.* Hellebore, any of certain dried roots of medicinal property identified with L *helleborus*, *hellebore* ‖ **blāk e.** Black hellebore ‖ **whīt e.** white hellebore
elebur (4×), *ellebur* (6×), *ellybur* (5×), *olebur* (1×)
elles, *adv.* Otherwise; in addition, also
elles (1×)
elycumpana, *n.* Elecampane, horseheal
elycumpana (1×)
emma, *n.* The hemina, an ancient measure
emma (2×)
emoraudes → **emoroyd**, *n.*
emoroyd, *n.* Hemorrhoids, esp. the bleeding kind
emoraudes (1×), *emoroydes* (2×)
empices, *n.* Empyics, persons suffering from empyema, a collection of pus in the cavity of the pleura, suppuration
empices (1×)
emplastre, *n.* Plaster, a salvelike preparation used in the form of a plaster
emplaster (1×), *emplastre* (4×)
emplastren, *v.* To plaster; to treat medically by applying a plaster

emplasterd (1×), *emplastre* (3×), *emplastred* (15×), *emplastrye* (1×)

encense, *n.* Incense; smoke or fragrance of burning incense
encense (14×)

encrescen, *v.* To increase, become great
encrescyth (1×)

ende, *n.* End, conclusion
ende (2×)

enden, *v.* To end, finish
endyth (3×)

Eneas, *n.* Aeneas
Eneas (1×)

enemy, *n.* Enemy
enemyes (1×)

Englisshe, *n.* The English language
englysse (1×), *englysshe* (1×)

entrayl, *n.* Viscera, the organs enclosed in the trunk of man or animals
entrales (2×), *entrall* (1×), *entrayles* (10×), *entraylles* (1×), *entrayls* (1×)

Enula, *n.* Elecampane, horseheal
enula (1×)

ere, *n.* Ear
eere (2×), *ere* (28×), *eres* (10×), *erys* (1×), *hyr* (1×), *yere* (1×), *yeres* (1×)

erse, *n.* Anus, rectum
erse (7×)

erthe, *n.* Earth
erthe (4×)

eruca, *n.* White peper
eruca (1×)

esely, *adv.* Easily
esely (2×)

esen, *v.* To alleviate, soothe (pain, suffering, a disease, a morbid condition)
esen (1×)

esy, *a.* Easy, peaceful
esy (3×)

eten, *v.* To eat
eete (1×), *ete* (41×), *eten* (65×), *etet* (1×), *ethet* (1×), *ette* (1×), *etyn* (4×), *etyt* (2×), *etyth* (12×), *y eten* (1×)

eter, *n.* Eater
eter (2×), *eters* (1×)

etyng, *ng.* The act or habit of eating
etyng (2×), *etynge* (1×)

eucatesma †, *n.* Encanthis, a small red excrecence in the inner canthus of the eye
eucatesma (1×)

euȝimum †, *n.* White pepper
euȝimum (1×)

eve, *n.* Evening
eue (1×), *euen* (1×)

evel, *adv.* With bad results, disastrously, wretchedly
euel (1×)

evel, *n. / a.* A disease, sickness; harmful, hurtful, painful
euel (15×)

evel couloured, *a.* Evil-coloured
euel couloured (1×)

even, *a.* Even
euen (3×), *euene* (3×)

everyday, *adv.* Daily; continual, constant
eueryday (1×)

evisca †, *n.* Hibiscus
euisca (1×)

evotoycy, *n.* A person suffering from a disease characterized by bloody sputum
euotoycy (1×)

exantimata †, *n.* Eruption, or rash such as takes place in measles, small-pox, etc.
exantimata (1×)

excyten, *v.* To stimulate (an organ, a function or reaction of an organism, growth, etc.)
excyte (1×), *excytyth* (3×)

experyence, *n.* Experience
experyence (1×)

experyment, *n.* Observation, test

experyment (1×)

expownen, *v.* To explain, interpret

expowne (1×)

eye, *n.* Eye

eye (3×), *eyen* (40×), *eyes* (1×), *eyne* (1×), *yen* (5×)

eye, *n.* Egg

egges (1×), *eye* (3×)

eyelyd, *n.* Eyelid

eye leddes (1×), *eyelyddes* (1×)

eyeshelle, *n.* The hard outer shell of an egg

eye shelle (1×), *yee shelle* (1×)

eyre, *n.* Air

eyre (2×)

F

face, *n.* Face

face (11×)

faden, *v.* To grow pale, dim, or dull

fadyth (1×)

fallen, *v.* To fall, drop; to become; to happen as a result

fal (1×), *fall* (2×), *falle* (2×), *fallen* (8×), *fallyt* (1×), *fallyth* (5×), *fyll* (2×)

fallyng evel, *n.* Falling sickness, epilepsy, falling-evil

fallyng euel (6×), *fallynge euel* (1×), *fallynge euell* (2×)

faren, *v.* To travel, journey; to come or go

faryst (1×)

faste, *adv.* Fast; quickly

fast (5×), *faste* (9×)

fastnen, *v.* To make firm, stable

fastne (1×)

fastynge, *ng.* Dieting

fastyng (4×), *fastynge* (3×)

fatte, *a.* Fat

fat (1×), *fatte* (2×)

fayre, *adv.* Properly

fayre (7×)

fayrnesse, *n.* Beauty, pulchritude

fayrnesse (1×)

feble, *a.* Weak

feble (5×)

februfuga †, *n.* Feverfew, centory

februfuga (1×)

federfoy, *n.* Feverfew

federfoy (2×)

feld, *n.* Relatively flat open country

feldes (1×)

felen, *v.* To feel

fele (4×)

feloun, *n.* Some kind of suppurative sore

feloun (2×)

felynge, *ng.* The sense of touch, of movement, of temperature, and of pain and pleasure

felynge (1×)

female, *n.* Female; a female

female (2×)

femygreke, *n.* Fenugreek (Trigonella foenum graecum)

femygreke (4×), *ffemygreke* (1×)

femynyne, *a.* Female

femynyne (1×)

fenel, *n.* Fennel

feenel (1×), *fenel* (17×), *fenell* (2×), *fenyl* (1×), *ffenel* (1×)

fenel seed, *n.* Fennel seed

fenel seed (2×)

fer, *a.* Distant, far

fer (1×)

fervent, *a.* Hot, burning

feruent (4×)

fervour, *n.* Heat; pathological heat of the body or of one of its humours

feruour (1×), *feruours* (1×)

festre, *n.* Fistula or fistulous wound

festre (4×), *festres* (2×)

fetten, *v.* To fetch, bring

fette (1×)

fever, *n.* Fever, an attack of fever
febrys (1×), *feuer* (14×), *feuere* (8×), *feuers* (13×), *feuerys* (4×), *feure* (1×)

flanke, *n.* The soft portion of the body between the ribs and the pelvis
flanke (1×), *flankes* (1×)

flee, *n.* Flea
flees (1×)

flen, *v.* To retreat, run away, flee
fle (1×)

flesshe, *n.* Flesh
flesse (1×), *flesshe* (8×)

fleumatyke, *a.* Composed of the humour called phlegm
fleumatyke (1×), *flumatteke* (1×)

fleume → **flume**, *n.*

flexe, *n.* Flax
flexe (1×)

fleys → **flye**, *n.*

floure, *n.* Menstrual flow
flores (2×), *floure* (3×), *floures* (5×)

flouren, *v.* To bloom, blossom
flouryth (1×)

flowyng, *ng.* Flow, movement of blood or other humours within the body
flowyng (1×)

flumatteke → **fleumatyke**, *a.*

flume, *n.* Phlegm
fleume (4×), *flume* (7×)

fluxe, *n.* Pathological flowing of blood; disentery
flux (1×), *fluxe* (19×), *flyxe* (4×)

flye, *n.* Any insect that flies
fleys (1×), *flye* (1×)

flyxe → **fluxe**, *n.*

fnesynge, *ng.* Sneezing
fnesynge (1×)

folefote, *n.* A plant used in medical recipes, coltsfoot
ffolefote (1×)

folewen, *v.* To come or occur after (something) in time
folewe (1×), *folewen* (1×), *folewyth* (2×), *folowed* (1×), *folowyth* (1×)

folke, *n.* Folk, people
folke (2×), *folkes* (3×)

forbeden, *v.* To prohibit, forbid
for bedyth (1×)

formen, *v.* To give shape
formed (1×), *formeth* (1×)

formust, *a.* Foremost (in space), farthest forward, first, front
formust (1×)

forseyd, *a.* Afore-said
for sayd (1×), for *seyd* (2×), *for seyde* (1×), *forsayd* (1×), *forseyd* (3×), *forseyde* (1×)

forsothe, *adv.* Truthfully
for sothe (1×)

forthe → **furthe**, *adv.*

foot, *n.* Foot
feet (3×), *foot* (1×)

footen, *v.* To walk or travel on foot
footed (1×)

foule, *a.* Dirty, filthy
foule (11×)

foxe, *n.* Fox
foxe (1×)

frakelyd, *a.* Freckled, pimply; speckled
frakelyd (1×)

frakles, *n.* Freckles; pimples
fracles (1×), *frakeles* (2×), *frakles* (7×), *frekles* (1×)

frankencense, *n.* Frankincense, olibanum
ffrankencense (1×), *frankencence* (1×), *frankencense* (2×)

Fraunce, *n.* France
fraunce (1×)

frekles → **frakles**, *n.*

frely, *adv.* Freely

frely (1×)

frenesy, *n.* Insanity, madness

frenesy (1×)

frentyke, *a.* Phrenetic; delirious, crazed, frenzied

frentyke (1×)

fresshe, *a.* Newly inflicted or suffered, unhealed

fresse (4×), *fresshe* (12×)

freten, *v.* To corrode, destroy

frete (1×), *freten* (1×)

fretyng, *ng.* Ache, gnawing or rankling pain

fretyng (4×), *fretynge* (4×), *fretynges* (1×)

frosshe, *n.* Frog or toad

frosshe (2×)

froten, *v.* To rub (with a medicating or treating substance); to apply by rubbing

ffrote (2×), *frote* (3×), *froted* (3×), *frotyth* (1×), *yfroted* (1×)

froth, *n.* Foam, spume, froth

froth (2×), *frothe* (1×)

frount, *n.* The forehead

front (1×), *frount* (2×), *frounte* (1×)

ful, *a. / adv.* Full; fully loaded

ful (8×), *full* (3×)

fully, *adv.* Fully, completely

fully (1×)

furfur, *n.* Bran

furfur (1×)

furniculus, *n.* A boil, furuncle

furniculus (1×)

furthe, *adv.* Forward, onward, ahead

forthe (2×), *furthe* (4×)

further, *adv.* To a more advanced position in space, forward; farther

further (1×)

furwith, *adv.* At once, immediately

furwith (1×)

fyala †, *n.* The white water lily

fyala (1×)

fygge, *n.* The fruit of the fig tree, especially the common fig

fyge (1×), *fygges* (7×)

fyghten, *v.* To fight

fyghte (1×)

fygure, *n.* Shape, form

fygure (1×)

fyllen, *v.* To fill

fylle (3×), *fyllyth* (1×)

fylthe, *n.* Putrid or decomposed matter, anything material that is considered foul, unclean, impure

felthe (1×), *fylthe* (2×)

fyne, *a.* Of supreme or select quality; excellent, superior

fyne (4×)

fynden, *v.* To find || **f. up** to originate or introduce formally

founde (3×), *funde* (1×), *fynde* (1×), *y founde* (1×), *yfunde* (1×)

fynder, *n.* Finder

fyndrys (1×)

fynen, *v.* To purify or clarify

y fyned (1×)

fynger, *n.* Finger

fynger (2×), *fyngers* (1×)

fyre, *n.* Fire

fyre (4×)

fyssh, *n.* Fish

fysshes (1×)

G

gaderen, *v.* To gather

gadre (2×), *gadred* (3×), *y gadred* (1×)

gaderyng, *ng.* Assembling

gaderyng (1×)

Galien, *n.* Galen

Galien (2×), *Galion* (1×), *Galyen* (2×)

galle, *n.* Gall, bile; the gall bladder of man or animal; the secretion of the liver, bile
gal (1×), *galle* (5×)
galyngale, *n.* The roots of various plants of the genera Alpinia
galyngale (3×)
garden, *n.* Garden, cultivated piece of land
garden (1×), *gardeyn* (1×), *gardyenes* (1×)
garlyk, *n.* Garlic (Allium sativum)
garlycke (8×), *garlyk* (14×)
gendren, *v.* To bring forth (offspring), beget (a child), produce
gender (1×), *gendre* (1×), *gendryd* (1×)
generaly, *adv.* Generally, usually
generaly (1×)
gentel, *a.* Courteous, polite
gentel (1×)
genytrall, *n.* Genital, the reproductive organs
genytrall (1×)
germandrya, *n.* A plant of the genus Teucrium
germandrya (1×)
ȝerna, *n.* Impetigo with ulceration, a pustular skin disease
ȝerna (1×)
geten, *v.* To obtain
gete (1×), *getyth* (1×)
getynge, *ng.* The act of getting something
getynge (1×)
gilofre, *n.* Clove
gilofre (1×), *gylofre* (1×)
glad, *a.* Glad
glad (1×)
glad chered, *a.* Glad-cheered
glad chered (1×)
gladen, *n.* A plant of any of several species of the genus Iris
gladen (9×), *gladyn* (1×)
gladen, *v.* To gladden
gladen (1×), *gladyth* (1×)
gladly, *adv.* Willingly, with good will
gladly (1×)
glas, *n.* Glass as substance
glas (1×)
glatte, *n.* Earthy filth
glatte (1×)
glatty, *a.* Viscous
glatty (1×)
glewe, *n.* Glue
glewe (1×)
gleyre, *n.* The white of an egg
gleyre (1×)
glyteren, *v.* To sparkle, glitter, shine
glytere (1×)
gnat flye, *n.* Any of various small, flying insects; esp. the European gnat
gnattes flyes (1×)
gnawen, *v.* To gnaw; to bite, chew
gnawe (1×)
gnawyng, *n.* Act of gnawing, chewing or biting
gnawyng (4×), *gnawynge* (1×)
gobet, *n.* Fragment; bit of flesh
gobet (1×), *gobettes* (1×)
good, *n.* Benefit, a good thing
good (47×)
good, *a.* Good
best (3×), *better* (18×), *good* (1×)
golden, *a.* Golden
golden (1×)
gome, *n.* The flesh surrounding the teeth
gomes (2×), *gommes* (3×)
goon, *v.* To go ‖ **g. away** to go away, disappear
go (1×), *gon* (2×), *goo* (3×), *goth* (1×), *goyn* (1×)
gose, *n.* Goose
gose (4×)

got, *n.* Male goat
gotes (3×)
goute, *n.* Attack of gout; painful swelling
goute (6×), *goutes* (1×)
goyng, *ng.* The act of traveling, passing, or going from place to place
goyng (1×), *goynge* (1×)
grape, *n.* Grape
grapes (1×)
graunten, *v.* To permit (sth.), allow or grant; to concede
graunt (1×), *graunte* (1×)
gravely, *a.* Gravelly; sandy
grauely (1×)
grece, *n.* The fat of an animal, adipose tissue
grece (20×), *grese* (3×), *gresse* (1×)
greef, *n.* Sickness, disease; pain, suffering
greef (3×), *gref* (1×)
greenesse, *n.* Green colour
greenesse (1×)
Greke, *n.* / *a.* A Greek, inhabitant of Greece; Greek, the Greek language
greke (29×), *grekes* (4×)
grene, *a.* Green
grene (32×)
gret, *a.* Great
greet (4×), *gret* (30×), *grete* (3×), *gretter* (1×), *gretyst* (2×)
gretly, *adv.* Greatly
gretly (4×)
grettnesse, *n.* Great size, great quantity
grettnesse (1×)
greven, *v.* To cause physical injury
greue (5×), *greued* (4×), *greuen* (1×), *greueth* (3×), *greuyth* (1×)
grevaunce, *n.* Sickness, disease
greuance (2×), *greuans* (1×), *greuaunce* (4×), *greuaunces* (3×), *greuonce* (1×), *grevance* (1×)
greuonce → **grevaunce**, *n.*
grevuse, *a.* Grave, serious
grouuse (1×)
grevyng, *ng.* Pain, causing injury (physical or otherwise), offending, oppressing
greuyng (1×)
groos, *a.* Large, thick
groos (1×)
grounde, *n.* Ground, soil
grounde (1×)
groundeswely, *n.* The common European groundsel
groundeswely (2×)
growen, *v.* To germinate; to grow, cultivate
grewe (1×), *growe* (2×), *growen* (1×), *growith* (1×), *growyht* (1×), *growynge* (1×), *growyth* (6×)
grydyng, *ng.* Pain, gripes
grydyng (1×)
grynde, *n.* Groin
grynde (5×), *gryndes* (1×)
grynden, *v.* To break (sth.) into small particles
gronde (2×), *gronden* (1×), *ground* (1×), *grounde* (23×), *grounden* (16×), *grunde* (5×), *grunden* (4×), *grynde* (22×), *grynden* (1×), *y gronde* (1×), *y grounde* (3×), *y grounden* (2×), *y grunden* (1×), *ygrounde* (1×)
gutte, *n.* Stomach or belly
gutte (1×), *guttes* (2×)
gwaisdo → **gwayde**, *n.*
gwayde, *n.* The plant woad (Isatis tinctoria) or the blue dyestuff prepared from the leaves of this plant
gwaisdo (1×), *gwayde* (1×)
gyngyver, *n.* Ginger, the root of the plant Zingiber officinale or of a related species

gyngyuer (1×)

gyrden, *v.* To encircle the waist of (sb. with a belt or girdle)

gyrde (1×)

gyth, *n.* A plant whose seeds were used as a condiment

gyth (2×)

H

half, *n. / adv.* A half part of an object, a quantity, a unit of measurement; half

half (1×), *halfe* (1×)

halvendele, *n.* A half portion of anything

haluendele (2×)

handlen, *v.* To touch with the hands

handeleth (1×), *handle* (1×), *handled* (1×)

hangen, *v.* To hang; to suspend

hange (5×), *hanged* (2×), *henge* (1×), *honged* (4×)

hangynge, *n.* The action of suspending somebody or something

hangynge (1×)

harde, *a.* Hard

hard (2×), *harde* (10×)

harden, *v.* To harden

hardded (1×), *harde* (2×)

hardenesse, *n.* Morbid hardening or hardness of a bodily substance, tissue, or structure; induration

hardenesse (5×), *hardnes* (2×), *hardnesse* (5×), *harnes* (1×)

hare, *n.* The common European hare

harys (1×)

harme, *n.* Harm, injury

harme (6×)

harmen, *v.* To harm

harme (1×), *harmeth* (1×)

harre → **hoos**, *a.*

hastely, *adv.* Speedily, quickly

hastely (3×), *hastyly* (1×)

haven, *v.* To have, possess ‖ **h. out** remove (sth.), drive (sb.) out

hadde (1×), *han* (28×), *hat* (6×), *hath* (22×), *haue* (12×), *hayth* (1×)

haven, *va.* To have

had (1×), *hadde* (3×), *hadden* (1×), *hade* (1×), *han* (11×), *hat* (1×), *hath* (30×), *haue* (25×)

heed, *n.* Head

hed (4×), *heddes* (1×), *heed* (57×), *heed* (1×), *heede* (1×)

heedache, *n.* Headache

hed ache (1×), *heed ache* (12×)

heer, *n.* Hair

heer (5×), *heere* (1×), *heres* (4×)

heet, *n.* Heat

heet (6×), *heete* (6×), *het* (1×), *hete* (10×), *hetes* (2×)

hele, *n.* Cure, heal; health

hele (2×), *helys* (1×)

helen, *v.* To cure, heal

heele (10×), *hele* (125×), *heled* (4×), *helen* (1×), *helle* (1×), *helyt* (1×), *helyth* (13×)

helpe, *n.* Help, assistance, succour, benefit

helpe (2×)

helpen, *v.* To help; to give aid or assistance to (sb. or sth.) ‖ **h. up** help (sb.) up

helpe (42×), *helped* (1×), *helpen* (1×), *helpet* (1×), *helpeth* (1×), *helpyn* (1×), *helpyng* (1×), *helpyt* (2×), *helpyth* (56×), *hepe* (1×), *hylpeth* (1×), *hylpyth* (3×)

helpyng, *ng.* Aid, assistance

helpyng (1×)

helthe, *n.* Health

helthe (1×)

helum †, *n.* Chyle, stick liquorice

helum (1×)

hemlok, *n.* The poisonous plant, hemlock

hemlok (12×), *hemloke* (1×)

henne, *n.* Hen

hennes (2×)

hennebane, *n.* Henbane

henne bane (1×), *hennebane* (2×)

hepeta mordax → **herpeta mordax**, *n.*

herbe, *n.* A non-woody plant

herbe (276×), *herbes* (14×), *herbys* (1×)

heren, *v.* To hear

heere (1×), *here* (1×)

herpeta mordax †, *n.* A skin disease, herpes; biting, gnawing herpes

herpeta (2×), *hepeta mordax* (1×), *herpeta mordax* (1×)

hert, *n.* Heart

hert (3×), *herte* (2×)

hervest, *n.* The season of autumn, fall, harvest

heruest (1×)

heryng, *ng.* The action of hearing; listening; the sense of hearing; the sense of hearing, capacity for hearing

heryng (1×), *hyryng* (1×)

hevy, *a.* Heavy; weighty

heue (2×), *heuy* (3×)

hevyen, *v.* To make (sth.) heavy in weight

heuyed (1×)

hey, *n.* Hay, grass cut or mowed and cured (usually as feed for livestock)

hey (1×)

heyght, *n.* Height, altitude

heyght (1×)

heyhony, *n.* The herb ground ivy (Nepeta hederacea), often used medicinally

hey hony (1×)

hocke, *n.* Any of several plants of the related genera Malva and Althæa; esp. the common mallow

hocke (6×), *hockes* (1×)

holden, *v.* To hold, keep

helde (2×), *helden* (2×), *hold* (1×), *holde* (9×), *holden* (2×), *holdyth* (1×), *y helde* (2×), *y holden* (1×), *y holdyn* (1×)

holsom, *a.* Healthful; healing

holsom (1×)

holsomlyche, *adv.* Healthfully; medicinally

holsomlyche (1×)

holowe, *a.* Hollow

holowe (2×)

holy fyre, *n.* Erisipelas; St. Anthony's fire

holy fyre (9×)

holy hocke, *n.* The Marsh Mallow, Althæa officinalis. Any of several plants of the related genera Malva and Althæa; esp. the common mallow

holy hocke (1×)

honde, *n.* Hand

honde (2×), *hondes* (1×)

hony, *n.* Honey

hony (82×)

honysoucle, *n.* Honeysuckle; clover; esp. the common red clover (Trifolium pratense); also, the flower of clover

hony soucle (1×), *honysoucle* (1×)

hool, *n.* External bodily orifice

hool (1×)

hoole, *a.* Healthy, cured, healed

hole (2×), *hool* (5×), *hoole* (6×), *hoolle* (1×)

hoos, *a.* Harsh, ungrateful to the ear; of the voice: husky, cracked, hoarse

harre (1×), *hoos* (2×), *hors* (1×)

hope, *n.* Hope; trust, confidence

hope (1×)

horehounde, *n.* The common herb horehound

horehonde (1×), *horehounde* (3×)

horn, *n.* Horn

hornes (1×)

horsehelne, *n.* Elecampane, horseheal

horsehelne (1×)

hose, *n.* A legging or stocking of woven cloth or leather, with or without feet

hosen (1×)

hoot, *a.* Hot to the touch or taste

hoot (63×), *hoote* (4×), *hot* (2×), *hote* (3×)

hound, *n.* A dog

hound (1×), *hounde* (1×), *houndes* (5×), *houndys* (1×)

hour, *n.* Hour

houres (1×)

house, *n.* House

house (1×)

housebonde, *n.* Husband

housebonde (1×)

hoveren, *v.* To stand protectingly (around sb.); to wait, stay

houere (1×)

huge, *a.* Huge; numerous

huge (5×), *hugest* (1×)

hugely, *adv.* Abundantly, copiously

hugely (14×)

humour, *n.* One of four fluids (blood, phlegm, choler, melancholy) which form and nourish the body

humers (1×), *humores* (1×), *humors* (1×), *humorus* (1×), *humorys* (1×), *humour* (2×), *humoure* (1×), *humoures* (3×), *humours* (23×)

hurten, *v.* To injure, wound, hurt; to afflict (sb.) with disease

hurte (7×), *hurtyng* (1×), *hurtyth* (1×), *y hurte* (1×)

hylpeth/hylpyth → **helpen**, *v.*

hype, *n.* Hip

hype (1×)

hyr → **ere**, *n.*

hyrere, *n.* Gray, grayish white hair

hyreres (1×)

hyve, *n.* Beehive

hyue (1×)

I

iaundyse, *n.* Jaundice

iaundese (2×), *iaundse* (1×), *iaundys* (3×), *iaundyse* (13×), *iayndys* (1×)

idelnesse, *n.* Inactivity, lack of employment

idelnesse (1×)

idem, *adv.* The same, the above-mentioned

idem (1×)

id est, *adv.* That is, that is to say

i (1×), *id est* (1×)

ierobothanum †, *n.* Vervain

ierobothanum (1×)

ignys sacer → **sacer ignis**, *n.*

illirica, *n.* A plant of the genus Iris associated with Illyria

illirica (1×), *illurica* (1×)

illurica → **illirica**, *n.*

impetigo, *n.* A skin disease characterized by small white spots or scabs and by itching

impetigo (1×), *inpetigo* (1×)

Inde, *n.* A broad geographical term for much of southern Asia, often including part of China or islands to the south and southeast of Asia

Inde (2×)

ioynen, *v.* To join, unite, combine

ioyned (2×)

ioynt, *n*. A joint between bones
ioyntes (2×)
Ipocras, *n*. Hippocrates, the physician
Ipocras (2×), *ypocras* (2×)
iris, *n*. The plant Iris germanica, used medicinally
iris (1×)
iubarbe, *n*. Houseleek
iubarbe (3×)
iusqiamus †, *n*. Henbane
iusqiamus (1×)
iuys, *n*. Juice of a plant, flower, or tree; sap
iuis (1×), *ius* (5×), *iuys* (159×), *yuys* (2×)

K

kebe, *n*. Chilblain
kebe (2×)
kepeman †, *n*. Keeper
kepemen (1×)
kepen, *v*. To keep (sth.) in one's possession; to retain, hold ‖ **k. away** to keep away, prevent from coming
kepe (9×), *kepte* (2×), *kepyt* (2×), *kepyth* (1×)
kerfe, *n*. Incision, a wound, gash
kerfe (1×)
kernel, *n*. Swollen gland; any pathological lump or growth; a tumor
cornels (1×), *kernel* (2×), *kerneles* (1×), *kernelles* (2×), *kernels* (1×)
kersoun, *n*. A plant of the mustard family, a cress
kersen (1×), *kersoun* (3×)
kervyng, *ng*. The action of cutting, rending
keruyng (1×)
knobbe, *n*. A lump in the skin or flesh; thickened and hardened skin, a pustule
knobbe (2×), *knobbes* (3×)
knowen, *v*. To know
knowe (7×), *knowen* (3×)
knowhers → **kowher**, *n.*
kocke, *n*. Cock, rooster
kocke (1×)
kockull, *n*. Corn cockle
kockul (3×), *kockull* (4×)
kowe → **cowe**, *n.*
kowhe, *n*. Cough, coughing
cowe (3×), *cowhe* (16×), *kowe* (1×), *kowhe* (9×)
kowher †, *n*. One who coughes
knowhers (1×), *kowhers* (1×)
kunte, *n*. A woman's private parts
cunte (2×), *kunte* (6×), *kuntes* (1×)
kutten, *v*. To cut
kutte (3×), *kutten* (1×), *y kutte* (1×)
kychen, *n*. Cooking
kychen (1×)
kynde, *n*. Kind, type
kynde (6×), *kyndes* (1×)

L

labore, *n*. Labour, work
labore (1×)
lamb, *n*. Lamb, a young sheep
lambys (1×)
lanceolata, *n*. The greater spearwort (Ranunculus lingua); ?ribwort plantain (Plantago lanceolata)
lanceolata (1×)
langedebeef, *n*. A plant of the borage family, oxtongue, langue de bœuf (see also *oxe-tŏnge*.
langedebeef (3×)
lappacium, *n*. Lapacio
lappacium (1×)
lappen, *v*. To wrap

lapped (2×)
large, *a.* Large
large (1×)
largely, *adv.* Largely
largely (2×), *largyly* (1×)
lasse → **lytel**, *n.* / *a.*
laste, *a.* Last, final
laste (1×)
Latyn, *n.* Latin
latin (1×), *latyn* (30×)
lauryel → **lorer**, *n.*
laven, *v.* To wash (sb. or sth.); moisten (sth.)
laued (1×)
laxatyf, *n.* / *a.* Diarrhea, loosening or purging of the bowels; Causing looseness of the bowels or diarrhea
laxatyf (6×)
laxe, *n.* / *a.* Diarrhea; unconstipated, loose
laxe (4×)
laxen, *v.* To have a laxative effect, cause looseness of the bowels
laxe (1×), *laxyt* (1×)
lay(e) → **leyen**, *v.*
leche, *n.* Physician, surgeon
leche (3×), *leches* (40×)
lechecrafte, *n.* The art or science of medicine and/or surgery
leche craft (1×), *leche crafte* (2×)
lecherye, *n.* The habit or practice of adultery, fornication
lechere (1×), *lechery* (7×), *lecherye* (7×), *lechyre* (2×), *lechyry* (3×), *lechyrye* (1×)
ledyr color, *a.* Lead-coloured, dull, wan
ledyrcolor (1×)
leef, *n.* Leaf
leef (1×), *leues* (46×)
leef, *a.* Prized, precious ‖ **l. unto** pleasing, agreeable to somebody
leef (1×)
leeke, *n.* Leek
leeke (11×), *leke* (9×), *lekes* (2×)
legge, *n.* Leg
legge (1×)
lenchemon, *n.* White ox-eye, chrysanthemum leucanthemum
lenchemon (1×)
lende, *n.* Loin(s, the flesh of the lower back between the ribs and the hips
lender (1×), *lendes* (4×), *lyndes* (1×)
lene, *a.* Lean, spare, slender
lene (1×)
lenstil, *n.* Lentil
lens (1×), *lens til* (1×)
lenþen, *v.* To lengthen (sth.) in time; to prolong
lenþe (1×)
lepre, *n.* Leprosy or any of its four varieties; any of several skin diseases, having symptoms similar to some of those in leprosy
lepre (9×), *lepres* (4×)
lesen, *v.* To lose
lese (1×), *lost* (1×)
lesse → **lytel**, *n.* / *a.*
leten, *v.* To let; to allow, grant
leet (1×), *lete* (7×)
letten, *v.* To hinder (sb.), impede, delay
lette (1×), *letten* (1×)
letuse, *n.* Lettuce
letuse (7×), *leuse* (1×)
leuke, *a.* Lukewarm, tepid
leuke (26×), *luke* (3×)
leukewarme, *a.* Lukewarm, tepid
leukewarme (1×), *luke warme* (1×), *lukewarme* (1×)
leuse → **letuse**, *n.*
leven, *v.* To stop, cease
leue (2×), *leueth* (1×)
leyen, *v.* To put (sb. or sth.), place, set ‖ **l. upon** give (smth.) to (sb.)

lay (1×), *layde* (1×), *laye* (2×), *leey* (1×), *leeyde* (1×), *ley* (13×), *leyd* (5×), *leyde* (60×), *leye* (30×), *leyen* (1×), *leyeth* (1×), *y leyde* (2×), *yleyde* (2×)

leymes → **lym**, *n.*

lichene, *n.* A skin disease, characterized by an eruption of reddish solid papules over a more or less limited area

lichene (1×)

lightes, *n.* Lungs

lightes (1×)

ligustion †, *n.* The European honeysuckle

ligustion (1×)

lilifagus †, *n.* The herb sage

lilifagus (1×)

loken, *v.* To look

loke (3×), *lokyth* (1×)

lollyum †, *n.* Cockle

lollyum (1×)

longe, *a.* Long-lasting, long

longe (12×)

longe, *adv.* For a long time, long

long (1×), *longe* (11×)

lorer, *n.* The European laurel tree, bay tree (Laurus nobilis)

lauriall (1×), *lauryel* (1×), *lorer* (3×)

love, *n.* Love

loue (1×)

lude, *n.* The backbone, spine

ludes (1×)

lunatyke, *a.* Insane, suffering from a recurrent frenzy or madness, believed to vary with the phases of the moon

lunatyke (2×)

lung, *n.* Lung

longes (3×), *lunges* (14×)

lupinus, *n.* The European white lupine (Lupinus albus); the bitter seed of this plant

lupinus (2×), *lupyn* (1×)

lurken, *v.* To hide

lurkyng (1×)

lust, *n.* Desire, wish, will

lust (2×)

luxatura †, *n.* Luxation, dislocation

luxatura (2×)

lycoure, *n.* Liquid found in, or derived from, plants

lecour (1×), *lycore* (1×), *lycoure* (1×)

lyd, *n.* Eyelid

lyddes (1×)

lyen, *v.* To be placed or located

lye (3×), *lyeth* (1×)

lyfe, *n.* Life

lyfe (2×)

lyfte, *a.* Left

lyfte (1×)

lyght, *a.* Free of pain; relieved of an illness

lyght (2×), *lythe* (1×)

lyghten, *v.* To be relieved of an illness or pain

lyghte (1×)

lyghtly, *adv.* (a) Instantly, promptly; immediately, soon

lyghtly (4×), *lygthly* (1×)

lyke, *a.* Like (sb. or sth.); similar to (sb. or sth.)

leche (1×), *lyke* (7×)

lyke, *adv.* Like, similarly to

lyke (1×)

lyknen, *v.* To resemble (sb. or sth.)

lykned (1×)

lykynge, *ng.* A feeling or experience of pleasure, enjoyment

lykynge (2×), *lykynges* (1×)

lylye, *n.* Lily

lilye (1×), *lyly* (4×), *lylye* (11×)

lym, *n.* Member, Any constituent part or organ of the body
leymes (1×), *lymes* (4×), *lymmes* (1×)

lyme, *n.* Lime
lyme (1×)

lynnyn, *a.* Cloth woven from flax, linen cloth
lynnyn (2×)

lynsede, *n.* The seed of flax, linseed
lynsede (1×)

lyppe, *n.* Lip
leppes (2×), *lyppes* (2×)

lyquoryce, *n.* The dried root of the plant Glycyrrhiza glabra, used in medicine and cooking; licorice
lyquorice (1×), *lyquoryce* (6×)

lytarge → **lytargicus**, *n.*

lytargie, *n.* Lethargy; a disease characterized by prolonged unconsciousness or coma; a mental disorder accompanied by passivity or stupor
litargia (1×), *lytargie* (1×)

lytargicus, *n.* / *a.* A person suffering from lethargy; afflicted with lethargy
lytarge (1×), *lytargicus* (1×), *litargius* (1×)

lytel, *n.* / *a.* Little, not much; smaller in size or spatial extent, less in quantity or amount
lasse (15×), *lesse* (1×), *lytel* (10×), *lytyl* (1×)

lyven, *v.* To live
lyue (2×)

lyver, *n.* Liver
lyuer (6×)

M

Macer, *n.* Macer
Macer (6×)

maken, *v.* To make, construct, produce
maad (5×), *mad* (2×), *madde* (2×), *made* (26×), *make* (97×), *maken* (6×), *makyn* (1×), *makyst* (1×), *makyt* (8×), *makyth* (36×)

maladye, *n.* Disease
malady (2×), *maladye* (5×), *maladyes* (2×)

male, *n.* Male human being
male (4×), *males* (1×)

malefaccio †, *n.* Malefaction, injury
malefaccio (1×)

malencolyke, *a.* Consisting of, or mixed with, black bile; of a humor other than melancholy
malencolyke (2×)

malencolyous, *a.* Having a pathological condition of the black bile
malencolyous (1×)

malowe, *n.* The common mallow (Malva sylvestris); also, the marsh mallow (Althaea officinalis); rarely, the Syrian mallow (Hibiscus syriacus)
malowe (2×), *malowes* (2×), *malua* (1×)

malyce, *n.* Harmful or dangerous quality
malyce (2×)

man, *n.* Man
man (15×), *manneys* (1×), *mannys* (5×), *mans* (2×), *manys* (5×), *men* (87×)

mankynde, *n.* Mankind, the human race
mankynde (1×)

maner, *n.* Kind, sort
maner (39×), *manere* (3×), *maneres* (10×), *maners* (3×), *manerys* (2×)

manya, *n.* Mental derangement characterized by frenzy, delusions, and violence
manya (1×)

maratrum, *n.* Fennel; the European marten (a member of the genus Martes); the European polecat (Mustela putorius)
maratrum (1×)
marubium, *n.* The common or white horehound
marubium (1×)
Mars, *n.* The god Mars
Mars (1×)
matre, *n.* A piece of business, affair
matre (1×)
matryce, *n.* Uterus, womb
matryce (29×), *matryces* (1×), *matryse* (1×)
maturen, *v.* To encourage suppuration in (sth.) by the application of maturatives
mature (1×)
maturyng, *ng.* Treatment to induce suppuration; bringing a morbid swelling to a head by medical treatment
maturyng (1×)
mawe, *n.* Stomach
maw (2×), *mawe* (19×)
mayde, *n.* Woman
mayde (1×)
mayst → **mowen**, *va.*
maystely, *adv.* Skillfully
maystely (1×)
mede, *n.* Meadow; clearing, open field
medes (1×)
medlen, *v.* To blend, mix
I medled (1×), *meddled* (1×), *medlde* (1×), *medle* (34×), *medled* (57×), *melde* (5×), *meldle* (1×), *mele* (1×), *meled* (4×), *melle* (2×), *melled* (1×), *nedled* (1×), *y meled* (1×)
medycynable, *a.* Medicinal, healing, therapeutic
medycynable (4×)
medycynall, *a.* Medicinal, healing
medycynal (3×), *medycynall* (4×)
medycyne, *n.* A medicine, medicament; a medicinal potion or plaster
medcynes (1×), *medycen* (1×), *medycyn* (6×), *medycyne* (28×), *medycynes* (23×), *medycyns* (4×), *medycynys* (2×)
mele, *n.* Meal made by grinding grain (usually wheat)
mele (2×)
mellisophilos †, *n.* Honeysuckle
mellisophilos (1×)
Mellitus, *n.* Meletius
Mellitus (1×)
membre, *n.* Sex organ; a bodily limb or organ
member (1×), *membre* (2×), *membres* (3×), *menbres* (1×)
memorie, *n.* Memory or recollection
memorie (1×)
Menacus, *n.* Menemachus
Menacus (1×)
mencyoun, *n.* Description, account, narration
mencyoun (1×)
mene, *a.* Common. Also inferior in rank
mene (1×)
menison, *n.* Dysentery; severe diarrhea
menson (1×), *menyson* (3×), *menysone* (2×), *menysoun* (1×), *nenyson* (1×)
mercuryal, *n.* A plant; prob. chenopodium
mercuryal (1×)
mery, *a.* Merry, mirthful, blithe
mery (1×)
meschyf, *n.* Misfortune, affliction, trouble
meschyf (1×)
mesel, *n.* One who is afflicted with any of various disfiguring skin diseases, such as, leucoderma, psoriasis, vitiligo
meseles (1×), *mesels* (1×)
mesure, *n.* Measure

mesure (2×)

mete, *n.* Food, nourishment, sustenance
mete (2×), *metes* (6×)

methe, *n.* Mead
methe (2×)

Metrydates, *n.* Mithridates
Metrydates (1×)

meven, *v.* To move
meue (3×), *meued* (2×), *meueth* (1×)

miconium †, *n.* Poppy
miconium (1×), *myconye* (1×)

millemorbia †, *n.* Millemorbia, fig-wort
mille morbia (1×), *millemorbia* (1×)

mirtus → **myrte**, *n.*

moder, *n.* Mother; the uterus of a woman, womb
moder (6×), *moders* (6×), *modrys* (1×), *mother* (1×)

moderat, *a.* Moderate, temperate, sparing
moderat (1×)

moderwort, *n.* Any of several medicinal herbs, including the mugwort
moderwort (1×), *moderworte* (1×)

moisten, *v.* To make (sb. or sth.) moist or wet
moste (1×)

moleyne, *n.* The herb mullein
moleyne (2×)

mollyfyen, *v.* To soften
mollyfye (1×)

monesten, *v.* To warn (sb.); to give warning; to condemn (sth.)
moneste (1×), *monestyth* (1×)

moor, *a.* More in quantity or amount
moor (1×)

moost → **moten**, *va.*

morell, *n.* Any of several herbs of the Solanum family; esp. black solanum, belladonna; black Nightshade
morell (2×), *morella* (1×)

morter, *n.* Mortar, bowl used for grinding and mixing ingredients in preparing food or medicaments
morter (2×)

morwe, *n.* Morning
morowe (1×), *morwe* (7×)

moste → **moisten**, *v.*

moten, *va.* To be allowed, be permitted, may
moost (1×), *must* (1×)

motthe, *n.* Worm, maggot, grub, the larva of various moths, beetles or other insects
motthe (1×)

moule, *n.* Sore spot on the heel, a chilblain on the heel
moule (1×), *mula* (1×)

mouse, *n.* Mouse
mouse (1×), *mys* (1×)

mouthe, *n.* Mouth
mothe (10×), *moþe* (1×), *mouþe* (2×), *mouthe* (29×)

mowen, *va.* May; to be able to (+ infinitive); to be allowed, be permitted, may
may (27×), *mayst* (7×), *mou* (1×), *mowe* (2×), *my* (1×), *myast* (1×), *myght* (2×)

moyst, *a.* Moist, wet
moyst (10×)

moysture, *n.* Moisture, wetness
moysture (1×)

mugwort, *n.* Mugwort
mogwort (1×), *mugwort* (3×), *mugworte* (1×)

mula → **moule**, *n.*

mulsa, *n.* Medicional beberage
mulsa (28×)

mundyfyen, *v.* To cleanse a wound or infection
mudyfyeth (1×)

muscelly †, *n.* Jussel, in ancient cookery a name including various forms of mince or hotch-potch
muscelly (1×)

must → **moten**, *va.*

must, *n.* Must, the juice of grapes, unfermented or undergoing the process of fermentation
must (2×)

my → **mowen**, *va.*

myast → **mowen**, *va.*

myconye → **miconium**, *n.*

myd day, *n.* The middle of the day
myd day (1×)

myddel, *n.* / *a.* The middle; middle
meddel (2×), *myddel* (3×), *mydel* (1×)

myght, *n.* Might, power
myght (12×), *myghte* (1×), *mygth* (1×)

myghty, *a.* Powerful, mighty
myghty (7×)

myghtyly, *adv.* Powerfully; strongly, vigorously
myghtyly (1×)

mylfoyle, *n.* Milfoil, yarrow (Achillea millefolium)
mylfoyle (1×)

mylke, *n.* Milk
melke (1×), *mylk* (1×), *mylke* (25×)

mylke warme, *a.* Warm as milk fresh from the cow
mylke warme (2×)

mynucen, *v.* To reduce, diminish
mynuce (1×)

mylte, *n.* Spleen
mylte (1×)

mynde, *n.* Mind, memory
mynde (4×)

mynte, *n.* A plant of the genus mentha
mynt (1×), *mynte* (14×), *myntes* (3×)

myre, *n.* Bog, marsh, swampland
myres (1×), *myry* (1×)

myrre, *n.* Myrrh
myrre (4×)

myrte, *n.* Myrtle, a shrub of the genus Myrtus
mirtus (1×), *myrte* (1×), *myrtus* (1×)

N

name, *n.* Name
name (7×)

namely, *adv.* Especially, in particular
namely (4×)

namen, *v.* To name, designate
ynamed (1×)

narde, *n.* Nard, the East Indian spikenard; also, any medicinal plant of the genus Valeriana ‖ **n. celtike** Celtic spikenard
narde (3×), *uarde* (1×), *nardus celtica* (1×)

nattercoppe, *n.* Spider
nattercoppe (1×)

naturium †, *n.* A name for various types of orchid
naturium (1×)

nature, *n.* Nature
nature (1×)

naturel, *a.* Normal, customary
naturel (1×)

navel, *n.* Navel, umbilicus
nauel (1×)

nayle, *n.* Fingernail or toenail
nayle (2×), *nayles* (5×)

necke, *n.* Neck
neck (1×), *necke* (4×), *neckes* (2×), *nek* (6×)

neden, *v.* To be necessary, needed, required
nede (1×), *need* (1×)
nefresis, *n.* Nephritis
nefresis (1×), *neufresys* (1×)
nepe, *n.* The turnip plant (Brassica rapa), a turnip
nepe (4×), *nepes* (1×)
nepte, *n.* Catnip, catmint (Nepeta cataria), often used in cooking or in medecines
nepte (2×)
nesse → **nesshe**, *a.*
nesshe, *a.* Physically soft in texture; pliant or yielding, not hard or stiff
nesse (2×), *nesshe* (18×), *nysshe* (1×)
nesshen, *v.* To make (sth.) soft; soften (sth.)
nesshyt (1×)
nether, *a.* Low, lower, under; downward
nether (2×)
nettel, *n.* Nettle
netel (1×), *netell* (1×), *nettel* (8×), *nettell* (6×), *nettelles* (2×), *nettels* (2×), *nettles* (1×), *nettls* (1×), *netyl* (1×)
neufresys → **nefresis**, *n.*
newe, *a.* New
newe (11×)
nex, *adv.* In the nearest position, immediately after in space
nex (1×)
ney, *a.* Near
ney (1×)
nigella, *n.* Cockel, fennel-flower (Nigella sativa), used medicinally; also, one of two plants: corn cockle (Agrostemma githago) or darnel (Lolium temulentum)
nigella (1×)
niter → **nytrum**, *n.*
noble, *a.* Efficacious
noble (2×), *nobler* (2×)
nombre, *n.* Name
nombre (3×)
northe, *n.* The northern cardinal point
northe (1×)
noryce, *n.* Nursemaid, governess; foster mother
noryce (4×), *norce* (1×)
norysshen, *v.* To feed, nourish
norysshed (1×), *norysshyt* (1×)
nose, *n.* Nose
nose (13×), *nosse* (1×)
nostrelle, *n.* Nostril
nesestrelles (1×), *nosestrelles* (3×), *nosstrelles* (2×), *nostrelles* (3×), *nostrellys* (1×)
notable, *a.* Worthy of note, important; praiseworthy
notable (1×)
note, *n.* Nut
nottes (1×)
noteful, *a.* Useful; beneficial
noteful (1×)
notemygge, *n.* Nutmeg; the seed of the kernel of the tree Myristica fragrans; nutmeg in powdered form; used as spice in cookery or medicinally
notemygge (3×)
noten, *v.* To take mental note of (sb. or sth.), give heed to
note (1×)
noyen, *v.* To harm (sb. or sth.), injure
noye (1×), *noyen* (2×), *noyeth* (4×)
noynted → **anoynten**, *v.*
noyous, *a.* Harmful, injurious, noxious
noyose (1×), *noyous* (13×), *noyus* (2×)
nyght, *n.* Night, nightfall
nyght (6×)
nyght tyme, *n.* Night-time
nyght tyme (1×)
nymfee, *n.* The white water lily (Nymphæa alba)

nymfee (1×)
nysshe → **nesshe**, *a.*
nytrum, *n.* Natron (used in medicaments)
niter (1×), *nitrum* (1×), *nytrum* (2×)

O

obolus, *n.* A small measure of weight; a weight used to balance a scale
obolus (1×)
observen, *v.* To observe
obseruyth (1×)
odour, *n.* Odour
odour (5×), *odoure* (2×)
ofgrowen, *v.* To proceed from (a source), be derived from
of growyth (1×)
often tyme(s), *adv.* Frequently, many times
of tyme (4×), *of tymes* (1×), *oft tyme* (1×), *ofte tyme* (1×), *ofte tymes* (3×), *often tyme* (1×), *often tymes* (2×), *oftentymes* (2×), *oftyme* (1×), *oftymes* (2×)
olde, *a.* Old, near the end of the normal span of life
olde (35×), *oode* (1×), *oold* (1×), *oolde* (1×), *wolde* (1×)
olebur → **ellebur**, *n.*
oleum rosaceum, *a.* Olive oil
oleum rosaceum (1×)
olyf, *n.* Olive tree
olyf (1×)
olyfaunt, *n.* Elephant
olyfaunt (1×)
only, *adv.* Solely, only, exclusively
only (6×), *onlyche* (1×), *oonly* (3×)
onyment → **oynement**, *n.*
onynement → **oynement**, *n.*
oon, *a.* Their, his, or its own
oon (1×)
open, *a.* Known; well-known, familiar
open (2×)
openen, *v.* To open
open (1×), *opene* (4×), *openyth* (1×)
opium, *n.* Leaves of the opium poppy
opium (4×)
oponly, *adv.* Plainly, clearly, distinctly
oponly (1×)
ordeynen, *v.* To regulate, control, or govern (sb. or sth.)
ordeyned (1×), *ordyne* (1×)
ordyne → **ordeynen**, *v.*
ornement, *n.* Ornamental apparel, trapping(s, etc.
ornement (1×)
orthononicus/orthonoici → **ortononicus**, *n.*
ortononicus, *n.* Orthopnoic, affected with orthopnoea, a form of asthma
ortonoici (1×), *orthonoici* (1×), *ortononicus* (1×), *orthononicus* (1×)
oryganum †, *n.* Pulliol
oryganum (1×)
osterlagya → **aristologia**, *n.*
ounnethe → **unnethe**, *adv.*
ountaken, *p.* With the exception of (sb., a place), except, except for
oun taken (1×)
overcomen, *v.* To be victorious, conquer
ouercome (2×)
overcomere, *n.* Victor; conqueror
ouercomeres (1×)
overmuche, *a.* Excessive, immoderate, superfluous
ouer muche (5×), *ouermuche* (2×)
overmuche, *adv.* Excessively, immoderately, superfluously
ouer muche (1×), *ouermuche* (1×)
overpassen, *v.* To surpass
ouerpasse (1×)

oxe, *n.* Ox
oxe (2×)
oxetonge, *n.* Oxtongue, a plant of the borage family, either Anchusa officinalis or Lycopsis arvensis (see also *lange-de-bēf.*
oxe tonge (1×)
oxiniel, *n.* A preparation of vinegar and honey, often with other herbal ingredients, principally used as a medicinal drink
oxiniel (1×)
oyle, *n.* Oil
oyle (64×), *oyly* (1×)
oynement, *n.* Medicinal ointment, medicinal salve prepared or used for external application
onyment (4×), *onynement* (1×), *oyenement* (1×), *oynement* (24×), *oynementes* (1×), *ynement* (1×)
oynoun, *n.* Onion
oynouns (24×), *oynous* (1×)

P

pacyent, *n.* Patient
pacyent (17×), *pacyentys* (1×)
padstol, *n.* Toadstool, mushroom
padstoles (4×)
palat, *n.* Palate, the roof of the mouth of man or animal
palat (1×)
pale, *a.* Light, pale
pale (1×)
palesye, *n.* Palsy; the failure of a part of the body to function properly; loss of tactile sensation
palesey (2×), *palesy* (1×), *palesye* (2×)
Palladius, *n.* Palladius
palladius (1×)
palme, *n.* The breadth of the palm of the hand as a unit of measure, a hand's-breadth
palme (1×)
pannaricum, *n.* Whitlow; an inflamed swelling around a fingernail
pannaricum (1×)
par, *n.* Counterpart or mate (of a joint or sinew)
pares (1×)
paradilla, *n.* Sorrell docke
paradilla (1×)
parodyda → **parotida**, *n.*
parotida, *n.* Tumor or sore located near an ear, inflammation of the parotid gland
parodycas (1×), *parodyda* (2×), *parotida* (1×), *peryodyda* (2×)
party, *n.* Part, division, or section
parte (1×), *partes* (6×), *party* (1×), *partye* (1×), *partyes* (8×)
passen, *v.* To leave, go away ‖ **p. away** to cease to exist, die
passe (3×), *passyth* (2×)
passyoun, *n.* Ailment, disease, affliction; also, an attack of fever
passyo (1×), *passyon* (1×), *passyons* (3×), *passyoun* (3×)
pastinaca, *n.* Parsnip
pastinaca (1×)
peletre, *n.* Common pellitory, pellitory of the wall (Parietaria officinalis); a spicy herb often used in cookery
peletre (4×), *pelletre* (2×)
peny, *n.* The value of a penny
peny (1×)
penydy, *n.* Barley sugar, often used medicinally; a piece or stick of barley sugar
penydyes (1×)
peper, *n.* The dried berries of the pepper plant (Piper nigrum), usually

ground and used as a condiment in cooking or in medicines; the dried berries of the pepper plant

peper (16×), *pepyr* (4×), *pyper* (5×)

peple, *n.* People

peple (3×)

peraventure, *adv.* Perhaps, possibly, maybe

perauenture (2×)

peryodyda → **parotida**, *n.*

perell, *n.* Peril, danger; exposure to physical injury, death, or destruction

perell (2×)

perelouse, *a.* Perilous

perelouse (1×)

pernio †, *n.* Kibe, chilblain

peruyo (1×)

persely, *n.* Parsley

persely (11×)

Persin, *n.* The Persians

Persins (1×)

person, *n.* Person

person (1×)

peruyo → **pernio**, *n.*

peryodica febre †, *n.* Periodic fever

peryodica febrys (1×)

perysteryon †, *n.* Vervain

perysteryon (1×)

pessarye, *n.* Suppository; esp. one inserted in the vagina to cure disease or draw out a dead fetus

pessarye (2×)

petrocylyum †, *n.* Parsley, saxifrage

petrocylyum (1×)

peyne, *n.* The action of punishing

peyne (1×)

phylosopher, *n.* Scholar, learned man; wise man

phylosophers (1×)

pia mater, *n.* Soft inner membrane covering the brain, the pia mater

pia mater (2×)

piche, *n.* Residue of the distillation of wood tar (as an ingredient of medicinal preparations)

piche (1×), *pycche* (1×), *pycke* (1×), *pykes* (1×)

pille, *n.* Husk or hull of grain; peel or rind of a fruit or vegetable

pilles (2×), *pylees* (1×), *pyles* (2×), *pylle* (1×)

pilyoll → **pulyoll**, *n.*

place, *n.* Place

place (45×), *places* (5×)

planteyn, *n.* A plant of the plantain family

planteyn (14×), *planteyne* (2×), *playnteyn* (2×), *playnteyne* (1×), *playntyne* (1×)

plastre, *n.* Plaster, poultice, or compress made from herbs, meal, or other substance, often applied on a cloth to the affected area for a variety of medicinal purposes

paster (1×), *plaster* (45×), *plastre* (30×), *plastres* (3×), *playster* (2×), *playstre* (1×)

plastren, *v.* To cover (a sore, part of the body) with a plaster or poultice

plastred (4×), *y plastred* (1×)

plastrewyse, *adv.* In the manner of a plaster or poultice

plaster wyse (2×)

playster/playstre → **plastre**, *n.*

plente, *n.* Abundance

plente (3×)

pleuresis, *n.* Pleurisy, inflammation of the membrane surrounding the lungs and lining the thoracic cavity

pleuresis (1×), *pleuresys* (1×)

Plinius, *n.* Pliny

Plinius (25×), *Pliuius* (1×)

Plybo, *n.* Plibus
plybo (1×)
pock, *n.* Skin eruption, sore, pustule, pimple
pockes (2×)
pocyoun, *n.* Potion, a medicinal drink
pocyoun (4×)
podadre → **podagre**, *n.*
podagre, *n.* Gout in the foot, podagra; gout in general
podadre (1×), *podagre* (13×), *potagre* (1×)
poet, *n.* Poet; any ancient writer
poetes (2×)
pollucyoun, *n.* Desecration, profanation
pollucyouns (1×)
polluten, *v.* To violate the sanctity of
pollute (1×)
polypus, *n.* Polyp, a small tumor in the nose
polypus (1×)
popye, *n.* Opium poppy
popy (5×), *popye* (5×), *popyes* (1×)
porcyoun, *n.* Portion, amount or quantity of something
porcion (1×), *porcyoun* (1×)
pore, *n.* An internal channel for bodily fluids
pores (1×), *poures* (1×)
pose, *n.* Catarrh, a head cold
pose (4×)
postome, *n.* Morbid swelling or inflammation in any part of the body
postemes (3×), *postome* (1×), *postomes* (3×)
pot, *n.* Vessel, pot, container
pot (1×)
potage, *n.* Porringer, a dish from which pottage or stew is eaten
potage (3×)
potagre → **podagre**, *n.*
pouder, *n.* Powder, pulverized or particulate substance
pouder (40×), *poudre* (3×), *poudres* (1×)
pounde, *n.* A pound, one of several measures of weight containing different numbers of ounces
pounde (1×)
poune garnet, *n.* Pomegranate
poune garnet (1×)
pownen, *v.* To pulverize
powned (2×)
poynte, *n.* A round spot or growth visible on the surface of the eye
poyntes (1×)
poysenen, *v.* To give poison to
poysened (1×)
poyson, *n.* Poison
poyson (1×)
prassion, *n.* The common or white horehound
prassion (1×)
precordya, *n.* The part of the abdomen close to the upper aperture of the stomach
precordya (1×)
precyouse, *a.* Valuable, precious
precyouse (3×)
pressen, *v.* To press against (sth.); to exert pressure, push
pressyd (1×)
presyd → **preysen**, *v.*
presynges → **preysynge**, *n.*
preue → **pryve**, *a.*
preven, *v.* To test, prove
preue (1×), *preued* (7×), *preueth* (1×), *preueyt* (1×), *preuy* (1×), *preuyth* (1×), *prevyd* (1×), *proued* (1×)
preysen, *v.* To praise
preysed (1×), *presyd* (1×)

preysynge, *n.* The act of praising someone or something; the fact of being praised
presynges (1×), *preysynge* (1×)
processe, *n.* Process
processe (1×)
profyt, *n.* Benefit, advantage, interest
profyt (4×), *profyte* (2×), *profyth* (2×)
profytable, *a.* Physically beneficial, advantageous, helpful
profytabele (1×), *profytable* (16×), *profytabler* (1×), *profytabyle* (1×), *prophetable* (1×), *prophytable* (2×), *prophytabler* (1×)
profyten, *v.* To be helpful or useful, be beneficial or useful to (sb.)
profyte (4×), *profyten* (1×), *profytyth* (1×), *prophytyth* (1×),
prophytable → **profytable**, *a.*
prophyten → **profyten**, *v.*
propryte, *n.* Property, quality
proprytees (1×), *propyrtes* (1×)
propyrly, *adv.* In proper terms, in strict terms
propyrly (3×)
provoken, *v.* To induce, cause
prouoke (1×), *prouoken* (1×), *prouokyth* (4×)
pryck, *n.* A pointed object, spike
pryckes (1×)
prycken, *v.* To pierce, stab
prycke (1×), *prykyth* (1×)
prykyng, *ng.* Pricking
pryckynges (1×)
pryse, *n.* Price
pryse (1×)
prysen, *v.* To value (sb. or sth.) highly, esteem, praise
prysen (1×)
pryve, *a.* Private, personal
preve (1×), *pryue* (2×)
ptisan, *n.* Shelled or cooked barley, ptisan; a medicinal tea or infusion made from herbs.
ptisan (1×), *ptisane* (1×), *ptysan* (1×), *tisane* (1×)
ptisyk → **tysyk**, *n. / a.*
ptysan → **ptisan**, *n.*
ptysyk → **tysyk**, *n. / a.*
pulyoll, *n.* Wild thyme; wild marjoram (Origanum vulgare)
pilyoll (1×), *pullyol* (1×), *pullyoll* (2×), *pulyol* (1×), *pulyoll* (19×),
pulyoll haunt, *n.* Wild marjoram (Origanum vulgare)
pulyol haund (1×), *pulyol haunt* (1×), *pulyoll haunt* (1×)
pullen, *v.* To uproot (a plant, tree, stake, etc.)
pulled (1×)
purgacion, *n.* Cleansing, purification
purgacion (3×)
purgen, *v.* To purify or cleanse; to purge (sb., the body) by a laxative, a diuretic
purge (21×), *purgen* (6×), *purgeyt* (1×), *purgyd* (1×), *purgyt* (4×), *purgyth* (33×)
purgynge, *ng.* The expulsion of evil or excess humors
purgynge (1×)
purselane, *n.* The European purslane
purselane (1×), *purslane* (1×)
purpul, *a.* Purple colour
purpel (1×), *purpul* (3×)
pusca, *n.* Mixture of water and vinegar or wine
pusca (5×)
putten, *v.* To push; to put ‖ **p. away** to purge (venom); of the large intestine: to excrete, expel ‖ **p. out** to expel, discharge

put (14×), *putt* (1×), *putte* (49×), *putten* (2×), *puttet* (1×), *puttyht* (1×), *puttyt* (3×), *puttyth* (16×), *putyth* (1×), *y putte* (2×), *yput* (1×)

pycke → **piche**, *n.*

pyement, *n.* Sweetened, spiced wine used for refreshment and in medical recipes

pyement (1×)

pykes → **piche**, *n.*

pyles/pylees → **pille**, *n.*

pylle → **pille**, *n.*

pylowe, *n.* Cushion, pillow

pylowe (1×)

pyone, *n.* A plant of the genus Pæonia, esp. male or entireleaved peony (P. mascula) and common peony (P. officinalis); peony

pyone (4×), *pyony* (2×), *pyonye* (1×)

pyppe, *n.* A disease of poultry in which a white scale forms around the tongue

pyppe (1×)

pysse, *n.* Urine

pysse (3×)

pyssen, *v.* To urinate

pysse (20×)

Q

quaken, *v.* To tremble with cold

quaken (1×)

quakyng, *ng.* Trembling, quivering, or shivering because of illness

quakyng (1×), *quakynge* (1×)

quantyte, *n.* Amount, quantity

quantyte (2×)

quarele, *n.* Illness

quareles (1×)

quarteyn, *n.* Intermittent fever with attacks recurring every third day, quartan fever

quarteyn (4×), *quarteyne* (1×)

quellen, *v.* To kill

quellyth (1×)

quenchen, *v.* To extinguish

quenche (3×), *quenchyth* (1×)

quyete, *n.* Peace, rest, quietness

quyete (1×)

quyk, *a.* Quick

quyk (1×)

quynse, *n.* The fruit of the quince tree

quynsys (1×)

quyteren, *v.* To form pus, suppurate

quytre (1×)

quytter, *n.* Pus, suppuration, a discharge of pus or matter

quytter (2×)

quotydyan, *a.* Daily; continual, unceasing

quotydyan (3×)

R

radiche, *n.* The radish plant

radiche (2×)

ragged, *a.* Tattered, ragged

ragged (1×)

raphane, *n.* The radish plant

raphanus (2×)

ratte, *n.* Rat

ratte (1×)

rawe, *a.* Uncooked, raw

rau (1×), *raw* (2×), *rawe* (16×)

recadyas, *n.* Recadias

recadyas (1×)

redde, *a.* Red colour

red (5×), *redde* (3×), *reed* (2×)

reden, *v.* To read

radde (2×), *y radde* (1×)
reformen, *v*. To restore
reformyth (1×)
regendren, *v*. To regenerate, cause flesh or skin to grow again
regendre (1×)
regnen, *v*. To reign, rule
regnyth (1×)
regyoun, *n*. Region, a part of the body
regyon (1×), *regyoun* (1×), *rygyon* (1×)
rehersen, *v*. To narrate
reherse (1×)
relaxen, *v*. To lose tension
relaxyth (1×)
relessen, *v*. To alleviate
relesse (1×), *relessyth* (1×)
releven, *v*. To relieve, alleviate
releue (2×), *releuyth* (1×)
remedye, *n*. Medical remedy, cure
remedye (1×)
remeven, *v*. To remove, take away
remeue (1×)
remyng → **rennyng**, *ng*.
renewen, *v*. To bring (a living thing) to a vigorous or flourishing state; revive
renewed (1×)
renmynges → **rennyng**, *n*.
rennen, *v*. To flow (blood, etc.) ‖ **r. out (of)** to flow from a body
renne (5×), *rennen* (1×), *rennyth* (4×)
rennyng, *ng*. The flowing of blood or bodily humour; also of tears
remyng (1×), *rennyng* (1×),
rennyng, *n*. Rennet; curdled milk from the intestines of various animals used as rennet
renmynges (1×), *rennynges* (1×)
repressen, *v*. To counteract (venom, pain, morbid conditions), overcome
represse (12×), *repressyth* (2×), *reprysse* (1×), *repryssyth* (1×)
reren, *v*. To raise, lift; to lift (the uvula) by reducing swelling
rere (1×), *reryth* (1×)
resceyven, *v*. To receive, catch
resceyueth (1×)
reserven, *v*. To preserve
reserue (1×)
resolven, *v*. To cause softening or dissolving of hard tumors, apostemes, etc.; of matter: soften, dissolve, dissipate; to diminish
resolue (6×), *resolued* (6×), *resoluyth* (3×)
resoun, *n*. Grape, raisin
resons (1×), *resouns* (1×)
rest, *n*. Rest
rest (1×)
restoren, *v*. To restore; to cure, heal
restore (3×)
restreynen, *v*. To prevent or staunch bleeding
restreyne (2×), *restreyneth* (1×), *restreynyt* (1×)
resvyour, *n*. Person on whom something is bestowed, passive recipient
resuyour (1×)
reverse, *a*. The opposite of something
reuerse (2×)
rewe, *n*. A plant of the genus Ruta, esp. common rue; the plant rye
rew (1×), *rewe* (25×), *rye* (1×)
rewme, *n*. Watery fluid or humor conceived as draining from the higher parts of the body
rewme (1×), *rewmes* (1×)
reyn, *n*. Kidney
reyn (1×), *reynes* (14×)
reynbowe, *n*. Rainbow
reynbowe (1×)

reyne, *n.* Rain
reyne (1×)
reysen, *v.* To lift up, hold up
reyse (1×)
rollen, *v.* To roll
rolle (2×), *rolled* (6×)
Romain, *n.* Inhabitant of ancient Rome or the Roman Empire
romaynes (1×)
Rome, *n.* Ancient Rome; the Roman Empire
rome (2×)
rosa camina → **rosa canina**, *n.*
rosa canina †, *n.* Dog rose
rosa camina (1×)
rosa emoroda, *n.* Rose Hemorrhoids, esp. the bleeding kind
rosa emoroda (1×)
rose, *n.* Rose
roos (1×), *roose* (1×), *rose* (19×), *roses* (22×)
rose mary, *n.* Rosemary
rose mary (1×)
roset, *n.* Rosin
roset (1×)
rosten, *v.* To roast
rosted (4×), *yrosted* (1×)
rote, *n.* A root of a tree or other plant
root (31×), *roote* (5×), *rootes* (17×), *rote* (6×), *rotes* (27×), *rothe* (1×)
roten, *a.* Putrid, rotten
roten (2×)
roten, *v.* To undergo natural decomposition
roote (1×), *rote* (1×)
rotnesse, *n.* The process of deterioration of a structure
rotnesse (1×), *rotynesse* (1×)
rotynesse → **rotnesse**, *n.*
rotyng, *n.* The process of putrefaction or festering in body tissues or members; suppuration of a wound or an aposteme
rotyng (1×), *rotynge* (1×)
rounde, *a.* Spherical, circular
round (1×), *rounde* (8×)
roundenes, *n.* The quality of being spherical
roundenes (1×)
rownesse, *n.* A scabby condition of the skin
rownesse (1×)
rybbe, *n.* Rib; the side of the body
rybbes (2×)
rye → **rewe**, *n.*
ryght, *n.* Rule of conduct, law
ryght (1×)
ryght, *adv.* Very, extremely; also, fully, quite
ryght (30×), *rygth* (1×), *rytgh* (1×)
ryghtfully, *adv.* In fact, in truth
ryghtfully (1×)
ryghtly, *adv.* Uprightly, righteously, dutifully; properly, appropriately; adequately
ryghtly (1×)
rygyon → **regyoun**, *n.*
rynde, *n.* The bark of a tree or other plant
rynde (1×)
ryngyng, *ng.* The sensation of ringing in the ear
ryugyng (1×)
rysen, *v.* To emerge, come out
ryse (1×), *rysen* (2×), *rysyth* (2×)
rytgh → **ryght**, *adv.*
ryugyng → **ryngyng**, *ng.*
ryvelyng, *n.* Wrinkling of the skin
ryuelynges (1×)
ryven, *v.* To sew
ryue (1×)

S

sacer ignis, *n.* Holy fire, erysipelas
ignys sacer (2×), *sacer ignis* (1×)
sadde, *a.* Sated, surfeited; satisfied
sadde (1×)
sadden, *v.* To make (sth.) hard or stiff
sadde (1×)
safferoun, *n.* The saffron crocus
saferon (1×), *saferoun* (1×), *safferon* (2×), *safferoun* (1×), *safrom* (1×), *safron* (1×), *safroun* (1×)
safly, *adv.* In safety, safely; without harm
safly (1×)
salgia → **salvia**, *n.*
salimica †, *n.* Wild rose
salimica (1×)
salisea, *n.* Willow
salisea (1×)
salte, *n.* Salt
salt (4×), *salte* (19×)
salvia, *n.* The herb sage
salgia (1×), *saluia* (1×)
same, *a.* Same
saam (4×), *same* (138×)
sampen, *v.* To gather, collect
sampe (4×)
samrede, *a.* Half-red, partly red, reddish
samrede (1×)
sanicle, *n.* The European sanicle
sanicle (2×)
sapa, *n.* New wine boiled to a syrup
sapa (3×)
saturya, *n.* Savory, any plant of the genus Satureia, esp. the annual herb Satureia hortensis (garden, summer savory), or the perennial S. montana (mountain or winter savory), natives of the south of Europe
saturya (1×)
sauce, *n.* Sauce, condiment for meat, fish, fowl, etc.
sauce (1×)
sauge, *n.* The herb sage
sauge (7×)
saverey, *n.* A plant of the genus Satureia, esp. the garden or summer savory
sauerey (8×), *sauorey* (3×)
saveyn, *n.* The plant Juniperus sabina
saueyn (2×), *saueyne* (2×), *sauyen* (1×), *sauyn* (1×)
sauorey → **saverey**, *n.*
savoure, *n.* Taste
sauar (1×), *saueur* (1×), *sauor* (5×), *sauore* (2×), *sauorre* (1×), *sauour* (2×), *sauoure* (6×)
savouren, *v.* To have a flavor or taste
sauored (2×), *sauoured* (2×)
savoury, *a.* Tasteful, flavourful; delicious
sauory (1×)
sauyen → **saveyn**, *n.*
saxifrage, *n.* A plant of the genus Saxifraga, used medicinally
saxifrage (3×)
sayen, *v.* To say
sathe (1×), *say* (20×), *sayd* (8×), *sayde* (9×), *saye* (1×), *sayen* (9×), *sayn* (62×), *sayt* (5×), *sayth* (46×), *seyd* (21×), *seyde* (29×), *seyden* (3×), *seyth* (3×), *y seyde* (1×)
sayenge, *ng.* The act of saying; Something spoken or said, a speech, statement, report
sayenges (1×), *seynge* (1×)
saylen, *v.* To attack, assail
sayle (1×)
scabbe, *n.* Any of various skin diseases characterized by itching, pustules, ulceration, etc.; also, the pustule characteristic of such diseases
scabbe (8×), *scabbes* (2×)
scabiose, *n.* Any of the plants of the genus Scabiosa; the plant horseheal

(Inula helenium); the plant silverweed (Potentilla anserina)

scabiose (1×)

scaldyng, *ng*. Burning by fire or hot liquid; an injury from scalding water; also, a place on the body that has been scalded by hot liquid or fire, a burn

scaldyng (1×), *scaldynge* (1×), *scaldynges* (2×)

scalle, *n*. Any of several types of disease of the scalp, tinea, ringworm; a case of such a disease

scalle (1×)

scally, *a*. Of the suture between the temporal and parietal bones

scally (1×)

scietica, *n*. The disease sciatica; an attack of the disease; of an inflammation: affecting the sciatic nerve

ciatica (1×), *scietica* (1×)

scietica passio, *n*. The disease sciatica

sciatica pasio (1×), *sciatica passio* (2×), *scietica passio* (4×), *scyetica passio* (1×)

sclayre, *n*. The herb clary (Salvia sclarea)

sclayre (3×)

sclirosys, *n*. Sclerosis

sclirosys (1×)

scome, *n*. (a) Froth, foam; the impure foam that rises to the surface when a liquid boils or is heated

scome (1×)

scoryth → **scuren**, *v*.

scorpyoun, *n*. Scorpion

scorpyon (1×), *scorpyoun* (1×)

scrabro, *n*. Hornet

scrabro (1×)

scrapen, *v*. To remove

scrape (2×)

scroof → **scrophee**, *n*.

scrophee, *n*. Scrofula, swelling of the glands

scroof (1×), *scrophee* (1×)

scruple → **scrypul**, *n*.

scrypul, *n*. A unit of apothecary's weight of one twenty-fourth of an ounce

scripules (1×), *scruple* (1×), *scrybulus* (1×), *scrypules* (2×)

sculle, *n*. Skull

sculle (1×)

scuren, *v*. To move rapidly

scoryth (1×), *scure* (9×), *scuryt* (1×), *scuryth* (3×)

sechen, *v*. To look for

seche (2×)

secundyne, *n*. Fetal membranes; the afterbirth

secundina (1×), *secundyna* (1×), *secundyne* (1×)

sedewale, *n*. The root of a plant of the species Curcuma, esp. the long zedoary (Curcuma zedoaria); also, the plant itself

cedewale (3×), *sedewale* (1×)

see, *n*. Chair

see (2×)

seed, *n*. Seed

sed (1×), *sedes* (2×), *seed* (92×), *seedes* (1×)

seen, *v*. To see

see (1×), *seest* (2×), *seie* (1×)

seeve, *n*. Sieve

seeue (1×)

sege, *n*. Seat; a chair, stool, bench ‖ **goon to s.** to ease oneself

sege (1×)

selde, *adv*. Seldom

selde (1×)

selinon, *n*. Smallage, wild celery

selinon (1×), *solumem* (1×)

seluel → **selver**, *n*.

selver, *n*. Silver

seluel (1×), *seluer* (2×)
selverne, *a*. Made of silver
seluerne (1×)
seme, *n*. Suture, esp. of the skull
seme (1×)
semen, *v*. Appear to be
seme (2×), *semed* (1×), *semeth* (5×), *semyth* (4×)
senacion †, *n*. Groundsel
senacion (2×)
senuey → **synvey**, *n*.
sephalargya, *n*. Constant headache
sephalargya (1×)
sercle, *n*. Circle
sercle (2×)
serpent, *n*. Serpent, snake
serpent (2×), *serpentes* (9×)
serpigo, *n*. A skin disease distinguished by scaling or eruption and a tendency to spread, as herpes or eczema
serpigo (1×)
serpillum, *n*. Parsley
serpillum (1×)
sethen, *v*. To boil, seethe, be heated to the boiling point
sethe (39×), *sode* (1×), *soden* (65×), *soiden* (1×), *y soden* (1×), *ysoden* (1×)
setten, *v*. To set
set (2×), *sette* (6×)
sextarye, *n*. A measure of dry weight or capacity, often equal to two pounds
sextarye (1×)
Sextus Niger, *n*. Sextus Niger
Sextus Niger (1×)
seynge → **sayenge**, *n*.
shadowe, *n*. Shadow
shadowe (1×)
shafte, *n*. Splinter
shafte (1×)
shapen, *v*. To give (sb. or sth.) a specific shape, form, fashion
shapen (1×)
shappe, *n*. Shape
shap (1×), *shappe* (2×)
share, *n*. Share; the division or fork of the body
share (5×)
sharpe, *a*. Strong; irritating, corrosive
sharpe (8×), *sharper* (1×)
sharpen, *v*. To intensify (heat, a color, etc.); to increase
sharpyth (1×)
shaven, *v*. To shave
shaue (1×)
shelle, *n*. Shell
shelle (1×)
shep, *n*. Sheep
shepes (2×)
sheten, *v*. To shoot
y shot (1×)
shewen, *v*. To show
shewe (2×), *shewyth* (1×)
sho, *n*. Shoe
shone (1×)
short, *a*. Short
short (1×), *shrot* (1×)
shorten, *v*. To decrease in duration
shorte (1×), *shorted* (1×), *shortes* (1×)
shortly, *adv*. For a short time, briefly; in few words; concisely
shortly (2×)
shrot → **short**, *a*.
shulen, *va*. Shall; as modal auxiliary expressing what is appropriate, reasonable, right, prudent, etc.: shall
schal (4×), *schalt* (1×), *shal* (76×), *shall* (2×), *shalt* (31×), *shold* (1×), *shul* (5×), *shuld* (11×), *shulde* (4×), *shull* (1×)

shylle, *a.* Loud, resounding
shylle (1×)
shynen, *v.* To shine
shyne (1×)
siasis, *n.* Siasis
siasis (1×)
simbria, *n.* Mint (of the genus Mentha), horse-mint (miswritten for sisymbrium)
simbria (1×)
siringa, *n.* A kind of fistula or fester
siringa (2×), *siringam* (1×), *syrynge* (1×), *syrynges* (1×)
Sirius, *n.* Sirius
Sirius (1×)
siroyne, *n.* Shoot, sprout
siroyne (1×), *syroyne* (1×)
sken → **skyn**, *n.*
skyn, *n.* Skin
sken (2×), *skyn* (16×), *skynne* (2×)
skyrwyt, *n.* Parsnip or water-parsnip plant
skyrewyt (1×), *skyrwyt* (4×)
slen, *v.* To destroy (a sore, tumor, dead flesh, etc.), remove
sle (13×), *sleeth* (4×)
slepe, *n.* The state of sleep
slepe (4×)
slepen, *v.* To sleep, be asleep
slepe (8×), *sleppe* (1×), *slepyng* (1×)
slomberynge, *ng.* Sleep, dozing
slomerynge (1×)
slowly, *adv.* Slowly
slowly (1×)
slyme, *n.* Mud, slime
slyme (1×)
smalache, *n.* A plant of the genus Apium, esp. wild celery
smalache (5×), *smaleache* (1×)
small, *a.* Small
smal (32×), *small* (29×)
smel, *n.* Smell
smel (1×)
smellen, *v.* To smell
smelle (1×), *smelled* (1×), *smellen* (1×), *smellyd* (1×)
smellyng, *ng.* The sense of smell
smellyng (2×), *smellynge* (1×), *smelynge* (1×)
smereworte, *n.* One of several kinds of plants, including Aristolochia rotunda, Chenopodium Bonus-Henricus, and Mercurialis annua
smere worte (2×), *smereworte* (1×)
smoke, *n.* Smoke
smoke (4×)
smytyng, *ng.* The action of striking
smytynges (1×)
snake, *n.* Snake
snake (1×), *snakes* (2×)
snesen, *v.* To sneeze
snese (2×)
Socrates, *n.* Socrates
Socrates (1×)
sodenly, *adv.* Suddenly
sodenly (1×)
sodeyn, *a.* Sudden
sodeyn (3×)
softe, *a.* Soft
softe (2×)
soken, *v.* To soak, moisten
soke (3×), *soked* (1×), *soken* (1×)
sole, *n.* Sole (of the human foot)
soles (1×)
soluble, *a.* Unconstipated, lax
solubles (1×)
solumem → **selinon**, *n.*
solven, *v.* To relieve; to dissolve, melt
solue (4×), *soluen* (2×)
somdele, *n.* / *a.* Part, portion; some degree or amount of, some
somdele (5×)
somwhat, *adv.* Considerably, fully

somwhat (1×)
sone, *adv.* Soon
sone (14×), *soon* (1×), *soune* (1×)
sone, *n.* Male son
sone (1×)
sonn rysynge, *n.* Sunrise
sonn rysynge (1×)
sonne, *n.* Sun
sonne (9×), *soune* (2×)
sool, *n.* Rope, esp. one used to tether cattle
sool (1×)
soor → **sore**, *n.*
soper, *n.* Evening meal, supper; the time at which this meal is eaten
soper (1×), *sowper* (1×)
sore, *n.* / *a.* Pain in bodily parts or organs; painful
soor (8×), *sore* (6×), *sores* (16×)
sorel, *n.* Sorrel
sorel (7×), *sorell* (6×), *sorer* (1×), *surell* (1×)
sorer → **sorel**, *n.*
sotell, *a.* Manifest, clear, evident
sotell (1×)
soth, *n.* Faithfulness, trustworthiness
soth (2×)
souken, *v.* To draw liquid by sucking
souke (2×)
soupen, *v.* To drink, swallow
soupe (1×)
souple, *a.* Relaxed
souple (1×)
souplen, *v.* To soften, promote softness of the skin, body, etc.
souple (1×)
souredocke, *n.* A plant of the genus Rumex; the plant sorrel
soure docke (1×), *souredocke* (1×)
soure dough, *n.* Leaven; leavened bread
soure dowe (1×)
southe, *n.* South
southe (1×)
southernewode, *n.* The plant southernwood
southernewod (1×), *southernewode* (2×), *southernwode* (1×), *southerwode* (2×)
soveraynly, *adv.* To a great extent, very much, highly, extremely; supremely
soueraynly (2×), *souereynly* (1×), *souerynly* (1×)
sovereyn, *a.* Distinguished, renowned, worthy
souereyn (1×)
sownen, *v.* To make or produce a sound
sowne (1×)
sownyng, *ng.* Sounding, ringing; a sound (perceived by the ear)
sownyng (3×)
sowper → **soper**, *n.*
sparclen, *v.* To throw out sparks
sparcle (2×)
specyal, *a.* Characteristic; exceptional
specyal (1×)
specyaly, *adv.* Particularly, especially
specialy (1×), *specyaly* (6×), *specyly* (1×)
spedy, *a.* Beneficial, helpful; efficacious
spedyer (1×)
speken, *v.* To speak
speke (3×)
spere, *n.* Spear
spere (2×)
sperme, *n.* Sperm, the male seminal fluid
sperme (1×)
sperren, *v.* To move quickly, rush
sperred (1×), *sperryd* (1×), *sperryth* (1×)
speten, *v.* To spit ‖ **s. out** to spit out
spete (1×), *speten* (8×), *spette* (1×), *spetten* (2×)

spettynge, *n.* The action of raising and ejecting phlegm or sputum
spettynge (1×), *spettynges* (1×)

spewen, *v.* To vomit; throw up (food, poison, etc.)
spewen (1×)

spiknarde → **spykenarde**, *n.*

spit, *n.* Saliva, spittle; sputum
spites (1×)

splene, *n.* Spleen
splen (1×), *splene* (24×)

spotel, *n.* Saliva
spotel (1×)

spotte, *n.* Morbid eruption on the skin, pimple; leprous lesion
spotte (1×), *spottes* (12×)

spotten, *v.* To create coloured spots
spotted (1×)

spotty, *a.* Spotty, having spots
spotty (1×)

spuynge, *ng.* Vomiting
spuynge (1×)

spyce, *n.* Spice (used as a medication or as a medicinal or an alchemical ingredient)
spices (1×), *spicys* (1×), *spyce* (2×), *spyces* (6×), *spycys* (1×)

spykenarde, *n.* A valerianaceous plant, prob. Valeriana officinalis
spiknarde (1×), *spyke narde* (1×), *spykenarde* (5×)

spreden, *v.* To spread, stretch || **s. abrood** to spread (sth.) out, stretch out, extend
sprede (2×)

spryngen, *v.* To come up, come out; to sprout, grow
spryngyth (1×)

spyder, *n.* Insect of the order Araneae, spider
spyder (1×)

stalke, *n.* Stalk
stalke (1×)

stampen, *v.* To pound or mash (an ingredient)
stampe (51×), *stamped* (46×), *stampyd* (7×), *stampyt* (1×)

staunchen, *v.* To be relieved of diarrhea; to stop bleeding
stanche (3×), *stanchyth* (1×), *staunche* (61×), *staunched* (1×), *staunchet* (1×), *staunchyd* (1×), *staunchyt* (15×), *staunchyth* (5×)

stede, *n.* Place
stede (2×)

stenche, *n.* Odour, smell
stenche (1×), *stynche* (1×)

stepen, *v.* To soak in liquid
steped (1×)

sterne, *a.* Harsh, severe; inflexible, rigid
sterne (1×), *storne* (1×)

stingen, *v.* To bite; to pierce, stab
y stong (1×), *y stunge* (1×)

stocosys, *n.* A kind of headache
stocosys (1×)

stok, *n.* The trunk of a living tree; the base of a tree
stok (1×)

stomak, *n.* Stomach
stomac (3×), *stomak* (55×), *stomake* (3×), *stomake* ys (1×)

stonden, *v.* To stand, assume or maintain a standing position
stonde (2×)

stone, *n.* Stone
ston (3×), *stone* (9×), *stoon* (3×)

stonynge, *ng.* Paralysis or cramping of a limb, tendon
stonynge (1×)

stoppen, *v.* To obstruct; to be afflicted with an obstruction
stoppe (1×), *stopped* (1×)

storclen, *v.* To ripen by drying, season
storcle (1×)
storne → **sterne**, *a.*
Strabus, *n.* Walafrid Strabus
Strabus (2×)
stranglen, *v.* To choke, be strangled, choke to death
strangly (1×)
strangurye, *n.* Strangury, disease characterized by difficulty of urination
strangurye (1×)
strecchen, *v.* To stretch out ‖ **s. out** to cause (sth.) to expand, distend
strecche (1×)
strengthe, *n.* Strength
strengthe (5×), *stryngthe* (2×), *strynthe* (1×)
strengthen, *v.* To strengthen; to reinforce; to make strong
strengthyth (3×), *strengyth* (1×), *strynthe* (1×)
streyght, *a.* Straight, not bent
streyght (1×)
streyghten, *v.* To straighten (a part of the body), stretch
streyght (1×)
streyghtnesse, *n.* Straightness
streyghtnesse (1×), *streytnes* (1×)
streynen, *v.* To stretch, extend
streyneyt (1×), *streynyth* (1×)
streynesse, *n.* Difficulty in breathing, constriction in the chest
streynesse (1×), *stryghtnesse* (1×)
streytnes → **streyghtnesse**, *n.*
strignum, *n.* Morel
strignum (1×)
stroke, *n.* Knock
stroke (1×), *strokes* (2×)
strong, *a.* Strong
strenger (2×), *strong* (2×), *stronge* (12×), *strongyst* (1×)
strongly, *adv.* Strongly
strongly (1×)
struccyon, *n.* Betony
struccyon (1×)
stryghtnesse → **streynesse**, *n.*
stryn(g)the → **strengthe**, *n.*
strynthe → **strengthen**, *v.*
sturdynesse, *n.* Physical strength; the intensity of a fever
sturdynesse (1×)
styf, *a.* Not flexible, not pliant, rigid
styf (1×), *styffe* (1×)
styfnesse, *n.* Pathological difficulty in moving
styfnesse (2×)
styk, *n.* Twig or slender branch on a living bush, shrub, or tree
styk (1×)
styken, *v.* To pierce
styked (3×), *stykyd* (2×)
styl, *a.* / *adv.* Motionless, without movement; silently, noiselessly
styl (2×), *styll* (1×), *stylle* (1×)
stynche → **stenche**, *n.*
styngkynge, *ng.* Disagreeable or foul odour, stench
styngkynge (1×)
styngyng, *ng.* Wound or pain caused by the biting of a snake or the stinging of a scorpion, bee, or wasp
stynggynges (1×), *styngyng* (2×), *styngynges* (1×)
stynken, *v.* To give off an odour
stynketh (1×)
subfumygacion, *n.* Suffumigation; treatment with aromatic fumes
subfumygacion (7×)
substaunce, *n.* A type or kind of thing
substaunce (1×)
suffren, *v.* To suffer
suffre (4×)

suffycen, *v.* To be adequate (in size, quantity, number, etc.) for a purpose
suffycyth (1×)
superflue, *a.* Immoderate, excessive
superflue (1×)
supposen, *v.* To suppose
suppose (1×), *supposen* (1×)
surell → **sorel**, *n.*
swagen, *v.* To relieve pain
swage (1×)
swalowe, *n.* A bird of the genus Hirundo, esp. the European swallow (Hirundo rustica)
swalowe (2×), *swalowes* (1×)
swayde, *n.* Seed pod, outer shell or husk of a pea, bean, etc.
swayde (1×)
swellyng, *n.* Increase
swallyng (1×), *swellyng* (1×), *swellynge* (2×), *swellynges* (3×), *swelyng* (1×)
swete, *a.* Sweet, having the quality of sweetness
soot (1×), *swete* (3×), *swettyst* (1×), *swote* (1×)
sweten, *v.* To perspire, sweat
swete (2×), *swete* (1×)
swetnes, *n.* The quality of being sweet or pleasant to the taste, inherent sweetness
swetnes (1×)
swnes → **swyn**, *n.*
swollen, *v.* To increase in size, swell
swol (1×), *swolle* (3×), *swollen* (2×)
swolwen, *v.* To swallow
swolewe (1×), *swolwe* (1×), *yswolewed* (1×)
swot, *n.* Perspiration, sweat
swot (1×), *swoot* (1×), *swote* (1×)
swote → **swete**, *a.*
swyft, *adv.* Swiftly, with great velocity, at a great speed
swyfther (1×)
swyn, *n.* Pig, swine
swnes (2×), *swynes* (12×)
syde, *n.* Side
syde (8×), *sydes* (8×)
syght, *n.* Sight
syght (7×)
syghyng, *n.* Rough or labored breathing
syghyng (1×), *syghynges* (3×)
sygne, *n.* Sign, indication
sygne (1×)
sygnifyen, *v.* To be an indication or symptom of (sth.), indicate
sygnyfye (1×), *sygnyfyeth* (1×)
syke, *a.* Sick
syke (11×)
syker, *a.* Free from danger, not at risk, in safety, safe
syker (1×)
sykerly, *adv.* In safety, in security, safely, securely
sykerly (1×), *sykerlyche* (1×)
syknesse, *n.* Sickness
seknesse (3×), *sykenes* (1×), *sykenesse* (7×), *sykenesses* (1×), *sykenysse* (1×), *syknes* (8×), *syknesse* (29×)
syler, *n.* A type of willow
syler (1×)
synegrene, *n.* Houseleek
synegrene (1×)
syngynge, *n.* Act of singing
syngynge (1×)
synow, *n.* A fibrous cord connecting a muscle to a bone or other bodily part, a tendon
synowes (9×)
synvey, *n.* (a) A plant of the genus Brassica, prob. the black mustard (B. nigra) or the white mustard (B. alba)
senuey (5×), *senueys* (1×), *synuey* (6×), *synueye* (2×)

syroyne → **siroyne**, *n.*
syrsty, *a.* Thirsty
syrsty (1×)
sytten, *v.* To sit
sytte (1×)

T

taken, *v.* To grip, take hold || **t. away** to deliver someone from danger
tak (1×), *take* (75×), *taken* (8×), *takyn* (2×), *takyt* (4×), *takyth* (2×), *toke* (2×), *ytake* (2×)
talowe, *n.* Fatty tissue of an animal
talowe (1×)
tansey, *n.* Tansy
tansey (2×)
tarte, *a.* Sharp to the taste, pungent, sour, acidic
tarte (1×)
taryen, *v.* To be delayed; to delay (sb.)
taryen (2×), *taryn* (2×)
tast, *n.* Taste
tast (3×)
tayl, *n.* Tail
tayles (1×)
techanus → **tethanus**, *n.*
techen, *v.* To give instruction, tell, say; to speak with authority
taught (2×), *techyth* (2×), *y taught* (1×)
techynge, *n.* The act of imparting knowledge or understanding
techynge (1×)
tellen, *v.* To speak, tell || **t. out** to talk unrestrainedly about sth.
tel (1×), *telle* (4×), *tolde* (1×)
temperat, *a.* Of an intermediate degree between extreme qualities; mild in effect; mild, gentle
temperat (2×)
tempernesse, *n.* Temperateness
tempernesse (1×)
temple, *n.* Temple, the flattened area on either side of the forehead between the eye and the ear
temples (2×)
tempren, *v.* To combine (ingredients), blend (a mixture of ingredients)
tempre (4×)
tenasmon, *n.* A medical condition characterized by a continual urge to defecate
tenasmon (1×)
tender → **tendre**, *a.*
tendre, *a.* Physically sensitive, esp. to pain; susceptible to injury
tender (1×), *tendre* (5×)
tercyan, *n.* / *a.* Tertiary; tercian
terciam (1×), *tercyam* (1×), *tercyan* (2×)
terrebentine, *n.* Turpentine, oleoresin of the terebinth tree
terrebentine (1×)
tete, *n.* Nipple, teat
tete (1×), *tetes* (5×), *tetys* (2×)
tethanus, *n.* Tetanus, a disease characterized by spasms and rigidity of muscles
techanus (1×), *tethanus* (1×)
þorfe → **thorugh**, *p.*
thorgh → **thorugh**, *p.*
þorne, *n.* Thorn, sharp-pointed spine or prickle on a plant
thorne (1×), *þorne* (2×)
thorugh, *p.* Through
þorfe (1×), *thorgh* (1×), *thorugh* (13×), *thurgh* (2×), *thurght* (1×), *thurglt* (1×)
threde, *n.* A piece of textile twine; cord made from fibrous material
threde (2×)

þrenosshe †, *n.* Groundsel
þrenosshe (1×)
throte, *n.* Throat
throte (1×), *throtes* (1×)
throw, *n.* Contraction of the uterus while giving birth; subsequent pain and discomfort
throwes (3×)
thrysten, *v.* To wring or squeeze out (a liquid)
thryst (1×), *y thurst* (1×), *ythurst* (1×), *ythursten* (1×)
thurgh(t) → **thorugh**, *p.*
thye, *n.* Thigh
thye (7×), *thyes* (3×), *thyghe* (1×)
thyghe → **thye**, *n.*
thyk, *a.* Thick, dense
thycke (1×), *thyk* (2×)
thyng, *n.* Thing
þyng (2×), *þynges* (4×), *thynges* (4×)
thynne, *a.* Thin
þynne (1×), *thynne* (1×), *tyn* (1×)
thynnen, *v.* To reduce the viscosity of (a humor, liquid, etc.)
thynnyth (1×)
timbria, *n.* Summer savory
tymbrya (1×)
tisane → **ptisan**, *n.*
togeder/togedre/togedyr → **togydre**, *adv.*
togydre, *adv.* Together, into a group
to geder (1×), *to gedre* (3×), *to gedyr* (3×), *to gyder* (12×), *to gydre* (24×), *to gydres* (2×), *to gydyr* (3×)
toon, *r.* The one, one; the very one
toon (1×)
top, *n.* The higher end of sth.
top (1×)
tothe, *n.* Tooth
teth (1×), *tethe* (7×), *toon* (2×), *toþe* (1×), *tothe* (4×)
totheache, *n.* Tooth-ache
toþe ache (1×), *tothe ache* (10×), *totheache* (1×)
touche, *n.* The making of physical contact
touche (1×)
touchen, *v.* To touch
touche (3×), *touched* (1×)
travaylen, *v.* To suffer from disease or injury, be afflicted with an illness or debilitating condition
trauayled (1×)
travelynge, *n.* The inflicting of damage; an attack from a pathological condition
trauelynge (1×)
tree, *n.* Tree
tre (1×), *tree* (1×)
tremelyng, *n.* Involuntary twitching or trembling of the body or a part of the body; a pathological condition characterized by muscle spasms; also, the phase of a fever characterized by shivering
tremelyng (1×), *tremlynge* (1×)
tremlynge → **tremelyng**, *n.*
trench, *n.* Parasite (an intestinal worm); sharp pain in the belly
trenches (3×)
treten, *v.* To deal with
treted (1×), *tretyth* (1×)
trowen, *v.* To have trust, be trustful
trow (2×), *trowe* (6×), *trowed* (1×), *trowen* (2×), *trowyth* (1×)
trusten, *v.* To trust, be confident
truste (1×)
tunge, *n.* Tunge
tonge (2×), *tung* (2×), *tunge* (5×)
turmentynge, *n.* Affliction, a source of distress
turmentynge (1×)
turnen, *v.* To turn
turne (2×)
tyme, *n.* Time

tyme (14×), *tymes* (2×)

tyme, *n.* Any plant of the genus Thymus, esp. wild thyme (Thymus serpyllum) or garden thyme (Thymus vulgaris)

tyme (3×)

tympana, *n.* Disease in which the abdomen is distended by gas

tympana (1×)

tyn → **thynne**, *a.*

tysyk, *n.* / *a.* A wasting disease of the lungs; phthisic

ptisyk (1×), *ptysyk* (1×), *tysyk* (4×)

U

unce, *n.* Ounce

unce (5×), *unces* (2×)

unclosen, *v.* To unlock

unclosed (1×)

underputten, *v.* To apply (medicament) to the lower part of the body or as a suppository

under put (3×), *under putt* (1×), *under putte* (4×), *underput* (3×), *underputt* (1×), *underputte* (3×), *unther put* (1×)

unknowen, *v.* To lack knowledge (of sth.), be unaware

unknowe (2×), *unknowen* (1×)

unkynde, *a.* Injurious to health, unwholesome

unkynde (1×)

unnethe, *adv.* With difficulty, not without effort, not easily

ounnethe (1×), *unneþe* (1×), *unnethe* (5×)

unwassen, *v.* Not to rinse in water, not to wash

unwasse (1×)

unwytyng, *ng.* State of being unaware or lacking in knowledge of something

unwytyng (1×)

Uribasius, *n.* Oribasius

uribasius (1×), *urybasyus* (1×)

urtica, *n.* Nettle

urtica (1×)

uryn, *n.* Urine (as a product of the digestive processes)

urym (2×), *uryn* (7×), *uryne* (3×), *urynes* (1×)

use, *n.* Use, the act of using or employing something

use (1×)

usen, *v.* To use

use (1×), *used* (6×), *usyth* (1×)

utmyst, *a.* Extreme, utmost

utmyst (1×)

uva, *n.* Uvula; epiglottis

uua (8×)

V

valeryan, *n.* A medicinal herb of the family Valerinaceae, esp. Valeriana officinalis; an extract made from this herb

ualeryan (2×)

vanysshen, *v.* To disperse (a group), scatter; to recede

uanysshyth (1×), *wanysshe* (1×)

vapur, *n.* Gas generated in the body, often with a debilitating effect upon the stomach, brain, or other organs; a gaseous substance formed within the body and often released through the pores or exhaled by the lungs

uapur (1×)

variole, *n.* Pustules, pocks

uariole (1×)

uenegre → **venygre**, *n.*

venemen, *v*. To poison, harm or kill (sb.) by inflicting a venomous bite, sting, etc.
uenemed (1×)
venemous, *a*. Venomous, deadly, capable of introducing or injecting a toxic substance by means of a bite, sting, etc.
uenemous (14×), *uenemouse* (4×), *uenomus* (1×)
ventosyte, *n*. Condition of gaseous pressure in the body, esp. of the ear or of the alimentary canal; an accumulation of gas in a bodily cavity or organ
uentosyte (1×)
venygre, *n*. Vinegar, usu. wine vinegar
uenegre (1×), *uenyger* (1×), *uenygre* (53×), *uynegre* (14×), *uynygre* (1×)
venym, *n*. Venom, a toxin produced or secreted by an animal, insect, etc.
uenenis (1×), *uenym* (25×), *uenymes* (1×), *uenymis* (1×), *uenyms* (1×), *uenymys* (1×)
vertu, *n*. Efficacious quality, medicinal potency
uertu (805×), *uertues* (14×), *uertuys* (1×)
vertygo, *n*. Condition or disorder known as vertigo; dizziness, giddiness
uertygo (1×), *uertylago* (1×)
uertylago → **vertygo**, *n*.
ver tyme, *n*. Spring time
uer tyme (1×)
verveyne, *n*. A plant of the genus Verbena, esp. Verbena officinalis, vervain
ueruenv (2×), *uerueyn* (2×), *uerueyne* (14×), *ueruyne* (1×)
vessel, *n*. A small, portable container (for food or drink)
uessel (1×)
veyne, *n*. Vein
ueyne (5×), *ueynes* (4×), *ueynys* (1×)
vinum passum †, *n*. Pass wine, raisin wine
uino passe (1×), *uinum passum* (1×), *uyno passo* (1×)
Virgil, *n*. Virgil
uirgil (1×)
vocale, *a*. Performed with the voice
uocale (1×)
vomyt, *n*. The act of regurgitation or an instance of it, emesis; an attack or a spell of vomiting
uomyte (7×), *uomytes* (1×)
voyce, *n*. Voice of a human being
uoyce (8×)
vulp †, *n*. An animal of the genus Vulpes, having an elongated pointed muzzle and long bushy tail
uulpes (1×)
vyce, *n*. Physical imperfection in a human or an animal body, physical flaw
uyces (5×)
vyctour, *n*. Winner
uyctours (1×)
uynegre → **venygre**, *n*.
vyolence, *n*. Physical force exercised injuriously, abusively, or with threatening or coercive intent, violence
uyolence (3×)
vyolent, *a*. Violent, forceful
uyolent (3×)
vyolet, *n*. Violet
uiolet (1×), *uyolet* (19×), *uyoletes* (1×)
vyrgyne waxe, *n*. Unused wax
uyrgyne waxe (1×)
vyscouse, *a*. Sticky, viscous
uyscouse (4×)

W

wall, *n*. Wall

walles (1×)

walowen, *v.* To writhe about while affected by grief
walowe (1×)

wanne, *a.* Grayish, leaden; also, dark, black and blue (as a bruise)
wanne (1×)

wannesse, *n.* A whitish gray colour
wannesse (4×)

ware, *a.* Aware
ware (1×)

warly, *adv.* Vigilantly, watchfully
warly (1×)

warmod(e) → **wermode**, *n.*

warysshen, *v.* To cure (sb.), heal
warysshe (1×), *warysshed* (1×)

washe(n) → **wassen**, *v.*

waspe, *n.* Wasp, an insect of one of the superfamilies Vespoidea and Sphecoidea, esp. a member of the genus Vespa
waspe (1×)

wassen, *v.* To cleanse oneself or a part of one's body with water, bathe, wash
washe (1×), *wasse* (4×), *wasshe* (1×), *wasshed* (1×), *wasshen* (1×), *wasshon* (1×), *wasshyth* (1×), *wassyng* (1×), *y wasshe* (1×)

wasshe(n) → **wassen**, *v.*

wasshynge, *n.* Bathing, cleasing
wasshynge (2×), *wasshynges* (1×)

wasten, *v.* To reduce (swelling, an inflammation, etc.)
waste (1×)

water, *n.* Water
water (60×), *wateres* (1×), *waterys* (1×), *watres* (1×)

watery, *a.* Watery
watery (4×)

waxe, *n.* Beeswax
wax (2×), *waxe* (3×)

waxen, *v.* To increase in size, swell; to grow, mature
waxe (2×), *waxen* (4×), *waxyn* (1×), *waxyth* (2×)

way, *n.* Way
way (1×), *wayes* (2×)

weght → **weyght**, *n.*

weherlebon → **whyrlebone**, *n.*

wel, *adv.* Good; well
best (1×), *better* (9×), *bettre* (1×), *wel* (101×), *well* (1×), *welle* (1×)

welke, *n.* A disease affecting the mucous membranes in the head
welkes (3×)

welken, *v.* To fade, droop, wither, dry up
welkyth (1×)

wellen, *v.* To emanate, to spring
wellyth (1×)

wel savourynge, *ng.* The act of tasting something
wel sauorynge (1×)

wenne, *n.* Lump or excrescence on the human body; a cyst; a wart
uennes (1×), *wennes* (2×)

weren, *v.* To wear
were (1×)

wermode, *n.* Wormwood
warmod (1×), *warmode* (2×), *wermod* (3×), *wermode* (17×), *wormode* (10×)

werplyng, *n.* Human embryo
warpelyng (1×), *werplyng* (2×), *werplynge* (2×)

wert, *n.* Wart, mole
wertes (1×)

wesel, *n.* Weasel
wesel (1×)

weten, *v.* To wet
wete (4×)

weyght, *n.* Weight; the physical property of heaviness

weght (1×), *weyght* (9×), *weyth* (1×), *wyght* (3×)

weyk, *a.* Flexible, pliant

weker (1×), *weyker* (2×)

whelke, *n.* Pimple, pustule, an eruption of the skin

whelke (1×), *whelkes* (2×)

whete, *n.* Wheat

whete (2×)

whyrlebone, *n.* Thighbone, hip or hip joint

weherlebon (1×), *whyrlebone* (3×), *wyrlebon* (1×)

whyte, *n.* / *a.* The colour white; white in colour

whyt (4×), *whyte* (25×), *wyt* (1×), *wyte* (1×), *wyth* (1×), *wythe* (6×), *wythy* (1×)

whyte ellebur, *n.* White hellebore, usu. the dried root of Veratrum album

whyt ellebur (1×), *whyte ellebur* (1×), *wythe ellebur* (1×)

whyte peper, *n.* The European white pepper plant

wythe peper (1×)

willen, *v.* To want

wol (1×), *wolde* (1×)

willen, *va.* To want

wol (662×), *wold* (2×), *wolde* (2×), *woldest* (1×), *wole* (1×), *woll* (7×), *wolle* (1×), *wolt* (11×)

witen, *va.* To know; to be certain about

wot (1×), *wote* (2×)

withdrawen, *v.* To withdraw; to depart from a place, move away, leave

with drawynge (1×)

withstonden, *v.* To oppose, resist (a disease)

with stonde (1×), *wyth stonden* (1×), *with stondyth* (2×)

wlgago †, *n.* Asarabacca

wlgago (1×)

wode, *n.* Madness

wode (1×)

wode, *a.* Insane, mentally deranged

wode (1×)

wodebynde, *n.* Woodbine

wodebynde (2×)

wodeman, *n.* Insane, lunatic

wodemen (1×)

wodenes, *n.* Madness

wodenes (1×)

wol → **willen**, *v.* / *va.*

wolde → **willen**, *v.* / *va.*

wolle → **willen**, *va.*

wolle, *n.* Wool

wolle (5×)

woman, *n.* Woman

woman (23×), *womans* (1×), *women* (2×), *womens* (1×), *womman* (1×), *wommans* (18×), *wommen* (3×), *wommens* (19×), *wommes* (1×)

wombe, *n.* Womb

wombe (62×), *wombes* (1×)

wombed, *a.* Having a large belly

wombed (5×)

wond, *n.* Wound

wonde (20×), *wondes* (38×), *woundes* (1×)

wonder, *n.* Extraordinary thing; cause for surprise or amazement

wonder (2×)

wonderfully, *adv.* Extraordinarily

wonderfully (1×)

wonderly, *adv.* Marvelously

wonderly (18×), *wonderlyche* (1×)

wonen, *v.* To live, exist ‖ **ben wont to** be accustomed, be inclined to

wont (12×), *wonte* (2×)

wont → **wonen**, *v.*

worchen, *v.* To perform, produce an effect
worche (1×), *worchyth* (2×)
worchynge, *n.* Performance
worchynge (1×), *workyng* (1×), *wyrchynge* (1×)
workyng → **worchynge**, *n.*
worle, *n.* World, the earth
worle (1×)
worm, *n.* Worm
wormes (22×)
wormode → **wermode**, *n.*
wort, *n.* Any plant or herb; an uncultivated grass, root, or vegetable
wortes (5×)
worþy, *a.* Significant; worthwhile
worþy (1×)
wot(e) → **witen**, *va.*
woundes → **wond**, *n.*
wryngen, *v.* To press (fruit, herbs, raw meat, etc.) so as to force out the juice or fluid, crush; to twist and squeeze ‖ **w. out** to squeeze
wrongen (1×), *wrynge* (1×)
wryten, *v.* To write, to put into written form
wrete (1×), *wreten* (1×), *wreton* (2×), *wretyn* (1×), *wroot* (1×), *wrote* (1×), *wryte* (1×), *wrytyth* (2×)
wycch, *n.* A witch, a practitioner of the occult arts, diviner; a maker of magical potions or poisons
wycches (1×)
wycked, *a.* Causing harm, pain, or injury; distressing; unwholesome, unhealthful
wycked (6×), *wyckyd* (2×), *wyckyt* (2×), *wyked* (1×)
wyckednes, *n.* Malignancy, disease, infirmity; the malignant portion of a diseased body part
wyckednes (1×)
wyckyd → **wycked**, *a.*
wyckyt → **wycked**, *a.*
wylde, *a.* Wild
wyld (1×), *wylde* (2×)
wylde malowe, *n.* Wild mallow
wylde malowe (4×)
wylnen, *v.* To wish, desire
wylnen (1×)
wylowe, *n.* Any tree or shrub of the genus Salix, characterized by pliant woody branches
uylowe (1×)
wynde, *n.* Wind
wynde (8×)
wyndy, *a.* Windy
wyndy (1×)
wyne, *n.* Wine
wyne (157×)
wynnen, *v.* To exert effort, struggle; to overcome; to suffer with an illness
wynne (1×)
wypen, *v.* To cleanse ‖ **w. away** to disappear
wype (2×)
wyrchynge → **worchynge**, *n.*
wyrlebon → **whyrlebone**, *n.*
wyse, *n.* Manner, custom
wyse (78×)
wyse, *a.* Wise
wyse (2×)
wysely, *adv.* Wisely, judiciously
wysely (1×)
wythe ellebur → **white ellebur**, *n.*
wytte, *n.* The mental capacity or inclination to do something; an inclination
wytte (1×)

Y

ycchen, *v.* To feel an itch
ycche (1×)
yche, *n.* Itching
yche (5×), *ycche* (4×)
ychynge, *ng.* Itch; a sensation or sensations of itching
ychynge (1×)
ydell, *a.* Futile, vain, worthless
ydell (1×)
yee shelle → **eye shelle**, *n.*
yelowe, *n.* / *a.* The colour yellow; yellow
yelow (1×), *yelowe* (3×), *yolow* (1×)
yelowenesse, *n.* Yellowness
yelownesse (2×)
yerde, *n.* Pennis
yerde (4×)

yere, *n.* Year
yere (4×), *yeres* (1×)
yere(s) → **ere**, *n.*
yeven, *v.* To give
eyue (1×), *y uethte* (1×), *yaf* (2×), *yeue* (24×), *yeuen* (2×), *yeueth* (1×), *yeuyth* (1×), *yone* (2×), *youe* (4×), *youen* (1×)
ylke, *adv.* In like or similar manner, in the same way, similarly, alike
yleke (1×), *ylke* (1×)
ynceste, *n.* Sexual relationship with one of one's kin to the fourth or fifth degree
ynceste (1×)
yncorporaten, *v.* To blend
yncorporat (1×)
yndusen, *v.* To bring about, bring on, produce, cause, give rise to
ynduse (1×)
ynement → **oynement**, *n.*
ynflammat, *a.* Inflamed, burning, itchy
yn flammat (1×)
ynke, *n.* Ink
ynke (2×)
ynmoderat, *a.* Lacking moderation, inordinate; excessive, extreme
yn moderat (1×), *ynmoderat* (3×), *ynmoderate* (1×)
ynner, *a.* Inner, internal; inmost
ynner (4×)
ynnumerable, *a.* Very great, numerous
ynnumerable (2×)
ynow, *a.* / *adv.* Plentiful, generous, abundant, plenty of; enough
ynow (4×), *y now* (3×)
ynstrument, *n.* A part or organ of the body performing a certain function
ynstrumentes (1×), *ynstrumentys* (1×)
yonge, *a.* Young
yong (1×), *yonge* (2×), *younge* (1×)
yongly, *a.* Having the characteristics of youth, youthful
yongly (1×)
yoxe, *n.* Hiccups
yoxe (3×)
yren, *n.* Iron
yren (1×), *yron* (1×)
ysaccis †, *n.* The plant woad (Isatis tinctoria)
ysaccis (1×)

ysope, *n.* Hyssop
ysope (12×)
yswolewed → **swolwen**, *v.*
yuys → **iuys**, *n.*

Z

Zenocates, *n.* Xenocrates
Zenocates (1×)

yongly, *a.* Having the characteristics of youth, youthful

yongly (1×)

yoxe, *n.* Hiccups

yoxe (3×)

yren, *n.* Iron

yren (1×), *yron* (1×)

ysaccis †, *n.* The plant woad (Isatis tinctoria)

ysaccis (1×)

ysope, *n.* Hyssop

ysope (12×)

yswolewed → **swolwen**, *v.*

yuys → **iuys**, *n.*

Z

Zenocates, *n.* Xenocrates

Zenocates (1×)

References

Alonso Almeida, Francisco 2002. Punctuation Practice in a Late Medieval English Medical Remedybook. *Folia Linguistica Historica* 22, 207-232.

Arakelian, Paul G. 1975. Punctuation in a Late Middle English Manuscript. *Neuphilologische Mitteilungen* 76, 614-624.

Barnhart, Robert K. 1988. *The Barnhart Dictionary of Etymology. The Core Vocabulary of Standard English*. New York: The H.W. Wilson Company.

Beck, Lily Y. (trans.) 2005. *De Materia Medica* by Pedanius Dioscorides. Hildesheim: Olms Weidmann.

Benskin, Michael 1991. The 'Fit'-technique Explained. In Felicity Riddy (ed.). *Regionalism in Late Medieval Manuscripts and Texts: Essays Celebrating the Publication of A Linguistic Atlas of Late Mediaeval English*. Cambridge: D.S. Brewer. 9-26.

Blake, Norman F. 1996. *A History of the English Language*. London: Macmillan.

Brook, George L. 1945. *Notes on Some English Sound-changes*. Leeds: Walter Gardham Ltd.

Calle-Martín, Javier 1996. Stereotyped Comparisons in the Language of Geoffrey Chaucer. *Selim* 6, 64-84.

Calle-Martín, Javier 2000. Written Variation in *A Treatise on the Mensuration of Heights and Distances* (MS Sloane 213): an Analysis of its Provenance. In Francisco J. Cortés et al. (eds.). *Variation and Variety in Middle English Language and Literature*. Barcelona: Kadle Books. 9-14.

Calle-Martín, Javier 2004a. A Codicological Description of British Library, Egerton MS 2622 (ff. 136-165). In Alicia Rodríguez Álvarez and Francisco Alonso Almeida (eds.). *Voices on the Past. Studies in Old and Middle English Language and Literature*. La Coruña: Netbiblo Publishers. 75-88.

Calle-Martín, Javier 2004b. Punctuation Practice in a 15th-century Arithmetical Treatise (MS Bodley 790). *Neuphilologische Mitteilungen* 4, 407-422.

Calle-Martín, Javier 2009. Line-final Word Division in Late Middle English *Fachprosa*: GUL MS Hunter 497 (V.7.24). In Javier Díaz Vera and Rosario Caballero (eds.). *Tectual Healing: Studies in Medieval English Medical, Scientific and Technical Texts*. Frankfurt: Peter Lang. 35-53.

Calle-Martín, Javier – Antonio Miranda-García 2005a. Aspects of Punctuation in the Old English *Apollonius of Tyre*. *Folia Linguistica Historica* 26.1-2, 95-113.

Calle-Martín, Javier – Antonio Miranda-García 2005b. Editing Middle English Punctuation. The Case of MS Egerton 2622 (ff. 136-152). *International Journal of English Studies* 5.2, 27-44.

Calle-Martín, Javier – Miranda-García, Antonio 2007. The Punctuation System of Elizabethan Legal Documents: the Case of G.U.L. MS Hunter 3 (S.1.3). *Review of English Studies* 59, 356-378.

Calle-Martín, Javier – David Moreno-Olalla Forthcoming. Body of Evidence: of Middle English Annotated Corpora and Dialect Atlases. In Laura Wright and Richard Dance (eds.). *Fourteen Essays on Middle English*. Frankfurt: Peter Lang.

Cappelli, Adriano 1990. *Dizionario di abbreviature Latine ed Italiane*. Milano: Editore Ulrico Hoepli.

Clemens, Raimond – Timothy Graham 2007. *Introduction to Manuscript Studies*. Ithaca and London: Cornell University Press.

Crespo, Begoña – Emma Lezcano 1999. A Preliminary Approach to Dialectal Localisation in Middle English. In Isabel Moskowich-Spiegel Fandiño (ed.). *Interpretations of English. Essays on Language, Linguistics and Philology*. La Coruña: University of La Coruña. 41-60.

Cross, Rowin 2004. *A Handlist of Manuscripts Containing English in the Hunterian Collection Glasgow University Library*. Glasgow: Glasgow University Library.

Cruz, Isabel de la – Francisco Javier Martín Arista (eds.) 2001. *Lingüística Histórica Inglesa*. Barcelona: Ariel.

Danchev, Andrei – Merja Kytö 2001. The Middle English '*for to* + infinitive' construction. In Dieter Kastovsky – Arthur Mettinger (eds.). *Language Contact in the History of English*. Frankfurt: Peter Lang. 35-55.

Dawson, Warren (ed.) 1934. *A Leechbook or Collection of Medical Recipes of the 15th Century: the Text of MS. no. 136 of the Medical Society of London, together with a Transcript into Modern Spelling*. London: Macmillan.

Denholm-Young, Noël 1964. *Handwriting in England and Wales*. Cardiff: University of Wales Press.

Derolez, Albert 2003. *The Palaeography of Gothic Manuscript Books. From the Twelfth to the Early Sixteenth Century*. Cambridge: Cambridge University Press.

Dobson, Eric John 1957. *English Pronunciation 1500-1700*. Oxford: Clarendon Press.

Fischer, Olga 1992. Syntax. In Norman Blake (ed.). *The Cambridge History of the English Language. Volume II 1066-1476*. Cambridge: Cambridge University Press. 207-408.

Fisiak, Jacek 1968. *A Short Grammar of Middle English I*. London: Oxford University Press.

Frisk, Gösta 1949. *A Middle English Translation of Macer Floridus De Viribus Herbarum*. Uppsala: Almqvist & Wiksells Boktryckery Ab.

Görlach, Manfred 1991. *Introduction to Early Modern English*. Cambridge: Cambridge University Press.

Hall, J.R. Clark 1894. *A Concise Anglo-Saxon Dictionary*. Toronto – Buffalo – London: University of Toronto Press.

Hamel, Christopher de 1992. *Scribes and Illuminators*. London: British Museum Press.

Hector, Leonard C. 1966. *The Handwriting of English Documents*. London: Edward Arnold.

Hogg, Richard and David Denison 2006. *A History of the English Language*. Cambridge: Cambridge University Press.

Horobin, Simon – Jeremy Smith 2002. *An Introduction to Middle English*. Oxford: Oxford University Press.

Jenkinson, Hilary 1926. Notes on the Study of English Punctuation of the Sixteenth Century. *Review of English Studies* 2, 152-158.

Johnston, Edward 1945. *Writing and Illuminating, and Lettering*. London: Pitman.

Jones, Charles 1989. *A History of English Phonology*. London: Longman.

Jordan, Richard 1974. *Handbook of Middle English Grammar: Phonology*. The Hague – Paris: Mouton.

Keiser, George R. 1998. *A Manual of the Writings in Middle English 1050-1500. Volume X. Works of Science and Information*. New Haven, Connecticut: The Connecticut Academy of Arts and Sciences.

Kurath, Hans – Sherman M. Kuhn – John Reidy – Robert E. Lewis (eds.) 1956-2001. *Middle English Dictionary*. Ann Arbour: University of Michigan Press. Electronic dictionary: <http://quod.lib.umich.edu/m/med/lookup.html>.

Lucas, Peter J. Sense-units and the Use of Punctuation-markers in John Capgrave's *Chronicle*. *Archivum Linguisticum* 2, 1-24.

Manitius, Max 1911. *Geschichte der Lateinischen Literatur des Mittelalters: Von Justinian bis zur Mitte des zehnten Jahrhunderts*. 2 vols. München: C.H. Beck'sche Verlagbuchhandlung.

Marqués-Aguado, Teresa – Antonio Miranda-García – Santiago González 2008. *The Middle English Ophthalmic Treatise on the Use of the Eye in G.U.L. MS Hunter 513 (ff. 1r-37r). An Annotated Edition*. Málaga: Servicio de Publicaciones.

Martin, Charles Trice 1910. *The Record Interpreter: A Collection of Abbreviations, Latin Words and Names Used in English Historical Manuscripts and Records*. London: Stevens and Sons.

McIntosh, Angus – M.L. Samuels – Michael Benskin 1986. *A Linguistic Atlas of Late Mediaeval English*. 4 vols. Aberdeen: Aberdeen University Press.

Mendez Naya, Belén 2007. *He nas nat right fat*: On the Origin and Development of the Intensifier *right*. In Gabriella Mazzon (ed.). *Studies in Middle English Forms and Meanings*. Frankfurt: Peter Lang. 191-207.

Molencki, Rafal 2005. The Confusion between *thurven* and *durren* in Middle English. In Nikolaus Ritt – Herbert Schendl (eds.). *Rethinking Middle English. Linguistic and Literary Approaches*. Frankfurt: Peter Lang. 147-160.

Moore, Samuel 1929. *Historical Outlines of English Phonology and Morphology*. Ann Arbor, Michigan: George Wahr.
Mooreman, Charles W. 1975. *Editing the Middle English Manuscript*. Jackson: University Press of Mississippi.
Moskowich Spiegel-Fandiño, Isabel – Elena Alfaya Lamas 1998. Translation in Middle English: A Problem of Scripts and Scribes. In Adolfo Luis Soto Vázquez (ed.). *Insights into Translation*. La Coruña: University of La Coruña. 101-111.
Mossé, Ferdinand 1968. *A Handbook of Middle English*. Baltimore and London: The Johns Hopkins University Press.
Mustanoja, Tauno 1960. *A Middle English Syntax*. Helsinki: Société Néophilologique.
Osley, A.S. 1980. *Scribes and Sources. Handbook of the Chancery Hand in the Sixteenth Century*. London: Faber and Faber.
Oxford English Dictionary. CD-ROM Version 3.1. Oxford: Oxford University Press.
Parkes, Malcolm B. 1992. *Pause and Effect. An Introduction to the History of Punctuation in the West*. Hants: Scolar Press.
Petti, Anthony G. 1977. *English Literary Hands from Chaucer to Dryden*. Cambridge, Mass: Harvard University Press.
Pollard, Graham 1976. Describing Medieval Bookbindings. In Jonathan J.G. Alexander – Margaret T. Gibson (eds.). *Medieval Learning and Literature. Essays Presented to Richard William Hunt*. Oxford: Clarendon Press. 50-65.
Raumolin-Brunberg, Helena 2000. *Which* and *the which* in Late Middle English: Free Variants? In Irma Taavitsainen et al. (eds.). *Placing Middle English in Context*. Berlin and New York: Mouton de Gruyter. 209-225.
Roberts, Jane 2005. *Guide to Scripts Used in English Writings up to 1500*. London: the British Library.
Roura Javier, María Isabel 1999. The Present Participle in Middle English: the Establishment of the Ending *–ng*. In I. Moskowich Spiegel-Fandiño (ed.). *Interpretations of English. Essays on Language, Linguistics and Philology*. La Coruña: University of La Coruña. 207-214.

Strang, Barbara M.H. 1970. *A History of English*. London and New York: Routledge.

Tannenbaum, Samuel A. 1930. *The Handwriting of the Renaissance*. New York: Columbia University Press.

Traugott, Elizabeth Closs 1992. Syntax. In Richard M. Hogg (ed.). *The Cambridge History of the English Language*. Cambridge: Cambridge University Press. 168-289.

Voigts, Linda Ehrsam – Patricia Deery Kurtz 2000. *Scientific and Medical Writings in Old and Middle English. An Electronic Reference*. Ann Arbor: Michigan University Press.

Wojtyś, Anna 2007. Middle English Prefixal Past Participle Marking in the Midlands. In Gabriella Mazzon (ed.). *Studies in Middle English Forms and Meanings*. Frankfurt: Peter Lang. 269-287.

Young, John – P. Henderson Aitken 1908. *A Catalogue of the Manuscripts in the Library of the Hunterian Museum in the University of Glasgow*. Glasgow: James Maclehose and Sons.